More praise for *Understanding West Africa's Ebola Epidemic*

'This comprehensive volume offers valuable analyses of the structural roots and social impacts of the West African Ebola outbreak. An excellent resource for anyone interested in learning about the history and political economy of this devastating epidemic.'

Adia Benton, Northwestern University

'This book successfully turns the neoliberal project on its head, forcing us to demand a different kind of development in contexts (such as Guinea, Liberia and Sierra Leone) where exclusion, exploitation and extraction reign supreme.'

Robtel Neajai Pailey, author and activist

Security and Society in Africa

The African Leadership Centre (ALC) is an educational Trust that has, since 2010, operated in Nairobi as a joint initiative of King's College London and the University of Nairobi. The ALC is guided by the promotion of African-led ideas and respect for independent thinking, with a core area of focus being issues at the intersection of security and development. This exciting and original series, a collaboration between the ALC and Zed, presents cutting-edge research into the society-based changes that are transforming our thinking about the practice and impacts of security in Africa.

UNDERSTANDING WEST AFRICA'S EBOLA EPIDEMIC

TOWARDS A POLITICAL ECONOMY

edited by Ibrahim Abdullah and Ismail Rashid

ZED

In association with the
African Leadership Centre

Understanding West Africa's Ebola Epidemic: Towards a Political Economy
was first published in 2017 by Zed Books Ltd, The Foundry,
17 Oval Way, London SE11 5RR, UK.

www.zedbooks.net

Typeset in Plantin and Kievit by Swales & Willis Ltd, Exeter, Devon
Printed and bound by CPI Group (UK) Ltd, Croydon, CR0 4YY
Index by Rohan Bolton
Cover design by Kerry Squires

A catalogue record for this book is available from the British Library

ISBN 978-1-78699-169-0 hb
ISBN 978-1-78699-168-3 pb
ISBN 978-1-78699-170-6 pdf
ISBN 978-1-78699-171-3 epub
ISBN 978-1-78699-172-0 mobi

To the heroines and heroes,
known and unknown
counted and uncounted
felled by the epidemic
and reposing now in graves,
marked and unmarked,
in the three lands
threaded together by
the river, Mano.

To the carers and healers,
who from places,
near and distant
compelled or called
by duty or compassion
who tended the afflicted
at great risk
to their life and health.

To the survivors and torch-bearers,
who overcame the Ebola's
murderous embrace,
but not its ugly stigma,
and the millions,
betrayed by
insouciant governments,
quarantined
from the world,
but never losing hope.

CONTENTS

PART THREE DEVELOPMENT, GENDER, AND ITS DISCONTENTS

PART FOUR TRANSNATIONAL ACTORS AND THE POLITICS OF CRISIS RESPONSE

ACKNOWLEDGMENTS

This project started as a two-pronged trans-Atlantic conversation between us (Ibrahim Abdullah and Ismail Rashid) on the one hand, and Ibrahim Abdullah, Jacques Depelchin and Pauline Wynter on the other, in the heat of the Ebola Virus Disease epidemic in mid-2014. Jacques and Pauline expressed solidarity with Ibrahim and his compatriots in the region, and offered advice on how he and his loved ones could protect themselves. They also urged Ibrahim to "bear witness" to the tragic consequences of a viral plague the world thought it understood. The tone and spirit of the exchanges between us were similar.

The conversation inspired us to be actively engaged instead of being helplessly resigned in the face of what then seemed like an unstoppable viral plague. By December 2014 Ibrahim had written three short articles on responses to Ebola, two for a local tabloid, *Awoko,* and one for a popular media website, Africa is a Country. Ismail had participated in two Ebola teach-ins at Rutgers University and Vassar College. It soon became evident that we were not alone. Other scholars across the Atlantic were also having conversations, writing short articles, and engaging the public on various aspects of the Ebola epidemic. Their enthusiastic response to our call to contribute to a collective project bearing witness to the unprecedented ravages of the deadly Ebola virus in West Africa is this anthology on the political economy of the epidemic.

We would like to express our sincere thanks to everyone who contributed to the realization of this project. Without the intellectual labor, commitment, and patience of all of the contributors, the anthology would not have been possible. The two anonymous reviewers selected by Zed offered positive and constructive comments. Jon Chenette, the Dean of Faculty, and Grants Office of Vassar College provided funds that supported research assistance, indexing, and maps. Lauren Fleming, Andrea Ditkoff, and Joseph Goakai assisted with research, collection of source materials, and proofreading. The unflinching support of family, fellow travellers, and friends kept us energized and focused on the project. In particular, we are thankful to Jacques, Pauline, and Stephan Palmie for their concern and prodding us to bear witness in this fashion. Finally, we are pleased that the African Leadership Centre made this anthology the first in their series on Security and Society in Africa.

ABBREVIATIONS

ADB	African Development Bank
AFRC	Armed Forces Redemption Council
AGOA	African Growth and Opportunity Act
APC	All Peoples Congress
ASEOWA	African Union Support to Ebola Outbreak in West Africa
AU	African Union
BDBU	Bundibugyo Ebolavirus
CBEP	Cooperative Biological Engagement Program
CDC (Liberia)	Congress for Democratic Change
CDC (US)	Center for Disease Control and Prevention
CFR	Case Fatality Rate
CHA	Community Health Attendants
CHW	National Health Worker
COMAHS	College of Medicine and Allied Health Sciences
DfID (UK)	Department for International Development
DHIS	District Health Information System
DHMT	District Health Management Team
DTRA	Defense Threat Reduction Agency
EBOV	Zaire Ebolavirus
ECOWAS/ CEDEAO	Economic Community of West African States
EHF	Ebola Haemorrhagic Fever
EMBO	European Molecular Biology Organization
ERC	Ebola Response Committee
ETC	Ebola Treatment Center
EVD	Ebola Virus Disease
FGD	Focus Group Discussion
FHCI	Free Health Care Initiative
GERC	Global Ebola Response Coalition
GOARN	Global Outbreak and Alert Response Network.
HDI	Human Development Index
ICG	International Crisis Group

IDSI	Integrated Disease Surveillance Information System
IFRC	International Federation of Red Cross and Red Crescent Societies
IHR	International Health Regulations
IHRIS	Integrated Human Resource Information System
IMATT	International Military Assistance Training Team
IMF	International Monetary Fund
IRC	International Rescue Committee
JIATF HQ	Joint Inter-Agency Task Force Headquarters
MARWOPNET	Mano River Women's Peace Network
MCHA	Maternal and Child Health Aides
MCHP	Maternal and Child Health Post
MDG	Millennium Development Goals
MMU	Monrovia Medical Unit
MOD (UK)	Ministry of Defence
MoHS	Ministry of Health and Sanitation
MRU	Mano River Union
MRU-LFN	Mano River Union Lassa Fever Network
MSF	Médecins Sans Frontières
NERC	National Ebola Response Center
NIAID	National Institutes of Allergy and Infectious Diseases
NIH	National Institute of Health
NPRC	National Provisional Ruling Council
OCHA	Office for the Coordination of Humanitarian Affairs
ONS	Office of National Security
PBF	Performance-Based Financing
PEPFAR	President's Emergency Plan for AIDS Relief
PHC	Primary Health Care
PHEIC	Public Health Emergency of International Concern
PHU	Peripheral Health Unit
PPE	Personal Protective Equipment
PPP	Public Private Partnership
PRSP	Poverty Reduction Strategy Paper
RESTV	Reston Ebolavirus
RT-PCR	Reverse transcriptase polymerase chain reaction
RUF	Revolutionary United Front
SAP	Structural Adjustment Program
SECHN	State Enrolled Community Health Nurses
SLPP	Sierra Leone People's Party

SSR	Security Sector Reform
SUDV	Sudan Ebolavirus
TAFU	Taï Forest Ebolavirus
TBA	Traditional Birth Attendants
TWP	True Whig Party
UFDG	Union des Forces Démocratiques de Guinée
UNAMSIL	United Nations Mission in Sierra Leone
UNDP	United Nations Development Programme
UNMEER	United Nations Mission for Ebola Emergency Response
UNMIL	United Nations Mission in Liberia
VHFC	Viral Hemorrhagic Fever Consortium
VVF	Vesical Vaginal Fistula
WAHO	West African Health Organisation
WANEP	West Africa Network for Peacebuilding
WARN	West Africa Early Warning and Early Response Network
WB	World Bank Group
WFP	World Food Programme
WHO	World Health Organization
WiPNET	Women in Peace Network
WRESL	Women's Response to Ebola in Sierra Leone Campaign

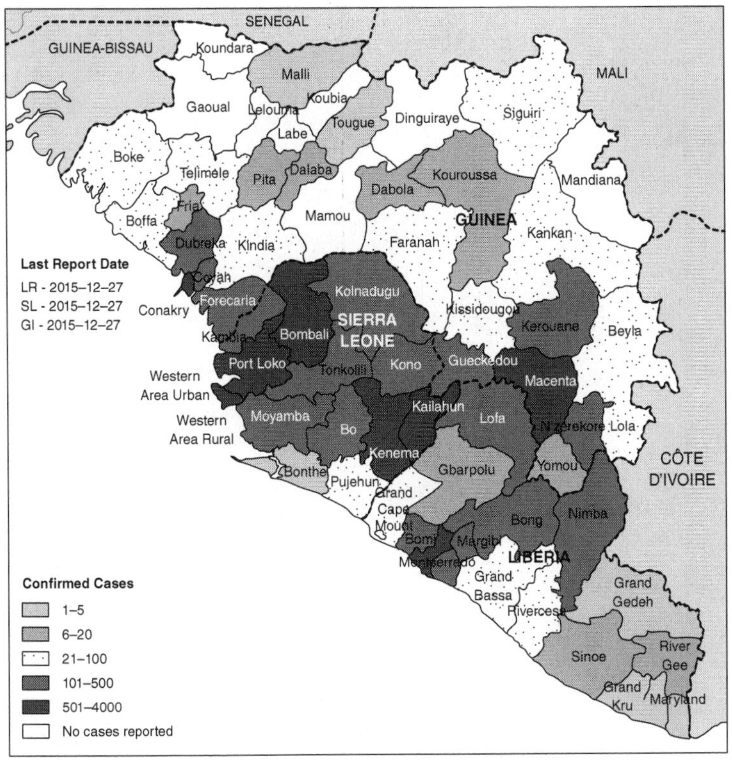

Map 1 Distribution of confirmed EVD cases in Guinea, Sierra Leone, and Liberia, 2013–2015 (*source*: adapted from WHO map on case count: http://apps.who.int/ebola/sites/default/files/thumbnails/image/sitrep_casecount_31.png?ua=1, accessed April 4, 2017)

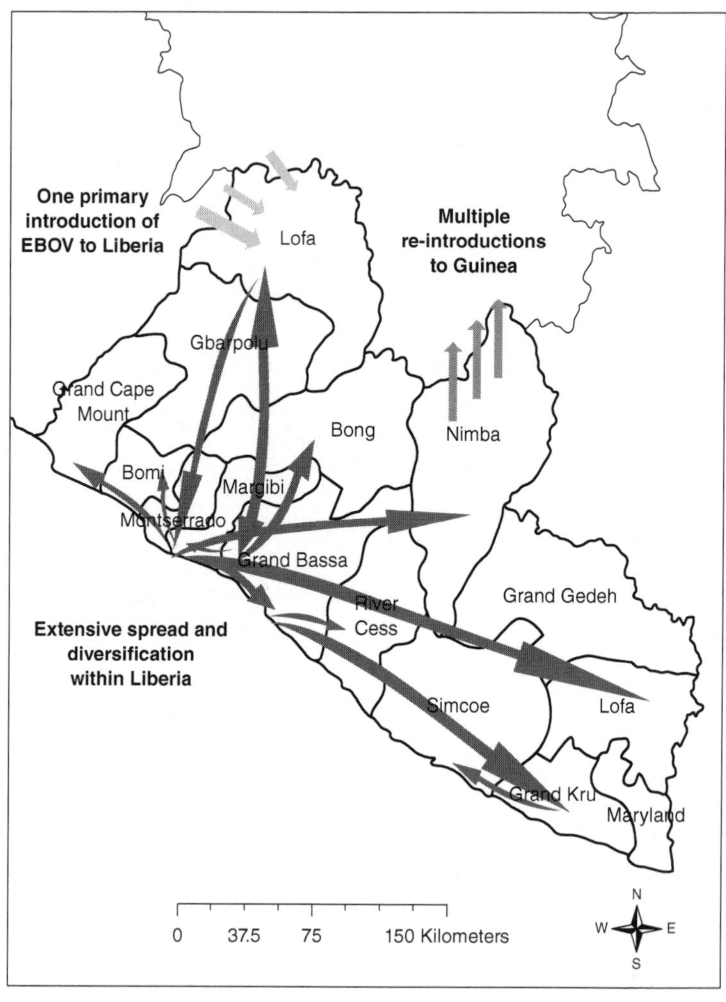

Map 2 Routes of EVD spread in Liberia (*source*: adapted from J.T. Ladner et al. (2015). "Evolution and Spread of Ebola Virus in Liberia 2014–2015," *Cell Host and Microbe*, 18, 6 (December): 659–669)

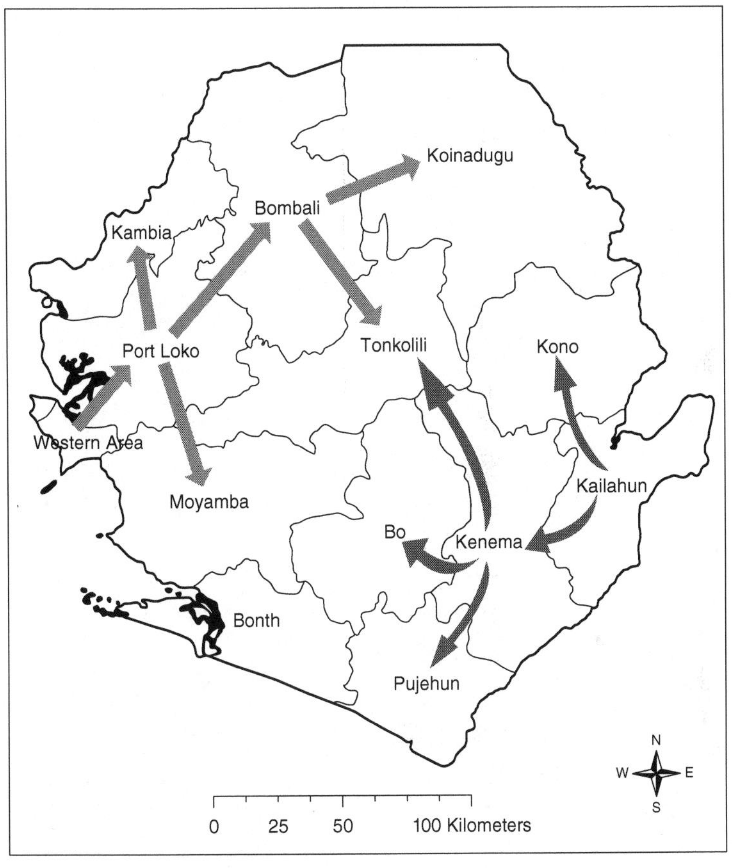

Map 3 Routes of EVD spread in Sierra Leone (*source*: adapted from W. Yang et al. (2015). "Transmission Network of 2014–2015 Ebola Epidemic in Sierra Leone," *Journal of the Royal Society Interface*, 12, 112: 20150536)

INTRODUCTION: UNDERSTANDING WEST AFRICA'S EBOLA EPIDEMIC

Ebola: an unknown enemy?

Between 2013 and 2016, the inhabitants of the three Mano River Union (MRU) countries of Liberia, Sierra Leone, and to a lesser extent, Guinea, relived a familiar nightmare. Like in the early 1990s, they were gripped with a pervasive sense of fear, insecurity, and uncertainty as they confronted a wily, ruthless, and seemingly unstoppable enemy. Initially, much was unknown about the pathways through which this enemy spread and attacked its victims. But, unlike the rebels and renegade soldiers of the recent past, this was an invisible enemy, and a completely unfamiliar one. Those at the forefront of the war against this unfathomable enemy – doctors, health care, and traditional healers – were at a loss and were either dying or being debilitated by it. People, therefore, filled their lack of knowledge about this enemy and its afflictions with myths, rumors, and innuendos (Epstein 2014). What was this enemy that not only snatches the life out of people in debilitating ways, but also makes pariahs out of individuals, communities, and whole countries?

We now know that this enemy was scientifically identified in March 2014 through samples sent to European laboratories by the Guinean government as Ebola Virus Disease (EVD). EVD, previously known as Ebola haemorrhagic fever (EHF), is a zoonosis; a disease caused by the spread of the *Zaire ebolavirus* (EBOV) from wild animals to humans, and then transmitted from person to person. EBOV is one of the five known subspecies of ebolavirus, the other four being *Bundibugyo ebolavirus* (BDBV), *Sudan ebolavirus* (SUDV), *Taï Forest ebolavirus* (TAFV), and *Reston ebolavirus* (RESTV). EVD, which takes between two to twenty-one days to incubate in humans, generates amongst many other symptoms: fever, muscle pains, vomiting, diarrhea, and in some instances, serious internal and external bleeding. EVD symptoms can be difficult to distinguish from malaria and typhoid, diseases prevalent in the MRU sub-region. The confirmation of EVD needs to be done using tests such as a reverse transcriptase polymerase chain reaction (RT-PCR) assay, an antibody-capture enzyme-linked immunosorbent assay (ELISA), or virus isolation through cell culture.[1] EVD spreads through the contact with bodily fluids, secretions, and blood of infected people. Stopping the transmission of the virus entails avoiding contact with fluids and secretions from an infected person or materials on which they are present. Death rates from the disease have varied widely from 25 to 95 percent in past outbreaks. The case fatality rate from the MRU epidemic was less than 50 percent. Even though a range of therapies is being developed, there is no cure for EVD, but early detection and the provision of palliative care, in particular oral rehydration, improves an infected person's chances of survival.[2]

When EBOV first emerged in the MRU sub-region, it may have been an unknown quantity for governments and inhabitants of the sub-region, but four decades of outbreaks in East and Central Africa have enabled virologists, geneticists, and epidemiologists to produce considerable knowledge about the virus and the disease it causes (Kangoy et al. 2006). From 1976, when the first incidence of EBOV was recorded, this growing library of knowledge (Ballabeni and Boggio 2015; Olinjnyk 2015) and field experience of dealing with ebolaviruses have ensured that outbreaks were usually stopped within seven months. EHF\EVD has historically been a rural disease, except for two outbreaks: the first in 1995 in Kikwit, a city in southwestern Democratic Republic of Congo and the 2000 to 2001 outbreak in Gulu, a city in northern Uganda. Both outbreaks were brought under control within seven months (Muyembe-Tamfum et al. 1999; Lamunu et al. 2004; Mbonye et al. 2014). The EVD outbreak in the MRU area fully traversed the rural and the urban divide, becoming the first epidemic of its kind.

The responsibility for responding to outbreaks of infectious diseases like EVD is shared by national governments, regional health agencies, and international organizations (WHO 2008). The communication and cooperation between these parties have been vital in containing previous outbreaks of EHF/EVD. The failure of communication, cooperation, and action in the MRU epidemic underlies some of the core questions of this anthology: Why, in this era of globalization, ubiquitous information, and super-fast communication, was the accumulated knowledge and expertise around EVD not quickly utilized in the case of the MRU countries?

Why were local communities, the national public health systems, and governments in Sierra Leone, Guinea, and Liberia unable to respond effectively to the spread of the outbreak? Why did international organizations, especially the World Health Organization (WHO), the US Center for Disease Control and Prevention (CDC), and Médecins San Frontières (MSF), which had been instrumental and relatively successful in curtailing previous outbreaks, fail to contain the initial outbreak in late 2013 and early 2014? What did it take to get the MRU governments, the international organizations, and the international community in general to respond more strongly to the epidemic? How did the EVD outbreak of 2013–2015 become the largest, most widespread and deadliest in history, infecting more than 28,616 and killing 11,310 people?[3] What was it about the MRU EVD outbreak that was different?

The starting point, perhaps, should be the frank acknowledgement that despite the publication of hundreds of scientific articles, there are still significant gaps in our knowledge of filoviruses, included that of *Zaire ebolavirus*. For example, the actual wild animal reservoir of the *Zaire ebolavirus* in Africa remains a mystery, despite the detection of the virus's presence in a wide range of dead or sick forest animals and its antigens in fruit bats (Porrut et al. 2005; Groseth et al. 2007). Up to this moment, there is no clear scientific evidence or indisputable explanation of how EBOV moved from wild animals to humans in the MRU sub-region. This lack of concrete knowledge about the real animal reservoir, the fact that previous outbreaks have largely been confined to Central and East Africa, and ongoing US Defense Department-sponsored bioterrorism viral research in the sub-region, raises the first set of puzzling questions that this anthology flags up (Campbell 2014; Kamara 2016).

In Chapter 2 of this anthology, Chernoh Bah, in his incisive critique of the findings of the German scientific team which identified a two-year child in Meliandou as the index case of EBOV in West Africa, foregrounds some of the still puzzling questions about the origin of the disease in the MRU sub-region. Why has the infelicitous conclusion of the German research team on the origin of the Ebola Virus Outbreak in West Africa been accepted so widely and uncritically? Why was it so certain that the two-year-old Guinean, later revealed to be Emile Ouamouno, was the index case of the outbreak? How did they arrive at the conclusion that the Ebola Virus Disease outbreak in Guinea could be traced to zoonotic causes even though it did not find evidence of the virus in the surrounding animal population? Bah's questions, which also find resonance in Bano Barry's discussion in Chapter 3 of the two theories of the origins of the disease, cannot be simply dismissed as the unsophisticated speculations of conspiracy theorists. These questions demand straightforward, transparent responses from the Western institutions and scientists engaged in research in the region, which can enable people to come to terms with the catastrophe and its traumatic legacy.

MRU, regionalism, and Ebola

The first overarching analytical approach that this anthology adopts is a sub-regional one, using the MRU as a unified and coherent spatial framework of analysis. Even though EVD appeared in Nigeria, Senegal, Mali, the UK, Italy, the United States, and Spain in late 2014, it was essentially an epidemic of the three core countries of the MRU.[4] Indeed, it could be argued that EVD, through its transmission chains, infections, and outbreaks, mapped out the basic spatial, political, and historical framework within which it should first be analyzed. It was tragic that the governments of Guinea, Sierra Leone, and Liberia only belatedly realized the spatial dynamics in the spread of the epidemic, and the need for a concerted sub-regional approach.[5] By the end of 2014 and early 2015, their actions to contain the outbreak began to mirror each other, and it was evident lessons were being learned and experiences shared. That EVD fanned out in chains of transmission from communities in the forested border zone of the three countries should not be surprising given the deep historical, ethnic, economic, and cultural connections between communities in the three countries.

As Allen Howard posits in the first chapter of this volume, Guinea, Liberia, and Sierra Leone constitute a single region with complementary ecologies, which has been integrated from the nineteenth century onwards by socio-cultural commonalities, flows of people and ideas, and commercial and socials exchanges. Howard draws attention to the similar historical processes – enslavement and slave trading, imperialism, and colonization – that have strongly influenced the developmental trajectories of peoples and their communities in this sub-region. Though Liberia remained nominally independent, its politics and economics had similar features to French-colonized Guinea and British-colonized Sierra Leone. All of the three countries had export-driven economies dominated by mineral and cash crops, with insufficient food crop production.

The post-independence trajectories of the three MRU countries have not been radically different, despite the slight variations in the political posturing that they adopted in the 1960s and 1970s, with Guinea being closer to the Soviet bloc, Liberia to the US, and Sierra Leone oscillating in between. Howard points out that all three of the countries experienced deepening rural impoverishment, burgeoning youth population, rapid growth of cities and urban slums, and high incidences of urban unemployment. They had also fallen prey to dictatorship, unbridled corruption, and recurrent military coups by the mid-1990s. These developments produced widespread distrust of government, youth disengagement and rebellion, and lack of popular participation.

Harsh structural adjustment programs (SAP), imposed by the World Bank and International Monetary Fund (IMF) on virtually every African country from the 1980s onwards, exacerbated the post-independence turmoil in the MRU sub-region. In Guinea, these developments resulted in an unstable political system characterized by periodic civil violence, while in Sierra Leone and Liberia they were partly responsible for triggering destructive wars, which displaced large numbers of people across the three countries and further afield. Billions of dollars and thousands of ECOWAS, and later UN peacekeeping troops had to be deployed to establish peace and security in the sub-region. The UN intervention in Sierra Leone and Liberia did not interrupt the neoliberalization of state, economy, and society in the MRU region; if anything, it deepened it through the governance, security sector reform programs, poverty reduction strategy programs, privatization, and civil society reform projects that it supported in partnership with the World Bank, IMF, and major Western donor countries. Much has been made of the democratic progress and the positive GDP growth rates of the three countries in recent years, yet high levels of impoverishment, social alienation, and elite misrule have persisted. When the EVD struck in 2013, the sub-region was still wrestling with the contradictions of neoliberal restructuring.

The neoliberal affliction: different countries, similar convulsions

Neoliberalism provides the second overarching analytical framework utilized in this volume. Understanding the transformation of EVD into a regional epidemic is not simply a scientific and medical matter; it is also about uncovering how governance, management of public health, resources, and ultimately human agency at local, national, and international levels intersected in dealing with the epidemic. In short, it is about understanding how the political economy of neoliberal restructuring of the MRU sub-region is implicated in the outbreak, spread, and eventual containment of the disease. Ebola was not simply a deadly viral disease; it was the manifestation of neoliberalism as an affliction, which wreaks havoc in the world's most vulnerable societies. The contributors to this volume are aware that "neoliberalism" is a much bandied and catch-all term used by scholars and activists to contest, critique, and organize against aspects of, or the totality of contemporary capitalism. Neoliberalism in this anthology refers to "new political, economic, and social arrangements within society that emphasize market relations, re-tasking the role of the state, and individual responsibility" (Springer et al. 2016, 2).

Emerging in the post-Second World War period and gaining ascendancy in the Washington Consensus of 1989, neoliberalism refers to a set of ideological assumptions, policy prescriptions, programs, and practices of how capitalist economic development should be conceptualized in relation to state authority, and how politics and society at all levels should be subjected to market forces. Of particular efficacy in this anthology is the conception of neoliberalism as governmentality (Peters 2001), the process by which the state and, to some extent, international agencies are limited in their power and ability to intervene in economics and society or are made to do so through the rubric of public private partnerships (PPP). For the MRU states, neoliberalism arrived with the World Bank and IMF-imposed structural adjustment programs of the 1980s, and the Poverty Reduction Strategy Papers (PRSP) at the dawn of a new millennium.

Neoliberal reforms have tended to deepen rather than ameliorate the structural legacies of historical violence and postcolonial authoritarianism in Africa. Chapters 3, 4, and 5 of this volume deal specifically with how the crisis of neoliberalism has played out in each of the three EVD-affected MRU states. The approaches adopted by our contributors differ from country to country, but not because of their different academic disciplines. The different perspectives adopted by our contributors underline the similarities that characterized the three countries: the emphasis on the peripheral capitalist state by George Kieh in Liberia could be applied to explain the situation in both Guinea and Sierra Leone. Similarly the empirical focus adopted by Ibrahim Abdullah and Abou Bakarr Kamara, concentrating on the analysis of health infrastructure, inadequate drugs and facilities, and lack of personnel, could also be employed to make sense of what happened in both Guinea and Liberia. Lastly, Bano Barry's sociological examination of state–society relations and popular repertoire in the time of Ebola is also efficacious in making sense of the damage wrought by EVD in both Liberia and Sierra Leone. Whether we are talking about broken health infrastructure and inadequate drugs or lack of qualified personnel, the role of the peripheral capitalist state in failing to meet the needs of the people needs to be explained. The reluctance or suspicion of citizens about going to the hospital, a place that they rarely ever visit, raises serious questions not only about the nature of health facilities in the MRU sub-region, but who gets to visit them, why, and when.

The chapter by Barry deals with a collapsed and compromised Guinean health infrastructure confronting a deadly virus in a context of intense multi-party competition in an environment with deep-seated political and ethnic cleavages. Unlike Liberia and Sierra Leone, where the epidemic engulfed the entire country, Guinean officials were able to contain the EVD largely within their Forestiere and Maritime regions, with certain portions of Moyenne and Haute regions remaining untouched by the disease. Barry explains how this containment played out in Guinea, which had a relatively low EVD infection rate and death toll.[6] As in Liberia and Sierra Leone, the broken health infrastructure, lack of qualified officials, inadequate drugs, and a total disconnect between state and society underlines the Ebola moment and the eventual containment of the disease.

What Barry documents as having played out in Guinea is not too dissimilar from the circumstances in Liberia and Sierra Leone: there was lack of information at the initial stage of the disease; partisan battles over so-called "sensitization"; and local cultures that were suspicious of health facilities, modern medicine, and its remedies. It is in making sense of the popular reaction – refusal to seek medical help; the need for community mobilization and its total involvement in tackling the disease; and the yanking of loved ones from a community when they fall sick and eventually die – that the chasm between the people and the state becomes evident. As in Sierra Leone, while people were dying, others were busy accessing funding for so-called sensitization. Decades of disconnect and top-down interaction between the people and health/state officials did not go away, even in the face of a national emergency that demanded trust on both sides. Barry neither dismisses nor unduly mystifies cultural practices – especially those pertaining to burial practices during the epidemic; instead, he emphasizes how they emblematized a deep distrust of the region's elite and outsiders.

This lack of trust, a product of the years of alienation, made the fight against Ebola much more difficult than it could have been. The chapter by Kieh on Liberia maps out the politics of a peripheral capitalist state that is programmed not to perform. Why this should be the case is tied up with the predatory politics of accumulation which makes it impossible for the state to perform qua state. Kieh traces the history of the state from its settler origin in the nineteenth century to its contemporary transformation into a liberal democratic project anchored in neoliberal market principles. As Kieh noted, there was no mechanism to deal with any medical emergency nor was there any institution designed to tackle anything close to an Ebola epidemic. Since the state was not designed to cater for the bulk of its citizens, it had to perforce turn to external forces at the first sign of a major crisis.

Abdullah and Kamara's empirical analysis of the decrepit state of health facilities in Sierra Leone, despite several reform efforts, is emblematic of the state of public health not only in the MRU region, but also in many parts of Africa. Like Liberia, Sierra Leone was recovering from a destructive rebel war that had virtually wrecked an already declining and dysfunctional health infrastructure. The infrastructure and new health initiatives had barely been cobbled together when EVD struck in 2014. With only one specialist in the area of haemorrhagic fever, who unfortunately perished as the disease engulfed the nation, Sierra Leone was left to face Ebola literally with bare hands. EVD was not simply about the lack of functional health facilities; it was also a case of the bulk of the population being cut off from access to modern public health services: 70 percent of the qualified medical officers and most of the health facilities were bunched in the Western Area of the country where the capital, Freetown, is located and where 21 percent of the population resides. The situation was eerily similar in Guinea and Liberia.

Development, gender, and its discontents

Whether viewed through the prism of the predatory peripheral capitalist state, dysfunctional public health facilities, or social alienation and suspicion of officialdom and modern medical practices, the EVD epidemic points to a continuing production of particularly deadly forms of structural violence rooted in the region's past as well as its present trajectory. Even international efforts to remake the Liberia and Sierra Leonean states, including their health care infrastructure, through international assistance have not broken this cycle of structural violence or public mistrust. As Julia Amos points out in Chapter 6, the militarization of post-war international development assistance, and the response to the EVD epidemic by the UK, the United States, and France have reinforced this violence and mistrust. She argues for a non-securitized and welfare-orientated approach to development and crisis that enables citizens in countries like Sierra Leone to trust those that govern them.

As the impact of EVD on women in Sierra Leone and the other MRU countries demonstrates, such trust is difficult to forge amidst deep-seated cultural, economic, and political inequalities. Aisha Fofana Ibrahim's chapter on gender performance addresses some of the structural inequalities that were played out when Ebola struck. She argues that the gendered structural inequalities, which were reproduced in the context of the Ebola scourge, are an indictment of the post-colonial state. Her analysis goes beyond the epidemiological data, which shows that EVD roughly infected and killed men and women in similar proportions, to mapping out the deep and unacknowledged ways in which the epidemic affected women because of their gender, place, and roles in society.

The relegation of women to second-class citizens in society together with their invention as vectors of culture, and "natural caregivers," placed them in the first line of the defense in the war against Ebola. As caregivers they nursed the sick, in community and the nation, with their bare hands, at a time when knowledge of the disease was hard to come by. As survivors they had to deal with the social abuse of stigmatization and exclusion as well as loss of livelihood as hairdressers, market women, sex-workers, or petty traders. The testimonies of women survivors from Kenema and Kailahun – the original epicenters – and Bombali and Port Loko – the later epicenters – are pointers to the multiple performances of gender in the death and destruction that characterized the Ebola epidemic. Much of Fofana's incisive observations and arguments have not made their way into the post-Ebola conversation. Nonetheless, she maps out unequivocally the need to privilege the voices, experiences, and interests of women in any post-Ebola restructuring in Sierra Leone and the two other MRU countries.

For the neoliberal regimes of the MRU, the tragedy of the EVD epidemic provided cover for corruption, containing dissent, and political entrenchment. However, in order to make sense of the tragedy, to challenge the official narrative from above, and to hold those in power accountable, a networked community of activists emerged in cyber-space. In Chapter 8 of this volume, Ibrahim Abdullah examines the making of a networked movement in cyber space, anchored in the use of WhatsApp as the medium of communication and choice. Transgressive communication under a state of emergency pooled in activists from all sectors: all were seemingly concerned with change broadly defined and the defense of the liberal principle of freedom of expression. The exclusivity and unfettered security that cyber activists had online made it possible for them to engage in the sharing of information and incendiary conversation, without interference from state officials and security agents. From parody to outright satire and lampoon to the use of video and audio clips, that occasionally go viral, cyber activists questioned state officials in all they did in the war against Ebola. This transgressive mode of engagement did not cease after the end of the epidemic. On the contrary, cyber activists stepped up their campaign with the establishment of more transcontinental WhatsApp groups stoutly defending their right to freedom of expression in cyber-space.

Transnational actors and the politics of crisis response

By August 2014, the three MRU countries had to rely on massive external assistance to contain the Ebola virus, and finally to bring the unprecedented epidemic to an end. As in the case of the responses of MRU governments, EVD exposed how the contradictions of neoliberalism shaped the responses of various transnational actors to the epidemic. Except for a few organizations, all the major transnational actors who could have helped nip the initial EVD outbreak in the bud in 2013 vacillated until it had become a raging sub-regional epidemic in late 2014. Until August 2014, the contradictory impulse, especially of high-income countries, to benefit from the profitable unfettered circulation of resources within a grossly unequal global economic system, while trying to curtail its undesirable consequences, was evident in the international attitude towards MRU countries. Nearly all of the major airlines and shipping lines stopped going to the affected countries. The wealthier actors in the international community only devoted significant financial, material, and human resources to stopping the EVD epidemic when it threatened to turn into a pandemic and had generated a sub-regional humanitarian crisis.[7] Even the description of the situation in the MRU sub-region had to be couched in highly securitized language to elicit international attention.

Like the governments of the MRU states, the international community also failed the people of the MRU sub-region spectacularly. By April 2014, the major organizations responsible for responding to the outbreak of infectious diseases, WHO and CDC, knew about the outbreak. So did the pan-African regional and continental organizations, ECOWAS and AU, the major financial institutions, the World Bank, IMF, and the African Development Bank (ADB), and leading Western countries, including the United States, UK, and France. WHO, in particular, has been harshly criticized for its initial tardiness and lack of decisive action. Meredeth Turshen and Tefera Gezmu consider this critique of the international response to the epidemic, especially that of WHO, which should have been the leading responder to the initial outbreak. Though informed of the EVD outbreak at the end of March 2014, WHO did not declare an international public health emergency or take decisive actions until August 2014. While not completely dismissing the widespread critique of WHO, Turshen and Gezmu point out that the organization is primarily designed to provide technical advice, not services. Most important, they maintain that the performance of WHO should be situated within the recent history of neoliberal budgetary constraints that were placed on the organization, which have enabled major donors to dictate its priorities. They argue that given the important role that the organization plays in the improvement of public health around the globe, high-income countries should increase their contribution to its regular budget.

The African response to the EVD epidemic also suffered from serious financial constraints. As a consequence, it demonstrated the gap between decades of aspirations and rhetoric about continental solidarity and integration, and the ability to operationalize them in a context in which regional and continental organizations were heavily dependent on the largesse of Western donors. To its credit, the Economic Community of West African States (ECOWAS) was one of the first international organizations to recognize the gravity of the unfolding Ebola crisis in the MRU, and to declare it a threat to regional security by March 2014. The African Union (AU) would also echo the security concern of ECOWAS. Within the still shaky framework of subsidiarity and complementarity, the two organizations tried to mobilize the necessary financial, material, and human resources to end the epidemic and to support the affected countries. The AU created the African Union Support to Ebola Outbreak in West Africa (ASEOWA), an unprecedented civilian–military mission, to help in the containment of the epidemic. According to Semiha Abdulmelik, however, these efforts continued to be embedded in, and mediated by an international political economy and architecture of humanitarian responses to "crisis" in Africa.

While the EVD epidemic did constitute a serious "human security" challenge, the extent to which it was a "hard" security threat to regimes in West Africa, Africa, or any Western nation is debatable. Nonetheless, as Fodei Batty points out in Chapter 11, the specter of a global Ebola contagion emanating from West Africa did offer an opportunity to see US relations with the region in action. The United States pledged over US$500 million to the response, and sent nearly 3,000 troops and medical personnel to Liberia. Looking closely at the media, debates, and legislation in Congress, and pronouncements by President Barack Obama, Batty argues that the efforts in Washington DC to stop Ebola in West Africa went beyond humanitarian intervention to addressing the shared consequences of global inequities.

The humanitarian and largely militarized US response, along with those of France and the UK, should be situated within the broader framework of the massive international response from August 2014 to contain the epidemic. Anchoring this massive international response was the unprecedented UN deployment of the United Nations Mission for Ebola Emergency Response (UNMEER) for ten months in the MRU region. The creation and deployment of this mission, according to Ismail Rashid, is recognition of the initial failure of WHO on the part of the UN Secretary-General Ban Ki-moon, and the recognition that the organization had invested considerable resources and energy to ensure peace and stability in the MRU region. Driven by security logic, UNMEER and the international responses against Ebola were conducted in militaristic fashion, with strong martial undertones in the language, strategy, and tactics that were used (Kamara 2016).

With the disappearance of the now known enemy into its deep and yet unfathomable wildlife recesses, the people of the MRU are left to grapple with the traumatic legacy and lingering questions of the EVD epidemic. We will never know exactly how many got infected, died, and fully recovered from EVD. We will probably never know why some people recovered and others did not. A numbers game pitting the deaths from the epidemic against infant mortality, malaria, and other diseases, which are much higher annually, will not take us anywhere. The crudely numbered graves behind an Ebola Treatment Center in Nzerekore, Guinea, and the rude crosses at Disco Hill graveyard in Monrovia, Liberia evoked an intense, public calamity that is not comprehensible on a quantitative scale. We are still trying to understand the lingering medical impact of EVD on survivors, and the continuing presence of the Ebola virus in breast milk, semen, and intraocular fluids of survivors. As Aisha Fofana underlines in her contribution to this volume, the region still has to reckon with the social cost, especially the impact on women, of EVD. From early 2015, there have been the usual raft of conferences, meetings, and commitment of resources to the rebuilding of health infrastructure of the MRU countries, but we will not know how robust these efforts are until the next crisis.

However, EVD has not left the MRU region with simply trauma, tragedy, and new questions, it has suggested possibilities of inculcating new forms of knowledge and techniques to tackle unfamiliar diseases. It has also, perhaps, widened the spectrum of political contestation in the region that is a source of trepidation for MRU governments. As Abdullah points out in his chapter, there is already evidence that the prevalence and dominance of cyber activism in the public sphere is provoking a strident official response from above. Some Sierra Leonean officials are already calling for a policy option along the lines of the Chinese government, enforcing total control of cyberspace. Others want to explore the use of technology to fish out those Sierra Leoneans that are covertly political. Whatever option is finally adopted, it is clear that the battle for freedom of expression in cyber-space may well determine the future of social movements in contemporary Sierra Leone as the country prepares for its fourth post-war elections in 2018.

Notes

1 See Ebola Virus Disease Fact Sheet. http://www.who.int/mediacentre/factsheets/fs103/en/ (last accessed on October 24, 2016).

2 In December 2016, WHO and *The Lancet* reported that an experimental vaccine, rVSV-ZEBOV, offered protection against Ebola (see Henao-Restrepo et al. 2017), and "Final trial results confirm Ebola vaccine provides high protection against disease" (http://www.who.int/mediacentre/news/releases/2016/ebola-vaccine-results/en/, last accessed February 6, 2017).

3 These figures based on actual, suspected, and probable cases of the disease continued to be refined by the World Health Organization. http://www.who.int/mediacentre/factsheets/fs103/en/ (last accessed October 24, 2016).

4 Côte D'Ivoire, the fourth member country and the last to join the MRU in 2008, was untouched throughout the epidemic; not a single case was recorded.

5 Well over a year after the EVD outbreak had started, the presidents of Guinea, Sierra Leone, and Liberia together with the Director-General of WHO met on August 1, 2014 to discuss experiences and coordinate their response strategies.

6 Guinea, where the EVD outbreak was first identified, reported at the end of the epidemic in 2016 the lowest number of infections, 3,804, and deaths, 2,536 of the three MRU countries. Liberia has 10,666 infections, and 4,806 deaths, and Sierra Leone, 14,122 infections and 3,955 deaths.

7 The US intervention and concern even in post-Ebola remained anchored on global security. See US documents on post-Ebola projects.

References

Ballabeni, A. and Boggio, A. (2015). "Publications in PubMed on Ebola and the 2014 Outbreak," *F1000Research*, 4: 68.

Campbell, Horace (2014). "Ebola, the African Union, and Bioeconomic Warfare," *Counterpunch*, October 10.

Epstein, Helen (2014). "Ebola in Liberia: An Epidemic of Rumors," *The New York Review of Books*, December 18.

Groseth, Allison, Feldmann, Heinz, and Strong, James E. (2007). "The Ecology of Ebola Virus," *Trends in*

Microbiology, 15, 9 (September): 408–416.

Henao-Restrepo, A. et al. (2017). "Efficacy and Effectiveness of an rVSV-vectored Vaccine in Preventing Ebola Virus Disease: Final Results from the Guinea Ring Vaccination, Open-label, Cluster-randomised Trial (Ebola ça suffit!)," *The Lancet*, 389, 10068: 508–518.

Kamara, Kewulay (2016). "Ebola: In Search of a Metaphor," *Futures*, June.

Kangoy, Aurielie Kasnagye, Muloye, Guy Mutangala, Avevor, Patrick Mawupemor, and Shixue, Li (2016). "Review of Past and Present Ebola Hemorrhagic Fever Outbreaks in the Democratic Republic of Congo 1976–2014," *African Journal of Infectious Disease*, 10, 1: 38–42.

Lamunu, M., Lutwama, J.J., Kamugisha, J., Opio, A., Nambooze, J., Ndayimirije, N., and Okware, S. (2004). "Containing a Haemorrhagic Fever Epidemic: The Ebola Experience in Uganda (October 2000–January 2001)," *International Journal of Infectious Diseases*, 8: 27–37.

Mbonye, A.K., Wamala, J.F., Nanyunja, M., Opio, A., Makumbi, I., Aceng, J.R. (2014). "Ebola Viral Hemorrhagic Disease Outbreak in West Africa: Lessons from Uganda," *African Health Sciences*, 14, 3: 495–501.

Muyembe-Tamfum, J.J, Kipasa, M., Kiyungu, R., and Coleblunders, R. (1999) "Ebola Outbreak in Kikwit, Democratic Republic of Congo: Discovery and Control Measures," *Journal of Infectious Diseases*, 179: S252–S262.

Olinjnyk, Nicholas V. (2015) "An Algorithmic Historiography of Ebola Research Specialty: Mapping the Science behind Ebola," *Scientometrics*, 105 (October): 623–643.

Peters, Michael A. (2001). *Poststructuralism, Marxism, and Neoliberalism: Between Theory and Politics*. Lanham, MD: Rowman and Little.

Pourrut, Xavier, Kumulungui, Brice, Wittmann, Tatiana, Moussavou, Ghislain, Délicat, André, Yaba, Philippe, Nkoghe, Dieudonné, Gonzalez, Jean-Paul, and Leroy, Eric Maurice (2005). "The Natural History of Ebola Virus in Africa," *Microbes and Infection*, 7, 7–8 (June): 1005–1014.

Springer, S., Birch, K., and MacLeavy, J. (eds) (2016). *The Routledge Handbook of Neoliberalism*. Abingdon: Routledge.

World Health Organization (2008). *International Health Regulations (2005)*, 2nd ed. Geneva: WHO.

PART ONE

THE REGIONAL HISTORY AND ORIGINS OF EBOLA

1 | EBOLA AND REGIONAL HISTORY: CONNECTIONS AND COMMON EXPERIENCES

Allen M. Howard[1]

Introduction

It is not surprising that the Ebola Virus Disease (EVD) spread fairly rapidly and easily among Guinea, Liberia, and Sierra Leone, or the countries faced similar difficulties responding to it. They long have constituted a region in several respects.[2] Four points emerge from a regional approach. Their similar histories – especially their histories of extractive economies and structural poverty, foreign intervention, colonial rule, patrimonial regimes, and, in the two cases of Liberia and Sierra Leone, civil wars – made each state ill prepared to address the Ebola crisis. Structural poverty grew out of the Atlantic slave trade, commodity trade, and other global economic relationships. On top of the impacts of long-existing extractive economies, all countries had by 2014 further depleted their educational and health systems because of externally imposed cuts in public spending (through Structural Adjustment Programs) and predatory and military regimes that drained national treasures. Together, those factors led to widespread distrust of government and youth disengagement and rebellion. Second, the three countries long have been and today are integrated by complexly ramifying social, economic, and cultural networks (nodes plus flows) that link individuals, places, communities, and institutions, facilitating communication and providing a basis for coordinated action. Third, in addition to their networks, peoples' patterns of movement within the region may help account for how the disease spread and how information was disseminated, while their history of social struggles may help explain how people at the grassroots level organized to combat the disease and overcome divisions. Finally, many factors suggest that future delivery of health services and responses to epidemic disease could be organized more efficiently with a regional approach – as could preparation for the challenges of climate change.

Yet, deep skill reservoirs exist throughout the region, and energy rises from below. Over the past 200 or more years, people throughout the region have resisted foreign oppression and struggled against internal structures of domination. And they have debated and created alternatives. Today, women's, youth, and environmental organizations dedicated to building a better future have launched projects that might serve as local and regional models to other communities and build new linkages among people of the three countries. They often generate imaginative ideas, political pressure, and alternative forms of action that complement and challenge the efforts of officials and health workers.

This chapter also poses questions that build upon the structural analysis provided here – and provides some speculations. I was prompted to write after attending a panel at the 2014 African Studies Association Annual Meeting in Indianapolis.[3] The panelists were experts on Ebola with field stays in the region. I asked them how historians, geographers, and other scholars of the humanities and social sciences might contribute background research that would help them address the crisis. They had no suggestions and wanted to know about concrete things that would enable their day-to-day work, such as how people in the region handled bodies of the deceased. While it is totally understandable why field workers would want information directly useful in their frontline campaign against EVD, I thought a deeper and wider background would also be valuable in both short- and long-term struggles against Ebola and other diseases.

Pre-colonial commonalities and integration: continuities

Guinea, Sierra Leone, and Liberia lie within an area where rainfall averages 1,500 mm (59 inches) per year, or more (Brooks 1993, 13). They all contain both lowland rain forests and drier highlands, but the environmental gradient has meant that historically forest covered a great share of Liberia, and a much smaller portion of Guinea, with Sierra Leone in between.[4] Futa Jallon and the Guinea Highlands are the sources of rivers that cut through all three en route to the Atlantic (Clarke 1966, 12–13). Each year rainfall patterns into a wet season and a dry season with the interior areas having a shorter period of rainfall.

In the pre-colonial past, the region was socially, culturally, and politically dynamic. People were affected by many of the same forces of change and had similar, though not identical, beliefs and practices, many of which continue today in modified form. People did (and do) speak languages from the Mande, West Atlantic (Fula or Pular and Mel), and Kruan groups (Brooks 1993, 27–33). Within each group there is considerable but not full inter-intelligibility. Because of migration, trade, and social inter-mixing, many people learned and still learn languages of different groups. Thus, Krio became the lingua franca of much of Sierra Leone in the twentieth century.

Age initiation associations were widespread, as were masking arts. In the deep past, the male *Poro* power association and its variants had spread over much of the region (Brooks 1993, 43 ff.).[5] Comparable female associations, especially *Bondo* and *Sande*, also have been long present. Masking arts are renowned, and people have created and shared rich dancing, singing, story-telling, and genealogical practices. People freed from slave ships in Sierra Leone, especially Yoruba-speakers, also have introduced beliefs, social practices, rituals, and associations, as well as masking and dancing practices, which have been borrowed by others (Cole 2013, 32–45, 155–163; Lamp 1996; Nunley 1987; Wyse 1989, 9–14).

The geographic distribution of languages seems to have been relatively stable over many centuries, but that does not mean that "ethnicity" or "ethnic" identity, however defined, has either coincided with language or remained stable. Though recent political leaders often have played up "ethnic" differences, "ethnic" lines have been fluid and blurred historically (Howard 1999, 13–40). Today, a great many people, perhaps most, have "ethnically" diverse ancestry and often live in "ethnically" varied households, especially in towns and cities (Harrell-Bond et al. 1978, 320–332 ff.; Cole 2013, 45–51).

Islam and Christianity have spread widely. The former has been established over many centuries through the influence of migrating Muslim traders and clerics, and through state-building, reformist, and expansionary movements (Barry 1998; Person 1968, 1015–1141; Skinner 1976). Christianity has been present along the Upper Guinea coast since the fifteenth century, but in its current forms is a nineteenth-century arrival, having been introduced and/or propagated by missionaries, repatriated and liberated Sierra Leoneans, and Americo-Liberians (Coifman 1994; Fyfe 1962; Wyse 1989, 33–39). The region long has had highly trained clerics and scholars of both "world" faiths, especially of Islam.

Nowadays, most people in the region claim to be members of a "universal" faith. One report states that Christians make up 86 percent of Liberians, about 21 percent of those in Sierra Leone, and 11 percent of Guineans, while, conversely, about 84 percent of those in Guinea and 78 percent in Sierra Leone are Muslims.[6] Such statistics fail to consider the strength of "indigenous" beliefs and practices, especially around healing and sacred places. Syncretism is widespread, and many have blended "universal" religions with "indigenous" beliefs and practices around naming, remembrance of the deceased, and so on (Cole 2013, 180–209; Ellis 2007, 220–280; Skinner 1976; Wyse 1989, 33–59 ff.). Despite religious chauvinism in some circles, people tend to be tolerant of religious difference.

Like religion, food, above all rice, has provided a shared set of deep beliefs and practices around which many people of the region might come together (Fanthorpe 1998). Rice historically has been the staple food crop for most (Currens 1979; Njoku 1979: 105 ff.). People tended and cultivated tree crops. Palm trees have been universally present in the lowlands and its margins, and palm oil has provided a nutritious base for soups with leaves and meat or fish (Holsoe 1979). Kola trees were scattered widely and dense stands were found around the lower Moa and Scarcies Rivers (Brooks 1993, 24; Howard 2007). In the drier uplands people raised cattle, most notably in Futa Jallon, where from the eighteenth century on large herds supported a hierarchical social order. Goats and sheep were kept by farming families nearly everywhere.

In the pre-colonial era, farmers, authorities, and traders organized exchange across the coastal, lowland, and inland zones of the region. Gold, mainly from Bure, circulated widely. The sea and coastal strip yielded fish and salt, the forest and its margin produced indigo, palm oil, and other products, especially kola, while the drier regions exported cattle, as well as shea butter and other things (Fyle 1979a; Fyle 1979b; Holsoe 1979, 66; Howard in preparation a). Women and men produced cloth, pottery, iron tools, jewelry, weapons, leather goods, wood carvings, and other manufactures for exchange (Holsoe 1979). Thus, although farming communities grew much of the food they needed and exchanged many things locally, a significant commerce existed within and across ecological zones. Traders also carried out an internal traffic in captives and other enslaved people, with Futa becoming a major recipient from the eighteenth century onward. Finally, from the 1400s, traders and others sold ivory, gold, manufactures, woods, and other commodities to Europeans and Eurafricans on the coast.

Once Atlantic demand for enslaved labor began to grow, and European, Eurafrican, and African traders along the coast organized to mediate that demand, the region became a supplier of captives. During the fifteenth through the eighteenth centuries, the overseas human traffic remained small in scale, relative to other areas of Africa and to later regional exports. It nonetheless was very harmful to people who came under attack and was instrumental in the rise of new classes of power holders, both those who specialized in trade and those who claimed political titles and established family dynasties, some of Eurafrican ancestry (located in what later became Guinea and Sierra Leone) (Rodney 1970). Starting in the mid-1700s, shipments rose rapidly and reached their highest levels by the late eighteenth and early nineteenth centuries. On January 1, 1808, the British began their campaign for abolition of the slave trade, with Freetown as the primary base. Exports from places near the Sierra Leone peninsula stopped but they remained quite high for the region as a whole into the 1840s and were not finally ended until the early 1860s.[7]

The impacts upon security and social life were devastating, though not evenly felt throughout. Southeastern Liberia seems never to have become an important source of enslaved people, whereas areas raided by Futa Jallon were hit hard and lowland Sierra Leone and southwestern Guinea were deeply affected (Barry 1998; Misevich 2008; Howard in preparation a). Many sections of the region underwent a transformation of the kind described by Paul Lovejoy, as slave holding became widespread, slave gathering mechanisms were developed, and political leaders geared up to participate (Lovejoy 2000). Regional economies were weakened and skewed toward exporting. Enslaved Africans laboring on American plantations contributed significantly to the enrichment and industrialization of Britain, the United States, and other northern countries (Fields-Black 2008; Blackburn 1997, 510–580; Solow 1991).

While the slave trade was stimulated by external demand, its organization in the region and often its impacts were connected with local and regional processes of social and political accumulation, power, and struggle (Howard in preparation a). Certain ruling groups, along with some other big men and women, professional war leaders, and traders built wealth, power, and influence through their participation in the slave trade (Rodney 1970; Mouser 1996). They also gained greater capacity to dominate those with fewer resources, especially those enslaved or otherwise under their patriarchal authority. The dominant classes, however, did not go unchallenged. Traders fought over control of towns; enslaved people and disgruntled wives took advantage of the presence of the colony and, later, European customs stations to escape (Howard in preparation a). States and decentralized polities organized to resist Futa Jallon (Barry 1998, 258–270; Hawthorne 2003). Enslaved people in Moria, now part of southeastern Guinea, and in nearby sections of contemporary Sierra Leone rose up against their masters, created Maroon settlements, and offered religious and other arguments against slavery (Mouser 1996; Mouser 2010; Rashid 2003).

In the nineteenth century, internal slaving and slavery itself expanded, in part because those with means put enslaved people to work as producers (Howard 2006; Klein 1998). In this so-called "legitimate" trade era, large numbers of free and enslaved farmers grew, harvested, and, often, processed palm oil and kernels, peanuts, and other commodities. Overseas and African demand, especially for cattle, kola, and imports, promoted economic and ecological integration. Professional traders spanned much of the region, and countless small traders and farmers carried commodities to exchange points. In the second half of the nineteenth century, traders, commodities, and information flowed widely through the "Sierra Leone–Guinea System," which comprised much of the upper Niger, southern Futa Jallon, and the highlands and plains of northwestern Sierra Leone and southeastern Guinea (Howard 1979). Traders also linked parts of interior Guinea and Liberia, and moved along coastal roads that ran from well north of what is now Conakry to near Monrovia. Various coastal areas, such as southeastern Sierra Leone, were tied into the world market (Hogg 2013). The integration that farmers, traders, and authorities forged involved protracted struggles over trade routes and sites of exchange (Howard 2003; Howard, in preparation a).

The "colonial" era: regional similarities and variations

People in all three countries experienced many commonalities in the era from 1900 to about 1960, with long lasting, often negative impacts. Politically, non-democratic regimes were established, and only late in the period were there limited moves toward wider participatory government. It is often said that Liberia and Ethiopia were the only African countries not colonized. While that is true in important ways, it obscures two realities in the Liberian case. First, the US has been a dominant foreign power in Liberia from that country's origins, and France and especially Britain have also exerted strong influence at times. Second the Americo-Liberian government based in Monrovia carried out an internal colonization of the hinterland, following a trajectory roughly parallel to that of the British in Sierra Leone and the French in Guinea. As one scholar has written: Liberia "was an active (albeit weaker) partner in the scramble for the hinterland. It made great efforts to demonstrate effective control in the hinterland territories it claimed" (Gershoni 1985, 35 ff.). All three conquered the interior, often with great brutality, and early on ruled autocratically through military officers (Abraham 1978; Barry 1998: 284–294; Denzer 1971; Ellis 2007: 208–209). All applied similar colonial techniques: defeating intransigent rulers, staging imperial events to demonstrate power, coopting "friendly chiefs" who ran patronage networks, dividing territory into administrative units headed by officers appointed from the center, and imposing taxes and forced labor.[8]

While there were certain differences in administrative methods, all three governed without democracy or popular participation, thus creating a model of top-down rule that carried over into the national period. In Liberia, the True Whig Party (TWP), run by a rather small group of Americo-Liberian elite men, had a monopoly of power from 1883 to 1980. Even though it was challenged on several occasions and coopted some from the majority, the TWP never undertook basic reforms and continued to run the country hierarchically (Dunn et al. 2001, 332–336). Because of the miniscule public treasury and the entrenchment of Americo-Liberians as district officers and county administrators, Liberia developed a particular form of administrative corruption while promoting tribalism. "Some district commissioners built personal fiefs in the hinterland by these means, accumulating money and private estate … In order to remain in power, they had to redistribute some of these resources through local patronage networks" (Ellis 2007, 214–215).

Throughout the region as a whole, chiefs and other local authorities varied greatly in their qualities and ability to maneuver and create autonomous spheres, but everywhere administrators used pressure and incentives to maintain a hierarchical order. No matter how selected or appointed, chiefs had to act in ways acceptable to officials or risk being replaced. Many were corrupt, extracting labor and "customary" fees. In the words of Elizabeth Schmidt,

> [f]or most Guineans, canton chiefs personified the evils of colonial rule. Appointed by the colonial administration, they served as intermediaries between the government and the rural population. As agents of the state, they collected taxes, recruited involuntary labor and military conscripts, and enforced the mandatory rendering of cash crops. They also transmitted the orders of European administrators to the local populace. (Schmidt 2007, 17)

In Liberia, senior government officials up to the president "manipulated the politics of chieftaincies ... supporting the opposition to any chief who did not conform" (Ellis 2007, 215). In all three territories, the system of "chiefly authorities" maintained patriarchy and promoted tribalism.

Cities and certain towns – especially those that were rail and administrative centers – grew during the "colonial era" and became the sites of most "modern" educational and health facilities and of wage or salary jobs – and thus magnets for youth. Capitals became primate cities where ruling groups, top-down institutions, headquarters of foreign firms, and salaried jobs were concentrated.[9] Their populations grew to be several times larger than any other center. City dwellers developed a wide variety of social associations concerned with housing, jobs, recreation, and other aspects of life. Generally, urban schools provided a higher quality of education than rural schools. Rural literacy levels remained low, and, generally, education of girls lagged seriously behind that of boys (Ojukutu-Macauley 1997; Dunn 2011, 360). For the most part, the curriculums were not geared to building agricultural or technical expertise.

All three countries developed export-oriented, extractive economies. Importing and exporting came to be dominated by large foreign firms, some the precursors of today's multinational food corporations (Goerg 1986, 337–367). In Liberia, officials alienated nearly a million acres to the Firestone Rubber Company.

Although Firestone devoted only a small portion of that acreage to rubber production, the enclave, plantation model became dominant. From the late 1930s to the 1960s, rubber was the "largest single sector" of the Liberian economy (Dunn et al. 2001, 134–135, 284). Although some Americo-Liberians and chiefs gained wealth through ownership of small rubber plantations, rubber did not result in a diversified rural economy and over 80 percent of the population remained subsistence farmers. Sierra Leone developed a different model. Small farmers produced a wide variety of export crops – palm oil, palm kernels, peanuts, kola, ginger, coffee, cocoa, and rice. While palm was the leading export, Sierra Leone did not become as monocultural as many West African countries. Guinea was somewhat of a mix. African small farmers contributed a significant share of exports, while Europeans established plantations. Though their acquisitions were tiny compared with land alienation in Liberia, they grew crops in competition with African farmers and were favored by authorities.

Traders who once had integrated complementary ecological zones were often thwarted or harassed after imperial rulers laid down territorial boundaries and enforced customs duties. What had once been normal commerce now was deemed punishable smuggling. Separate currencies, different legal systems, and incompatible laws further inhibited cross-border traffic. African traders countered by managing alternative commercial institutions and re-arranging their travel patterns and networks. Some of this re-orientation involved crossing colonial borders, for instance in the Kambia–Forekaria area (northeastern Sierra Leone–southeastern Guinea), and integrating new rail and administrative centers, for instance Mamou (Guinea) and Makeni (Sierra Leone). Thus Africans sought to sustain a wider commercial integration, while authorities opposed it (Howard 2014; Howard in preparation b).

Whatever their differences, all three export- and revenue-oriented regimes failed to promote economic diversification and regional integration. While there was growth as measured by expanding exports, the economies did not develop in ways that raised the standard of living of the vast majority. Administrations neglected the crucial role of women in agriculture and did little to advance food production that drew on local knowledge. Research, extension services, and other support for small farmers received little funding. Officials emphasized rail and feeder roads, thus installing a dendritic system to channel export crops overseas and manufactures inland. Only late in the colonial era did attention turn toward creating a reticulated national transport system and improving the connections with neighboring territories.

The Second World War increased pressures upon ordinary people in all territories. Freetown became a strategically critical convoy port enabling the Allies' victory over the fascists. To handle the vast number of ships entering the harbor, tens of thousands of men and women flocked to the city, which doubled in size in less than two years. Laboring under extremely arduous conditions, dockworkers went on strike, building upon the militancy of the mine strikes of the late 1930s but also responding to the needs of city living (Howard 2015). In Guinea, both the Vichy regime and the Free French extracted forced labor and requisitioned crops to support their war efforts (Schmidt 2015). To escape such pressures, vast numbers of people fled their home districts: by the end of the war, "some 7,000 to 8,000 people had migrated from N'Zerekore circle … to Liberia, depopulating all of the frontier cantons" (Schmidt 2015, 452).

Capital-intensive, foreign-owned mining began (in Sierra Leone) in the 1930s, and expanded during the war. By the early 1960s, each country was mineral dependent. In Sierra Leone, diamonds and iron together then accounted for over 90 percent of the overseas earnings. Rubber lost its position as the premier Liberian export when the Timbi Hills were discovered to be almost solid iron and companies vied for the right to exploit it and other rich sites. In Guinea, bauxite rose quickly to rank first among exports. Enclave operations prevailed. The owners built dedicated railways and ports, or, in the case of diamonds, airports, for taking the unprocessed minerals out of the country. Managers lived in protected, closed-off stations. Labor practices were backward especially in Liberia where the rubber industry provided the example. Generally, wages were low, work conditions dangerous, and bosses cared little about injured workers.

Workers took the lead in resisting top-down controls and racism. In Sierra Leone, some of the earliest strikes had been by civil servants and rail workers, who demanded fairness in wages and promotion. Ibrahim Abdullah has documented the fierce, sustained resistance offered by mine workers in Marampa in the late 1930s, in part inspired by I.T.A. Wallace-Johnson and the West Africa Youth

League (WAYL) (Abdullah 1995). The WAYL was a militant socialist, anti-imperial movement that responded to and mobilized popular antagonism to colonial rule. Its largest rallies in Freetown on the eve of the war drew 40,000 or more. Officials were extremely fearful of this movement's base support and the ideological challenge offered by Wallace-Johnson, whom they imprisoned for the duration of the Second World War (Spitzer and Denzer 1973). Historically, unions in Liberia have been nominal, controlled by the state and weak in comparison with employers. Important exceptions were the Mine Workers' Union and Dock Workers' Association, which flourished briefly in the late 1970s before authorities suspended them (Dunn et al. 2001, 199–200).

A strong, independent left grew up in late colonial Guinea, mainly based in the labor movement, but also involving peasants, veterans, and urban dwellers who were not organized workers, especially young men and women. During the war and immediately after, great resistance arose against forced labor. Once France ended its prohibition against labor organizing, workers quickly formed unions. A 1946 strike paralyzed Conakry and other important cities. Guinean rail workers joined the 1947–1948 rail strike that spanned much of French West Africa, and were supported by workers in other sectors and the general community. This led to the massive general strikes of 1950 and 1953, which included public and private sectors and skilled and unskilled workers (Schmidt 2005, 58–83). Guinea also experienced much rural unrest during this era and beyond. In part, this was manifested against chiefs; peasants had been resisting their pressures since the Second World War, when chiefs served as collectors of special levies and attempted to extract unpaid labor (Schmidt 2005, 91–111). In Sierra Leone rural dissatisfaction led to widespread uprisings against chiefs in 1954–1955 (Rashid 2009).

Women's base organizations were strong in Sierra Leone and Guinea.[10] They challenged colonial rule and gender-based injustices, and sought to advance women's interests. In Sierra Leone, during the period after the First World War, market women, petty traders, and others fought the efforts of large firms to commandeer urban spaces (Howard 2003). Later, Constance Cummings-John emerged as the principal leader of a cross-class alliance of Western-educated women and market women, an alliance that sought, among other things, fair prices for traders. Cummings-John was a feminist,

Pan-Africanist, member of the militant West African Youth League, and, later, leader in the Sierra Leone People's Party (SLPP), that headed the country at independence (Cummings-John and Denzer 1995). In Guinea, the Rassemblement Démocratique Africain (RDA), the primary nationalist party, took up women's campaigns over rice prices and urban water supplies, as well as education and health (Schmidt 2005, 116–126). During one anti-tax campaign in early 1955, a chief killed a woman leader, M'balia Camara. The RDA and others built momentum around this event, and M'balia Camara became a national heroine, with moving songs composed to honor her memory (Schmidt 2007, 86–87).

Economic crisis, dictatorship, war, and popular resistance in the post-colonial era

Liberia, always nominally independent, joined the United Nations when it was established in 1945; Guinea and Sierra Leone became independent in 1958 and 1961, respectively. The wave of African independence brought widespread optimism. From the 1970s, however, all three countries went through wrenching changes that greatly decreased their economic and political capacity to respond to the Ebola crisis: highly unfavorable global economic forces, heavy international debt, and imposed structural adjustment programs; dictatorship and corruption; military coups, destructive wars, and large numbers of refugees and exiles. Existing economic weaknesses continued, but were intensified by the oil price jolts of the 1970s and precipitous declines in world commodity prices. Especially harmful were the retrenchment programs imposed by the International Monetary Fund (IMF) and World Bank (WB) in the 1980s and 1990s, which led to reduced incomes for the poor and layoffs of teachers, nurses, and others who delivered medical services (Kamara 2008, 133–148). Economies were further undermined by corruption and mismanagement. Still, many people continued to organize energetically for a more just social, economic, and political order within each country and internationally.

By the 1980s, if not earlier, it was apparent that extractive mining under prevailing global forces brought vast human, environmental, and economic costs. Guinea is an instructive case. It has the world's largest supply of high-grade bauxite, and in 2005 contributed 40 percent of global trade in that mineral sector. During most of his leadership (1958–1984), Sekou Toure pressured companies to process bauxite to create aluminum within Guinea. The value added by selling finished aluminum rather than raw bauxite could then be channeled into other sectors, resulting in a more balanced development. At the heart of the strategy was a massive electricity-generating project on the Konkoure River. Yet, by his death, in 1984, companies had failed to carry out such plans, and Guinea suffered from external debt. Toure's successor through a coup, General Lansana Conteh, turned to the IMF and attempted to meet Structural Adjustment Program (SAP) conditionalities by reducing the public sector. He also opened the economy to foreign investment. In the 1980s and 1990s, state revenues from bauxite fell, making it impossible to meet IMF and World Bank loan repayments. Guinea lost its capacity to sustain income from bauxite because of international forces: low bauxite prices due to competition from other producers and, especially, weak bargaining position vis-à-vis mining companies (Campbell 2009).

Sierra Leone felt its vulnerability to world prices and corporate policies when Delco Mining unilaterally closed the Marampa mines in 1975. Marampa, known for its high-quality iron ore, was once a major employer and earner of foreign currency. Iron mining resumed at two sites in the twenty-first century, but company financing was weak. When world prices fell and the spread of Ebola affected operations, companies closed mines in 2015.[11] Liberia went from being dependent on rubber exports to being dependent on mineral exports. President William Tubman (1944–1971) advocated for an "Open Door Policy" that he claimed would bring increased foreign investment, economic diversification, revenue, and income for workers. During the 1960s, iron mining at Bomi Hills and elsewhere increased nearly seven times in volume. All ore was exported through dedicated rail lines. About 11,000 men were employed as unskilled or semi-skilled laborers in the iron mines by 1970 (von Gnielinski 1972, 88–91). In 1977 the mine at Bomi Hills was closed, and eventually the three other major mines shuttered (Chinese firms have recently re-opened two). Although iron brought jobs and revenue to the national coffers, it resulted in little economic integration or diversification.

A great austerity took hold of the region in the 1980s and 1990s, following on the oil price hikes, commodity price falls, and greater national indebtedness. In the aftermath of the Cold War, leaders of the countries sought new forms of external support and patronage. "Development aid" grew both absolutely and relative to national sources of revenue. In 1993, to pick a date after war had been ravaging Liberia and Sierra Leone, the former received development aid equivalent to 96 percent of its internal revenue and the latter 178 percent (Reno 1999, 115). This situation was unsustainable, and failed to "solve" the problem of structural poverty. By about 2000, the Extractive Industries Review (EIR) of the World Bank recognized the need for stricter guidelines in providing loans and risk insurance to logging and mining companies in order to reduce poverty; to protect poor people, local communities, and the environment; and to ensure that extractive companies honor basic human rights. Generally, in practice, the guidelines were only implemented in a minimal way or were not followed.[12]

Other large forces drained economic and social capacities and raised dissatisfaction with governments. Urban populations boomed because of a combination of relatively high birth rates, rural poverty, and insecurity resulting in the concentration in cities of better paying salaried jobs, wage work, and informal sector opportunities. Conakry, Freetown, and Monrovia tripled or quadrupled in size between 1960 and the 1990s. In all three countries 15–29 year-olds became a sizeable percentage of the population. Youth experienced very severe impacts from the era's economic downturn and environmental pressures, having especially high unemployment and urban and rural poverty rates (Abdullah 2004; Aning and Atta-Asamoah 2011).

All three countries became dictatorships. Early leaders of the newly independent Sierra Leone took steps to consolidate their power, which among other things entrenched ethnicity in politics and undermined national institutions. Albert Margai, the second prime minister, worked to ensure that the army, electoral commission, and Sierra Leone People's Party (SLPP) were dominated by Mende (Cartwright 1978). When Siaka Stevens became prime minister after a military coup, he "showed himself to be [even] more Machiavellian, practical, and 'effective' at power consolidation" (Conteh-Morgan and Dixon-Fyle 2005, 81). Within two years he fundamentally altered the ethnic makeup of the army and its officer corps, then went on to entrench minority northern groups that aligned with him and to forge a loyal paramilitary State Security Division that amounted to a "palace guard" (Conteh-Morgan and Dixon-Fyle 2005, 78–83).

In Guinea, the RDA moved from being a "highly democratic mass party to the ultimate source of power in a repressive authoritarian state" (Schmidt 2007, 184). The RDA took advantage of the sense of a state of siege felt by Guineans when France, the United States, and others isolated and rebuffed its overtures after the "no vote"; then and in subsequent years it cracked down on dissent within the party and outside it. Leaders accumulated political functions at several levels, from the local to the national, and concentrated power in their hands (Schmidt 2007, 184–186). A military coup, at the time of Sekou Toure's death, opened the way for decades of brutal and highly repressive military rule, culminating in 2009 when soldiers killed hundreds of citizens peacefully assembled to protest and raped scores of women.[13]

Liberia saw a more twisting path, but much the same results. The True Whig Party (TWP) was founded in 1869, and in the late nineteenth and early twentieth centuries TWP presidents accrued much power. Liberia gained a reputation for being "West Africa's first de facto one-party state" (Ellis 2007, 213). William V.S. Tubman, president from 1944 to 1971, consolidated an authoritarian regime through shrewd political manipulation and a cult of personality as a "powerful, stern, generous" father to "his people" (Ellis 2007, 215). Besides his familiarity with local politics throughout the country, his patronage machine stemmed from his ability to distribute contracts and largesse. His successor, William Tolbert, lacked the same personal and political capabilities. He held office during most of the 1970s, a time of economic difficulties that culminated in mass civil disobedience and his 1980 overthrow and assassination by enlisted members of the army, ending 133 years of political domination by Americo-Liberians. The military-run People's Redemption Council was headed by Samuel K. Doe, who ruled until 1990, when he too was ousted and killed. Doe increasingly resorted to violence and ethnic favoritism (as well as US backing) to maintain power, laying the basis for the bloody regime of Charles Taylor and the ethnic retributions of the civil war (Ellis 2007, 45–74, 211–219; Dunn et al. 2001, 111–113, 324–326, 332–338).

If dictatorship and violence thwarted the development of participatory democracy, all three countries were sapped by a patrimonialism that drew wealth into the center and re-distributed (part of) it outward to officials, chiefs, and other leading supporters. This was accompanied and followed by the IMF and WB retrenchment policies, which shrunk the national spending for health, education, and infrastructure, including the incomes of many thousands of rural and urban people. Patrimonialism in Sierra Leone depended upon a concentrated source of great wealth, diamonds, which political leaders could easily tap. Conteh-Morgan and Dixon-Fyle have aptly described and analyzed how the system operated. Siaka Stevens, who by 1971 had created the office of president and ruled unopposed, drained a share of the country's wealth into his own pockets and those of close supporters and held the country together by rechanneling state revenues. His successor, Force Commander Joseph Saidu Momoh, continued a similar system with much less skill – until the diamond supply ran down, foreign debt reached unsustainable levels, and massive public anger and opposition arose (Conteh-Morgan and Dixon-Fyle 2005; Reno 1999, 114–133).

Liberia had a much more limited patrimonial order until Charles Taylor expanded the system and ruled in a manner that combined violence and personal engagement with networks of supporters.[14] During the war era, he became the main global outlet for Sierra Leone diamonds obtained by the Revolutionary United Front (RUF) in Kono and Tongo Fields. Felix Gerdes estimates that in the five years between 1997 and 2001 the RUF exported between US$175 million and US$245 million worth of diamonds, and Taylor's "profits" were between US$91 million and US$129 million. "The revenue derived [from diamonds] was a major source of finance for Taylor's sovereign system of domination" (Gerdes 2013, 143–144). Once the RUF was defeated and the embargo against "blood diamonds" was installed, Taylor financed his regime through timber exports.

War tore Sierra Leone apart through much of the 1990s (actually March 1991 until January 2002). Over 50,000 people are estimated to have died, with vast disruption of the social fabric (Gberie 2005). The Liberian war lasted from 1989 to 2003 – although there was a two-year hiatus when Charles Taylor headed an elected government and became engaged in the Sierra Leone fighting. Reportedly 250,000 to 500,000 people were killed. While there was no direct fighting in Guinea during this era, Guineans went through great upheavals. The country was a staging ground for attacks into its neighbors, especially Liberia. It was a corridor for international smuggling, received several hundred thousand refugees, and saw its economy further damaged by the chaos around it. Finally, Guinea experienced intensified internal military oppression, partly justified by regional instability.

The war in Sierra Leone, following on decades of insufficient funding, resulted in destruction of the educational and health infrastructures. A joint report by the IMF and International Development Association drew special attention to

> disruptions to schooling owing to population displacements; a devastated school infrastructure, displacement of teachers and resulting difficulty in maintaining records and paying salaries on time; lack of basic furniture and teaching and learning materials; overcrowding in many schools in safer areas; disorientation and psychological trauma among a large segment of the population, especially children; and a weakened institutional capacity of the Ministry of Youth Education and Sports (MYES) to manage the education system. (International Monetary Fund/International Development Association 2002, 15)

The same report noted that the "health situation of the population is more critical than in other sub-Saharan African countries." The life expectancy at birth was only 38 years, and under-five infant mortality was 286/1,000 live births. Many health facilities had been destroyed and the sector's operations were severely weakened by lack of staff and disruptions in transportation, communications, electricity, and water supply. All in all, Sierra Leone ranked last among 174 countries on the United Nation's Human Development Index. According to the Index, Guinea ranked about the same as Sierra Leone in basic health and other measures, with Liberia only slightly better (IMF/IDA 2002, 5, 16 ff.).

During the era of warfare, cities again grew massively while social resources shrunk, making their populations especially vulnerable to contagious diseases. Freetown, in particular, may have doubled as refugees and people seeking safety flowed in. According to some estimates, over a few years in the 1990s, the city rose from about 500,000 to 1,000,000. By 2014, Sierra Leone and Guinea were nearly 40 percent urbanized, and Liberia was approaching 50 percent, according to United Nations data.[15] Youth unemployment skyrocketed in all three countries, leading – along with corruption, military abuses, and inadequate spending on education and social services – to widespread alienation of youth from government. Tens of thousands of young men and women were drawn into the Sierra Leone war as combatants and supporters of combatants, but also as its victims. In both Liberia and Sierra Leone, women and girls were subject to high levels of rape and other forms of sexual abuse and violence (O'Neill and Ward 2005).

When the RUF carried out its devastating attacks on Freetown, women stood out as protectors of the city and proponents of peace, none more so than Zainab Bangura. An NGO activist in the 1990s, she later would head the ministries of foreign affairs and health before being appointed as Special Representative on Sexual Violence in Conflict of the United Nations Secretary-General. During the war she challenged the RUF for its atrocities against civilians and was threatened with assassination on several occasions. Later, she targeted the national army for its abuses and the then ruling party for corruption. Many other Sierra Leonean women joined in her oppositional campaign.[16] In Liberia, the Association of Female Liberian Lawyers drew attention to sexual and other abuses of women and took the lead in bringing prosecutions of criminal acts. One of the standout figures was Leymah Gbowee, who in 2011 was awarded the Nobel Peace Prize. As a young woman she became a leader of the Women in Peace Network (WiPNET), consisting of mainly Christian women, and joined forces with Muslim women to form Liberian Mass Action. The group gained a face-to-face meeting with Charles Taylor, extracted his agreement to attend peace negotiations in Ghana, and then sent a delegation to keep pressure upon combatants.[17]

Throughout the region, women were actively engaged in reconstruction as well as peacemaking. Probably most important from a regional perspective has been the Mano River Women's Peace Network (Réseau des Femmes du Flueve Mano pour la Paix), started during the later years of the Liberian war. It sponsored peace tours around the region and held seminars in all three countries to represent and empower women and build gender into policy planning. Specific campaigns have focused on stopping the abuses and extractions that women traders have experienced when crossing borders and doing business in countries where they were not citizens.[18] It also has engaged in dialogue with youth organizations seeking to build social and economic skills among former combatants. Despite its potential, leadership cooptation could drain away the energies generated by the elite–mass linkages.

Rethinking regional history/networks in the context of Ebola: by way of conclusion

During the late decades of the twentieth century, elite leaders recognized the value of pulling their countries together and formed the Mano River Union (MRU). Sierra Leone and Liberia first created the compact in 1974, and Guinea joined in 1980. The MRU took some useful steps, such as reducing customs barriers as a move toward greater economic integration. It collapsed during the wars, but in 2004 was revived and has since expanded its objectives and membership by adding Côte d'Ivoire in 2008. In its first incarnation, it sought to build from the top, rather than from the bottom, and it remains to be seen if, now resuscitated, it will incorporate the energy and knowledge of the vast majority.

The movement of people within the region to trade, work, and settle is ancient and continues. Typically, people who migrate build ties in their new residences while retaining connections with their former homes. Their flows back and forth result in extensive transnational networks, while their settlement embeds them in dense, local networks. This is especially true for certain patterns of trade and migration. In the Guéckédou–Kailahun and the Forekaria–Kambia areas, large numbers of traders in rice, cassava, cattle, imported goods, and other things have been moving back and forth across the frontiers, sometimes illegally, from the establishment of colonial borders in the early twentieth century up to the present. They have focused their exchange in particular market centers. Those flows grew out of earlier, pre-colonial commerce, but were intensified by the growth of towns and modern motor roads within the countries and across borders. (Howard 2014; Bah 1998, 89 ff.) The same (or nearby) routes and towns were important during the crisis of the 1990s and early 2000s. When hundreds of thousands of people fled fighting in eastern Sierra Leone, they crossed into Guinea through Kailahun and Kono districts and wound up in camps near Guéckédou (in the so-called "parrot's beak," where the three countries meet). Later, many refugees from those camps and other locations in Guinea returned to Sierra Leone via the Guéckédou–Kailahun route, which early on included a dirt causeway across a branch of the Moa River. Or, they followed a roundabout way through Guinea to Forekaria then Kambia.[19] A 2013 study found many of the same roads in Guinea and across the borders were vital for commerce.[20] It is possible that the trans-border networks (nodes plus flows) established through trade and refugee movement were important in the transmission of Ebola in at least two time periods: first, during the rainy season of 2014 in the "parrots beak" zone where the first heavy outbreak of EVD occurred, and, second, during March and April 2015 in the Forekaria and Kambia districts.[21] The World Health Organization is aware of the importance of such regional factors: in an "Ebola Situation Report" issued late in the epidemic when new cases were few, WHO noted that its criteria for prioritizing support to other partner countries "include geographical proximity to affected countries, trade and migration patterns, and strength of health systems."[22]

Personal and institutional networks have long existed among members of so-called "universal" religions and across those faiths – and also among members of "ethnic" associations. Such networks also have linked emigrants to neighboring countries of origin (Sierra Leoneans in Guinea and Liberia, Liberians in Guinea and Sierra Leone, Guineans in Liberia and Sierra Leone) and linked immigrants living overseas with one another and with their homelands. Sometime such networks have promoted narrow national, ethnic or sectarian loyalties, but they have also been critically important in facilitating a flow of information and in rallying people. Such networks need much deeper study with regard to education about Ebola and other diseases, mobilization in times of crisis, and distribution of assistance. At an inter-faith training meeting in Bo, Sierra Leone, in mid-2014, as EVD was spreading rapidly, a prominent convener of the Religious Leaders Task Force on Ebola declared: "Ebola does not discriminate between Muslims and Christians ... When it strikes it kills anybody of any faith or political group."[23] The Ministry of Health called for religious networks to take a larger role in disseminating accurate information about EVD. It would be equally valuable to investigate how assistance funds from overseas were channeled, particularly if they were channeled in exclusive ways that led to division and antagonism, or thwarted efforts of more neutral agencies to coordinate responses regionally.

At the most applied level, this survey raises questions about ways that historical, geographic, and social research with a regional perspective might be of value to those providing medical services. Detailed information about people's migratory patterns and social, cultural, and commercial exchanges could assist officials seeking to stop the flow of contagion or responding to an environmental crisis – especially with the recent seaweed invasion off the coastline of the MRU states and the growing threat of climate change. There are many other cultural questions. For instance, how might knowledge of people's beliefs and practices and their communication networks provide understanding about how they perceive the etiology of disease and share those perceptions with others, and how they generate local responses to disease or other threats?

The kind of structural approach offered here prompts questions about how people recognize and express commonalities and come together around issues of health, disease, or economic advancement. Gender and class have intersected differently from place to place, yet women in all three countries have been affected by similar forces of patriarchy, colonialism, predatory government, war, environmental deterioration, and retrenchment of services. Those commonalities of experience provide a foundation for the sense of solidarity and kinds of organizations that women are building across borders. Youth, too, have a trans-regional foundation in experience and struggles. Needed are local, national, regional, and external policies and programs that promote rather than inhibit the strengthening of such ties. While organizations like MARWOPNET have modeled a regional approach, international agencies generally operate on a country-by-country basis. The major "northern" powers involved in the area (United States, Britain, and France), often seem to have continued a "neo-colonial" division of the region into spheres and distributed money to national branches of transnational organizations rather than promoting region-wide coordination. Continuation of state- rather than region-oriented planning is likely to generate costly redundancies, promote narrow nationalism, and serve politicians who take credit for projects. For example, while many basic health services may most efficiently be provided locally or nationally, no individual country can afford a full range of medical training and health delivery services. It makes economic sense for more costly training, equipment, and facilities to be supported on a regional basis with full access by citizens of all states, perhaps through a restructured Mano River Union.[24]

Most of all, history shows that common people need to forge a region that benefits them. A regional economy could be the framework for easier foreign access to resources; it could facilitate large corporations using the electricity generated in one country to extract minerals of another country at lower cost. Or it could provide the framework for building a sustainable economy based on complementary ecological zones and people's knowledge, skills, and contemporary education – an economy that allocates scarce resources justly. The similar experiences of ordinary people also demonstrate that they must organize and struggle economically and politically to have sufficient decision-making capacity and bargaining power to ensure their interests are protected and advanced.

Notes

1 This chapter honors four decades of work by Boubacar Barry, Professor Emeritus of History at Université Cheikh Anta Diop, Dakar, Senegal, to conceive and promote a more unified West Africa. Thanks to Ibrahim Abdullah, Sarah K. Howard, Ismail Rashid, and Elizabeth Schmidt for their very helpful comments on drafts of this chapter.

2 The three countries have constituted a "formal" region through their legal integration into the Mano River Union. They also have been and are part of different, overlapping interactive regions (social, political, cultural, and economic), shaped by flows of people, goods, and ideas. For definitions of "formal" and interactive regions in African history, see Howard (2005, 46–50 ff.).

3 Board-sponsored Round Table: Ebola: Exposing the Fault Lines, November 21, 2014.

4 The farthest interior areas of Guinea lie in the drier savanna/woodland zone.

5 Ellis presents a succinct overview of pre-Liberian politics, masking, and religion, and notes that the southeast, corresponding with the Kruan-speaking areas, lacked *poro* and masking (Ellis 2007, 191–206).

6 Pew Research Center, *The Future of World Religions: Population Growth Projections, 2010–2050* (April 2, 2015), 234–242, www.pewresearch.org (accessed December 9, 2015). This survey does not adequately indicate the widespread blending of "world" and local religious beliefs and practices.

7 For details on the organization of the Atlantic slave trade, see Hancock (1995); Mouser (1996).

8 Ellis has written the following about Liberia: "A description of a military expedition to put down a rising in the south-east, apparently in 1930, led by President Barclay in person, reveals it to have been a veritable plundering operation" (Ellis 2007, 210).

9 In Freetown, a system of "tribal" headmen and women emerged; some were close to "their people," assisted immigrants find jobs and housing, and promoted schools and other amenities (Harrell-Bond et al. 1978). Monrovia had certain parallels (Fraenkel 1964).

10 Little has been written about the resistance of peasant and market women's organizations in Liberia; elite women's groups existed in all three territories, but are not covered here.

11 *Bloomberg*, "Timis Misses Payment to Australian Backer after Mine Closes," June 23, 2015; *Mining*, "African Minerals Starts Temporary Shutdown at Sierra Leone Mine," December 1, 2014.

12 Mainhardt-Gibbs (2003); The World Bank Group in Extractive Industries, *2011 Annual Review*; Jubilee USA Network, "Debt and the Environment," www.jubileeus.org (accessed November 12, 2015).

13 "Guinea: September 28 Massacre Was Premeditated. In-Depth Investigation Also Documents Widespread Rape," Human Rights Watch report of October 27, 2009; "Guinea's Ex-Junta Leader Indicted over Stadium Massacre," *Reuters World*, July 9, 2015.

14 There is considerable debate as to whether or not Taylor ran a patrimonial order in the classic sense. Gerdes argues that a "considerable share" of funds derived from diamonds, timber, and so on were transferred abroad and not "used for consolidating authority"; Taylor's regime, he feels, depended on a personalistic use of power (Gerdes 2013, 152).

15 UN Department of Economic and Social Affairs, Population Division "World Urbanization Prospects: The 2014 Revisions, Highlights," New York: United Nations, 2014 ST/ESA/SER. A/352, p. 2, table "percentage of population residing in urban areas in 2014 ...."

16 Amedzrator (2014, 11–12); Sorie Sudan Sesay, "Zainab Bangura Gets Honorary Oxford Doctorate," *Awareness Time, Sierra Leone News and Information*, June 30, 2015.

17 Amedzrator (2014, 9–11); Nobel Peace Prize 2011, "Leymah Gbowee – Biographical," www.nobelprize.org/nobel_prizes/peace/laureates/2011/gbowee-bio.html (accessed November 14, 2015); "Saying 'Yes' to Peace: How the Women of Liberia Fought for Peace and Won," *Tavanna*, n.d., https://tavaana.org/sites/default/files/Liberia%20PDF.pdf (last accessed November 14, 2015).

18 Reseau des Femmes du Flueve Mano pour la Paix / Mano River Women's Peace Network, "MARWOPNET – Guéckédou: Solving Conflicts in the Marketplace," *Voices of Peace*, April 2004.

19 Ray Wilkinson, "Sierra Leone Refugees Return to Their Homes," November 27, 2001, http://www.unhcr.org/news/latest/2001/11/3c03a7664/sierra-leone-refugees-return-homes.html; Delphine Marie, "Fast Track Back to Sierra Leone Raises Hopes of Complete Repatriation by End of 2004," April 7, 2003, http://www.unhcr.org/news/latest/2003/4/3e91a6864/fast-track-sierra-leone-raises-hopes-complete-repatriation-end-2004.html; Rachel Goldstein-Rodriguez, "A Rough but Happy Journey Home for Sierra Leonean Refugees," UNHCR News Stories, June 7, 2004, http://www.unhcr.org/news/latest/2004/6/40c47fe84/rough-happy-journey-home-sierra-leonean-refugees.html; "Progress on Guinea Refugees' Plight," *BBC News*, February 15, 2001, http://news.bbc.co.uk/2/hi/africa/1171872.stm (all accessed November 14, 2015).

20 "Guinea Production and Market Flow Map Report," USAID FEWSNET, April 2013.

21 "Ebola-related Fears Disrupt Markets and Livelihoods; Elevated Levels of Food Insecurity Expected," USAID FEWSNET, September 8, 2014; World Health Organization, "Ebola Situation Report," April 15, 2015.

22 World Health Organization, "Ebola Situation Report," April 15, 2015.

23 Phileas Jusu, "Christians and Muslims Fight Ebola," July 28, 2014, The United Methodist Church, Michigan Area, http://news.michiganumc.org (accessed December 15, 2015).

24 Thomas Jaye and Fifi Edu-Afful, "Ebola Impact and Lessons for West Africa," Kofi Annan International Peacekeeping Training Centre, Policy Brief 4 / November 2014; World Health Organization, "Ebola Recovery Is Impossible Unless Resilient Health Systems Are Rebuilt in Guinea, Liberia, and Sierra Leone," July 6, 2015.

References

Abdullah, Ibrahim (1995). "'Liberty or Death': Working Class Agitation and the Labour Question in Colonial Freetown, 1938–1939," *International Review of Social History*, 40: 195–221.

Abdullah, Ibrahim (2004). "Bush Path to Destruction: The Origins and Character of the Revolutionary United Front (RUF/SL)," in Abdullah, Ibrahim (ed.) *Between Democracy and Terror: The Sierra Leone Civil War*. Dakar: CODESRIA, 41–65.

Abraham, Arthur (1978). *Mende Government and Politics under Colonial Rule*. Freetown: Sierra Leone University Press.

Amedzrator, Lydia Mawuenya (2014). *Breaking the Inertia: Women's Role in Mediation and Peace Processes in West Africa*. KAIPTC Occasional Paper no. 38.

Aning, Kwesi and Atta-Asamoah, Andrews (2011). *Demography, Environment and Conflict in West Africa*. KAIPTC Occasional Paper no. 34.

Bah, Mohammed Alpha (1998). *Fulbe Presence in Sierra Leone: A Case History of 20th Century Migration and Settlement among the Kissi of Koindu*. New York: Peter Lang.

Barry, Boubacar (1998). *Senegambia and the Atlantic Slave Trade*. Cambridge and New York: Cambridge University Press.

Blackburn, Robin (1997). *The Making of New World Slavery: From the Baroque to the Modern 1492–1800*. London and New York: Verso.

Brooks, George E. (1993). *Landlords and Strangers: Ecology, Society, and Trade in Western Africa, 1000–1630*. Boulder, CO: Westview Press.

Campbell, Bonnie (2009). "Guinea and Bauxite-Aluminum: The Challenge of Development and Poverty Reduction," in Campbell, Bonnie, *Mining in Africa: Regulation and Development*. London and New York: Pluto Press, 66–118.

Cartwright, John R. (1978). *Political Leadership in Sierra Leone*. Toronto: University of Toronto Press.

Clarke, J.I. (ed.) (1966). *Sierra Leone in Maps*. London: London University Press.

Coifman, Victoria Bomba (1994). "The Western West African and European Frontier: Contributions from Former Archbishop of Conakry Raymond-Marie Tchidimbo's Autobiography for West African History," in Harms, Robert, Miller, Joseph C., Newbury, David S., and Wagner, Michele D. (eds) *Paths Toward the Past: African Historical Essays in Honor of Jan Vansina*. Atlanta, GA: The African Studies Association Press, 273–292.

Cole, Gibril R. (2013). *The Krio of West Africa: Islam, Culture, Creolization, and Colonialism in the Nineteenth Century*. Athens, OH: Ohio University Press.

Conteh-Morgan, Earl and Dixon-Fyle, Mac (2005). *Sierra Leone at the End of the Twentieth Century: History, Politics, and Society*. New York: Peter Lang.

Cummings-John, Constance with Denzer, LaRay (1995). *Constance Agatha Cummings-John: Memoirs of a Krio Leader*. Ibadan, Nigeria: Sam Bookman for Humanities Research Center.

Currens, Gerald E. (1979). "Land, Labor, and Capital in Loma Agriculture," in Dorjahn, Vernon R. and Isaacs, Barry L. (eds) *Essays on the Economic Anthropology of Liberia and Sierra Leone*. Philadelphia, PA: Institute for Liberian Studies, 79–102.

Denzer, LaRay (1971). "Sierra Leone – Bai Bureh," in Crowder, Michael (ed.) *West African Resistance: The Military Response to Colonial Occupation*. New York: Africana Publishing Corporation, 233–267.

Dunn, D. Elwood (2011). *The Annual Messages of the Presidents of Liberia 1848–2010: State of the Nation Addresses to National Legislature: From Joseph Jenkins Roberts to Ellen Johnson Sirleaf*. Berlin and New York: Walter de Gruyter.

Dunn, D. Elwood, Beyan, Amos J., and Burrowes, Carl Patrick (eds) (2001). *Historical Dictionary of Liberia*, 2nd ed. Metuchen, NJ: Scarecrow Press.

Ellis, Stephen (2007). *The Mask of Anarchy: The Destruction of Liberia and the Religious Dimension*, 2nd ed. New York: New York University Press.

Fanthorpe, Richard (1998). "Limba 'Deep Rural' Strategies," *Journal of African History*, 39: 15–38.

Fields-Black, Edda L. (2008). *Deep Roots: Rice Farmers in West Africa and the African Diaspora*. Bloomington and Indianapolis, IN: Indiana University Press.

Fraenkel, Merran (1964). *Tribe and Class in Monrovia*. London: Oxford University Press.

Fyfe, Christopher (1962). *A History of Sierra Leone*. Oxford: Oxford University Press.

Fyle, C. Magbaily (1979a). *Oral Traditions of Sierra Leone*. Niamey, Niger: Centre d'Etudes Linguistique et Historique par Tradition Orale.

Fyle, C. Magbaily (1979b). *The Solima Yalunka Kingdom: Pre-Colonial Politics, Economics, and Society*. Freetown: Nyakon Publishers.

Gberie, Lansana (2005). *A Dirty War in West Africa: The RUF and the Destruction of Sierra Leone*. Bloomington and Indianapolis, IN: Indiana University Press.

Gerdes, Felix (2013). *Civil War and State Formation: The Political Economy of War and Peace in Liberia*. Frankfurt: Campus Verlag.

Gershoni, Yekutiel (1985). *Black Colonialism: The Americo-Liberian Scramble for the Hinterland*. Boulder, CO and London: Westview Press.

Goerg, Odile (1986). *Commerce et Colonisation en Guineé 1850–1913*. Paris: Harmattan.

Hancock, David (1995). *Citizens of the World: London Merchants and the Integration of the British Atlantic Community, 1735–1785*. Cambridge and New York: Cambridge University Press.

Harrell-Bond, Barbara E., Howard, Allen M., and Skinner, David E. (1978). *Community Leadership and the Transformation of Freetown (1801–1976)*. The Hague: Mouton.

Hawthorne, Walter (2003). "Strategies of the Decentralized: Defending Communities Slave Raiders in Coastal Guinea-Bissau, 1450–1815," in Diouf, Sylviane A., *Fighting the Slave Trade: West African Strategies*. Athens, OH: Ohio University Press; Oxford: James Currey, 52–169.

Hogg, Trina (2013). "'Our Country Customs': Diplomacy, Legality, and Violence on the Sierra Leone Frontier 1861–1896." Unpublished Ph.D. dissertation, New York University.

Holsoe, Svend E. (1979). "Economic Activities in the Liberian Area: The Pre- European Period to 1900," in Dorjahn, Vernon R. and Isaacs, Barry L. (eds) *Essays on the Economic Anthropology of Liberia and Sierra Leone*. Philadelphia, PA: Institute for Liberian Studies, 63–78.

Howard, Allen M. (1979). "Production, Exchange, and Society in Northern Coastal Sierra Leone during the 19th Century," in Dorjahn, Vernon R. and Isaacs, Barry L. (eds) *Essays of the Economic Anthropology of Liberia and Sierra Leone*. Philadelphia, PA: Institute for Liberian Studies, 45–62.

Howard, Allen M. (1999). "Mande and Fulbe Interaction and Identity in Northwestern Sierra Leone, Late Eighteenth through Early Twentieth Centuries," *Mande Studies*, 1: 13–40.

Howard, Allen M. (2003). "Cities in Africa, Past and Present: Contestation, Transformation, Discourse," *Canadian Journal of African Studies*, 37, 2/3: 197–235.

Howard, Allen M. (2005). "Nodes, Networks, Landscapes, and Regions: Reading the Social History of Tropical Africa 1700s–," in Howard, Allen M. and Shain, Richard M. (eds) *The Spatial Factor in African History. The Relationship of the Social, Material, and Perceptual*. Leiden: Brill, 21–140.

Howard, Allen M. (2006). "Nineteenth-Century Coastal Slave Trading and the British Abolition Campaign in Sierra Leone," *Slavery and Abolition*, 27, 1: 23–49.

Howard, Allen M. (2007). "Mande Kola Traders of Northwestern Sierra Leone, Late 1700s to 1930," *Mande Studies*, 9: 83–102.

Howard, Allen M. (2014). "Cross-Boundary Traders in the Era of High Imperialism: Changing Structures and Strategies in the Sierra Leone-Guinea Region," *Articulo: Journal of Urban Research*, 10 (online).

Howard, Allen M. (2015). "Freetown and World War II," in Byfield, Judith A., Brown, Carolyn A., Parsons, Timothy, and Sikainga, Ahmad Alawad (eds) *Africa and World War II*. Cambridge and New York: Cambridge University Press, 183–199.

Howard, Allen M. (in preparation a). *Spatial Strategies, Resources, and Power: Traders in the Sierra Leone-Guinea Plain.*

Howard, Allen M. (in preparation b). *Traders and Colonial Domination, Northwestern Sierra Leone, 1890–1920s.*

International Monetary Fund and the International Development Association (IMF/IDA) (2002). *Sierra Leone. Enhanced Heavily Indebted Poor Countries (HIPC) Initiative Decision Point Document*. February 15, 2002.

Kamara, Fouday S. (2008). *Economic and Social Crises in Sierra Leone: The Role of Small-Scale Entrepreneurs in Petty Trading as a Strategy for Survival 1960–1996*. Milton Keynes, UK: Authorhouse.

Klein, Martin (1998). *Slavery and Colonial Rule in West Africa*. Cambridge: Cambridge University Press.

Lamp, Frederick (1996). *Art of the Baga: A Drama of Cultural Reinvention*. Baltimore, MD: The Museum for African Art and Prestel Verlag.

Lovejoy, Paul E. (2000). *Transformations in Slavery: A History of Slavery in Africa*, 2nd ed. Cambridge and New York: Cambridge University Press.

Mainhardt-Gibbs, Heike (2003). *The World Bank Extractive Industries Review: The Role of Structural Reform Programs towards Sustainable Development Outcomes. Executive Summary*. Assets.panda.

org/downloads/eirsalsummary deco3.doc (accessed December 10, 2015).

Misevich, Phillip (2008). "The Origins of Slaves Leaving the Upper Guinea Coast in the Nineteenth Century," in David Eltis and David Richardson (ed.) *Extending the Frontiers: Essays on the New Transatlantic Slave Trade Database*. New Haven, CT: Yale University Press, 155–175.

Mouser, Bruce (1996). "Îles de Los as Bulking Center in the Slave Trade, 1750–1800," *Revue Française d'histoire d'Outre-Mer*, 83, 313: 77–90.

Mouser, Bruce (2010). "Insurrection as Socioeconomic Change: Three Rebellions in Guinea/Sierra Leone in the Eighteenth Century," in Knörr, Jacqueline and Filho, Wilson Trajano (eds) *The Powerful Presence of the Past*. Leiden: Brill, 55–74.

Njoku, Athanasius O. (1979). "The Economics of Mende Rice Farming," in Dorjahn, V.R. and Isaac, B.L. (eds.) *Essays on the Economic Anthropology of Liberia and Sierra Leone*. Philadelphia, PA: Institute for Liberian Studies, 103–120.

Nunley, John W. (1987). *Moving with the Face of the Devil: Art and Politics in Urban West Africa*. Urbana and Chicago, IL: University of Illinois Press.

O'Neill, April and Ward, Leora (2005). *Mainstreaming or Maneuvering? Gender and Peacekeeping in West Africa*. KAIPTC Monograph no. 1.

Ojukutu-Macauley, Sylvia (1997). "Religion, Gender, and Education in Northern Sierra Leone, 1896–1992," in Jalloh, Alusine and Skinner, David E. (eds) *Islam and Trade in Sierra Leone*. Trenton, NJ: Africa World Press, 86–117.

Person, Yves (1968). *Samori: Une révolution Dyula*, vol. 1. Dakar: IFAN.

Rashid, Ismail (2003). "'A Devotion to Liberty at Any Price': Rebellion and Antislavery in the Upper Guinea Coast in the Eighteenth and Nineteenth Centuries," in Diouf, Sylviane A., *Fighting the Slave Trade: West African Strategies*. Athens, OH: Ohio University Press; Oxford: James Currey, 132–151.

Rashid, Ismail (2009). "Decolonization and Popular Contestation in Sierra Leone: The Peasant War of 1955–1956," *Afrika Zamani*, 17: 87–116.

Reno, William (1999). *Warlord Politics and African States*. Boulder, CO and London: Lynne Reinner.

Rodney, Walter (1970). *A History of the Upper Guinea Coast, 1545–1800*. Oxford: Oxford University Press.

Schmidt, Elizabeth (2005). *Mobilizing the Masses: Gender, Ethnicity, and Class in the Nationalist Movement in Guinea, 1939–1958*. Portsmouth, NH: Heinemann.

Schmidt, Elizabeth (2007). *Cold War and Decolonization in Guinea, 1946–1958*. Athens, OH: Ohio University Press.

Schmidt, Elizabeth (2015). "Popular Resistance and Anti-Colonial Mobilization: The War Effort in French Guinea," in Byfield, Judith A., Brown, Carolyn A., Parsons, Timothy, and Sikainga, Ahmad Alawad (eds) *Africa and World War II*. Cambridge and New York: Cambridge University Press, 441–461.

Skinner, David (1976). "Islam and Education in the Colony and Hinterland of Sierra Leone, 1750–1914," *Canadian Journal of African Studies*, 10: 499–520.

Solow, Barbara L. (ed.) (1991). *Slavery and the Rise of the Atlantic System*. Cambridge and New York: Cambridge University Press.

Spitzer, Leo and Denzer, LaRay (1973). "I.T.A. Wallace-Johnson and the

West African Youth League," *The International Journal of African Historical Studies*, 6, 3: 413–452.

Von Gnielinski, Stefan (ed.) (1972). *Liberia in Maps: Graphic Perspectives of a Developing Country*. New York: Africana Publishing Company.

World Bank Group in Extractive Industries. *2011 Annual Review*. Washington, DC.

Wyse, Akintola (1989). *The Krio of Sierra Leone: An Interpretive History*. London: C. Hurst and Co.

2 | EUROCENTRIC EPISTEMOLOGY: QUESTIONING THE NARRATIVE ON THE EPIDEMIC'S ORIGIN

Chernoh Alpha M. Bah

In April 2014, a German scientific research team funded by the Robert Koch Institute in Berlin traveled to Guinea in West Africa following the World Health Organization (WHO) and Médecins Sans Frontières (MSF) announcement that a number of deaths in the southern region of Guinea had been caused by the Zaire Ebola virus. Led by wildlife epidemiologist Fabian Leendertz, the team aimed at investigating the origin of the 2014 West African Ebola outbreak, which WHO and other humanitarian agencies, at the time, believed was caused by the Zaire Ebola virus – one of the five known species of Ebola. It sought to find out "whether there was a larger Ebola virus outbreak happening in the wildlife in the region and how the index case might have gotten infected and sparked the epidemic that spread into other areas of Guinea and then Sierra Leone and Liberia, representing the largest ever recorded outbreak" (Saéz et al. 2015).[1] They focused on a small Guinean village named Meliandou in the Guéckédou prefecture.

Fabian Leendertz and his team spent eight days interviewing people and observing community behavioral patterns in Meliandou and several other surrounding villages. They also captured around 189 bats, which were subsequently tested for the presence of the Ebola virus or antibodies against the virus. In their report, "Investigating the Zoonotic Origin of the West African Ebola Epidemic" (Saéz et al. 2015), first published online in the *European Molecular Biology Organization (EMBO) Molecular Medicine Journal*[2] in December 2014, the team stated that they discovered "an entrenched tradition of hunting and eating of bats." They asserted,

> We investigated the zoonotic origins of the epidemic using wildlife surveys, interviews, and molecular analyses of bat and

> environmental samples. We found no evidence for a concurrent outbreak in larger wildlife. Exposure to fruit bats is common in the region, but the index case may have been infected by playing in a hollow tree housing a colony of insectivorous free-tailed bats. (Saéz et al. 2015)

The overall conclusion of the final report is less speculative, with the team emphatically stating, "the severe Ebola virus disease epidemic occurring in West Africa stems from a single zoonotic transmission event to a two year old boy in Meliandou, Guinea." This conclusion, based on circumstantial evidence, has dominated global understandings on the origin of the outbreak (Leendertz et al. 2016; Pigott et al. 2016).

Why has the infelicitous conclusion of the German research team, on the origin of the Ebola virus outbreak in West Africa, been accepted so widely and uncritically? Why was the team so certain that the two-year-old Guinean, later revealed to be Emile Ouamouno, was the index case of the outbreak? How did it arrive at the conclusion that the Ebola Virus Disease outbreak in Guinea could be traced to zoonotic causes even though it did not find evidence of the virus in the surrounding animal population? This chapter suggests three possible frameworks to begin to unpack and answer these questions. The first is that they reveal a pattern of faulty and highly problematic Western scientific practices that reproduces problematic understandings of Africans and their ecologies. Second, they draw from and reinforce (neo-)colonialist discourses of African cultural backwardness and barbarism. Third, they act as alibi or detractions from historical and contemporary phenomena which (re)produce patterns of domination, conflict, and security in which the West is deeply implicated.

The making of a faulty scientific narrative

The literature on past Ebola outbreaks, beginning in the Central African region in the 1970s, had always traced the disease to zoonotic origins created by major wildlife deaths (Georges et al. 1999; Khan et al. 1999). Researchers linked the Central African outbreaks of the 1970s to the exposure of hunters to dead animals (Walsh et al. 2003). They claimed that hunters in Central Africa had contracted the virus by handling and consuming the carcasses they found in the forests of the region. In West Africa, Leendertz and his team applied the same research methods used in Central Africa to identify the origins of the virus. They wanted to establish how the hunting and eating of animals caused the emergence of the Ebola virus in West Africa and its infectious transmission chains.

Indeed, insectivorous free-tailed bats (otherwise known as *Mops condylurus*) are a species of bats that scientists believed to be "potential sources for Ebola virus outbreaks" (Olival and Hayman 2014). Evidence from experimental studies in the past had shown this species of bats to survive experimental injections of the Ebola virus, thereby making them prospective reservoirs for transmissions and outbreaks. Yet, while the evidence collected by the German team failed to substantiate this theory, they nonetheless asserted that the insectivorous free-tailed bat had been the original reservoir for the virus. In other words, the West African outbreak, according to the team, represented a departure from the usual Western scientific script on the history of Ebola epidemiology in Africa.[3]

This departure from the usual scientific script becomes even more glaring if we consider the team's admission that they did not encounter any wildlife carcasses in their surveys and they discovered no evidence of recent decline in wildlife populations in the southern Guinean region. "This suggested that there was likely no amplifying epidemic in wildlife in the region, which could have enabled the virus to jump into the human population," they noted in their published report (Saéz et al. 2015). The researchers confirmed that carnivore and chimpanzee populations had, in fact, increased over the years in southern Guinea. This situation ultimately removed the possibility that the Ebola epidemic, then at its preliminary stages in the region, was caused by the same type of animal-to-human transmissions that occurred in the Congo in the 1970s, which were characterized by large wildlife die-off and hunter exposure to carcasses of large mammals. The epidemiological outbreak in West Africa represented a stark contrast with scientific observations supposedly made during previous Ebola epidemiological outbreaks in other parts of Africa where the heavy death tolls of wild apes were reported and where scientific claims of a zoonotic origin were easily established (Quammen 2014). Rather than concede that they could find no clear answers to their research questions and that more research needed to be done, the German scientific team proceeded with the predetermined conclusion that the 2014 West African Ebola epidemic was the result of a "zoonotic transmission."

It appears from the published report that the bat transmission story was advanced as part of the German scientific team's effort to resolve its own lack of real evidence to establish actual causative factors relative to its zoonotic assumptions. All experimental exercises carried out by the team clearly show that there was no evidence of the presence of Ebola amongst the local wildlife populations – bats and other animals. The researchers captured 88 bats in Meliandou and 81 from other surrounding villages in southeastern Guinea. These bats were said to belong to at least 13 different species. The team reportedly carried out several experimental examinations on these bats, but none tested positive for Ebola antibodies. Following these experiments and observations, the team stated clearly that they "found no evidence of additional zoonotic transmission events stemming from the consumption of these bats" (Saéz et al. 2015).

The German scientific team proceeded with the bat-to-human transmission claim although there was no evidence of additional Ebola infections stemming from the consumption of bats in Meliandou. They based their conclusions solely on the extant oral tradition in the area – that children in Meliandou are said to have regularly caught and played with bats from a particular tree housing a colony of fruit bats known as *lolibello*. They then latched on to this simplistic assumption as the evidence that the virus likely emerged out of the insectivorous free-tailed bats from the said tree. The tree itself was located some 50 meters from the home of the index case, and was reportedly burnt down a month ahead of the team's arrival in the village. "Under the assumption that the two-year-old boy was indeed the index case, a source of infection unrelated to food items consumed in the home might be more plausible," the Leendertz team claimed in a poor attempt to justify how Emile Ouamouno is the primary case of the outbreak (Saéz et al. 2015). "The close proximity of a hollow tree housing a large colony of free-tailed insectivorous bats, of a species for which serological evidence also suggests Ebola virus, provided opportunity for infection," they asserted (Saéz et al. 2015). The assertion was not supported by any tangible scientific data, but the German scientists implanted an originating narrative that lacks any corresponding scientific evidence.

Sadly, the conclusion in this report still serves as the official Western scientific explanation dominating the causative events responsible for the largest Ebola outbreak in recent epidemiological history. But this conclusion presents a major scientific problem. It is evident that Leendertz and his colleagues' deliberate insistence on establishing the same causative factors for the West African epidemic as the epidemics in the Central African region in the 1970s ignored all of geography, ethnography, and demographic variations between and among the various regions of Africa. Their investigation in Guinea clearly fails to consider the specificities of the region they were investigating. In particular, the landscape of the Congo basin and its population dynamics in the 1970s were completely dissimilar from the Mano River enclaves of Guinea in 2014. Meliandou, for instance, is a small village of 31 houses, surrounded by farmland and few large trees. "The landscape in that region is heavily human-modified, with Meliandou surrounded by plantations and bush land rather than tropical rainforests, as was the case for index villages in many previous Zaire Ebola virus outbreaks," the Koch Institute acknowledged (Saéz et al. 2015). Indeed, Meliandou is not located in a densely forested area like the communities of the Congo River Basin where the first Ebola epidemic reportedly erupted in the 1970s.

Though bat hunting is a common practice in the southern region of Guinea, in Meliandou and the six other villages studied by the scientists, only adult men reportedly engage in the hunting of bats. Even then, they only hunt *fruit bats* (as opposed to the *insectivorous bats* the team claimed as the reservoir of the virus) for meat. This practice existed in Guinea's southern region for decades, or even centuries, without any epidemiological consequences in the region. It must be reiterated that Leendertz and his team found no clear evidence the epidemic resulted from any animal or bird hunting practices in the indexed village. And, *if* the hunting of bats had been the cause of transmission, it is more likely that the index case of the virus would have been among the adult male rather than the infant population.

The omitted facts and ignored evidence The conclusion that the presence of the Ebola virus in Guinea was a "zoonotic transmission event" involving an infant raises serious questions about the integrity of the research and the broader motives of the report. It is now apparent that the report omitted significant information about the child who they determined as the "patient zero" of the outbreak. The determination was not based on any empirical or clinical evidence: no laboratory examination was carried out on the child's remains to determine his actual cause of death. Available medical records of the child at the Meliandou community health clinic in Meliandou only state that Emile Ouamouno was diagnosed with acute malaria in December 2013. Local health workers still think malaria may have been the actual cause of his death. The medical records also noted that he was 18 months rather than two years old at the time of his death, contradicting the information provided by the German scientists.[4] The age discrepancy calls into question the child's supposed ability to participate in the activities of hunting and grilling of the "insectivorous bats," which Leendertz and team speculated were the source of the viral infection that triggered the outbreak. The team also did not enquire about the fate of Emile's playmates whom the team also implicated in "child bat hunting" activities.

Also ignored by the German scientists in their investigation and their final report are the circumstances surrounding the death of Emile's mother and the survival of his father. Emile's immediate senior sister died around the same time as him. Emile's mother was eight months pregnant at the time of her children's death. The mother reportedly fell ill a few days after the funeral of the two children.[5] A doctor at the community health clinic in the village who treated Emile also diagnosed the mother with malaria. The doctor prescribed ten shots of anti-malaria medication. She complained of severe hip pains the very night she commenced the treatment prescribed by the doctor. The hip pains later developed into severe bleeding, and in the middle of the night the woman eventually miscarried and died in a pool of blood (Bah 2015). The circumstances of the woman's death – an eight-month pregnant woman receiving anti-malarial medication, suffering severe hip pains followed by profuse bleeding, then having a miscarriage and eventually dying – should have generated more questions rather than quick and simple conclusions.

In their published report, the German scientists never asked why the resident doctor (and other health care personnel) who treated both Emile Ouamouno and his mother never got infected. Their report also did not question or offer any explanation why Etienne

Ouamouno, the child's father who took care of all the so-called index cases, was not infected with the virus. He did not experience any fever or illness throughout the outbreak. The other family members of the supposed index case (child's other siblings –Victorienne, eight years old; Sergio, seven years old; Marie, six years old; and Kanih, 18 months old) also never got infected, despite the speculation that the outbreak, which spread across international borders and killed thousands, erupted in their household. With all of this conflicting evidence in the final published report and unanswered questions, why has the zoonotic transmission story generated by the German scientific team persisted as the dominant official narrative around the origin of the West African Ebola epidemic?

Historicizing the origin of the outbreak

An examination of the immediate post-war environment of the Mano River region of West Africa (the epicenter of the outbreak) will provide a clear context for the national and international events that preceded the outbreak. Such an examination will help contextualize how the post-9/11 security anxieties in Washington changed the health landscape of West Africa and generated renewed international interests in certain pathogens regarded or listed as potential bioweapons. This politics of *securitization*, necessitated by changing developments in the international political environment, opened up the global health landscape to an increasingly challenging security threat: the anticipated dangers of bioterrorism in the twenty-first century and the focus on previously disregarded pathogens as having potentials of weaponization. In West Africa, the Lassa fever virus, which has been present in the region since the early 1970s, was re-assessed and included on the list of notable diseases with potentials of weaponization (Garret 2011).

This development made the Mano River region of West Africa a part of the international discourse on existential threats to Western safety and security after the 9/11 attacks and anthrax incidents in the United States. This trend became increasingly common in the international geopolitical landscape, which was now feeling threatened by the adverse forces of globalization and new security concerns (Okeke 2011).

The re-assessment of the Lassa virus as a bioterrorist agent and its categorization by the US Center for Disease Control (CDC) and

US National Institutes of Allergy and Infectious Diseases (NIAID) as a *Category A* agent generated enormous international medical and security interests in the region (Khan et al. 2008). Lassa fever's *Category A* classification elevated it to the highest risk level of any pathogenic agent with potential for use in bioterrorism. Pathogens are classified as such only on account of their ability to spread easily and cause major public health impacts, including high mortality. Due to this security hysteria coming from Washington, Lassa fever, now included as a notifiable disease under the WHO's revised International Health Regulations (IHR), led Western nations to regard the Mano River countries of Sierra Leone, Liberia, and Guinea as significant bioterrorist breeding grounds (Baker and Fidler 2006). The civil wars of the 1990s had opened up the region to similar international policy concerns: the potential of terrorist investments in the wars for access to strategic resources.

In West Africa, the recalibration and reclassification of Lassa fever within the realm of bioterrorist concerns offered potential opportunities for resource mobilization and international funding. On the international level, networks of actors mobilized policy narratives and convincing storylines based on these new policy considerations. Lassa fever became an attractive investment for the political and institutional power sectors of the west. It created an assemblage of diverse biodefense interests, which opened-up funding incentives and research possibilities for Western scientists and biotech companies to work on what was before a neglected tropical disease in the rain forests of West Africa. This CDC classification, which turned Lassa fever into a threat against US national security interests, made the Mano River region a crucial site of the US war on terror. It eventually meant that a significant amount of the billions of dollars that were raised and set aside by the US government for biodefense efforts since the anthrax incident in 2001 were channeled towards laboratory research efforts in West Africa located at the Kenema Government Hospital in eastern Sierra Leone.[6] This research work was aimed at supposedly strengthening the United States' medical capacity to deal with a bioterrorist attack or outbreak intentionally unleashed against its military or civilian population.

This led the United States' National Institute of Health (NIH) to fund Tulane University's grant proposal entitled "Diagnostics for Biodefense,"[7] a proposal that regarded Lassa fever as having a potential to be used as a biological weapon directed against civilian or military targets. Tulane's proposal stated that the classification of the Lassa virus as a *Category A* pathogen necessitated the development of an "effective, highly sensitive, and cost-effective medical diagnostics for public health laboratories and hospital-based clinical laboratories to diagnose individuals exposed to and/or infected with the virus."[8] The proposal received a budget of US$10 million from the National Institute of Health and a further US$15 million five-year grant focusing on the study of the pathogenesis of Lassa. The Tulane grant was the largest biodefense allocation that opened up the Lassa Laboratory of the Kenema Government Hospital for field research. The portfolio of biodefense related projects in Kenema also included those of Metabiota, which had at least three grants from the Defense Threat Reduction Agency (DTRA) and Cooperative Biological Engagement Program (CBEP), both of which are US Department of Defense (DOD) agencies. Metabiota's efforts were concentrated primarily on the pathogenesis of Lassa fever, with applications for treatments and vaccines.

By 2010, the US-funded biodefense research on Lassa fever reached a climax: a centralized organization, the Viral Hemorrhagic Fever Consortium (VHFC),[9] was established to coordinate the various institutions trooping into eastern Sierra Leone to execute biodefense research-related projects. VHFC comprises researchers from Tulane University, Scripps Research Institute, Broad Institute, Harvard University, University of California at San Diego, University of Texas Medical Branch, Autoimmune Technologies LLC, Corgenix Medical Corporation, Kenema Government Hospital, and the Irrua Specialist Teaching Hospital in Nigeria. The biodefense dollars that flowed into Sierra Leone from 2009 to 2012 instantly transformed the once dilapidated and abandoned Lassa Ward of the Kenema Government Hospital, located on its small site in eastern Sierra Leone, into the recipient of a well-funded international research program. In February 2011, for example, the Reuters News Agency reported that the Lassa research project at the Kenema Government Hospital cost around US$40 million in biodefense funding.[10] This Reuters article described the Kenema laboratory as an outpost of the US government's "war on terror," funded by biodefense dollars with the purpose of limiting vulnerability of Western interests to biological agents. An American researcher, Matt Boisen told Reuters,

"There has been a renewed emphasis on those tropical diseases that government health officials consider bio-threats. It would be naive not to think some terrorist group could use one of these things to create terror."[11]

Western biodefense research and the outbreak

The driving forces behind these research efforts were entirely anchored on the security concerns of the United States and its European allies. Their objective was to understand mechanisms related to the human immune response to Lassa virus infections with the goal of developing treatments and vaccines. Although the recalibration of Lassa fever as a threat to international security necessitated the flow of several millions of dollars in biodefense funding, Western scientists (Yun and Walker 2012; Flatz et al. 2010; Russier et al. 2012) also debated the implications of the CDC's *Category A* classification. Some expressed doubts as to whether Lassa would make an effective bioweapon because, for such a thing to happen, contact with infected bodily fluids was needed to transfer the disease from one human host to another. These questions and uncertainties about Lassa created the need for additional scientific studies into the Lassa virus. This scientific enquiry applied DNA sequencing or the science of genomics. This inquiry also became a task of the VHFC, taken over by scientists at the Broad Institute of Harvard University. The researchers aimed at discovering the viral and host genetic factors that influence susceptibility and resistance to infection and disease. Pardis Sabeti, a specialist in reading and analyzing the genomes of organisms, led the genomics research conducted at the Broad Institute of MIT and Harvard University, exploring the way viruses change over time as they adapt to their environments. Sabeti and her team obtained blood samples of people infected with Lassa fever and read the genomes of whatever they could find in the patients' blood (Andersen et al. 2015; Yozwiak et al. 2015; Park et al. 2015).

At the Kenema Government Hospital, these efforts were coordinated in a ward with a 12-bed facility headed by Dr. Sheikh Umar Khan. Khan and Sabeti established strong friendship ties in the years ahead of the 2014 outbreak. Between October 2006 and October 2008, Dr. Khan received blood samples from patients with suspected Lassa fever submitted to the Lassa Diagnostic Laboratory in Kenema. The samples, collected from the 500–700 patients from Sierra Leone, Guinea, and Liberia annually admitted at the hospital, were processed as part of the ongoing research at the laboratory for other viruses of interest. These samples were also sent to the Broad Institute where Sabeti and her team conducted their genomic studies. Sabeti told *The New Yorker* that Khan was fascinated by genomics and was curious to find out how the sequencing was done at the Broad Institute. He had planned to visit Harvard to join Pardis Sabeti and her team a few months before he died in July 2014 as a victim of the EVD outbreak.[12]

In a research paper submitted to the United States' CDC documenting the outcome of this research, Khan and others revealed that over 25 percent of the suspected Lassa patients they studied showed evidence of infections similar to Ebola and Dengue fever. The findings of Khan and his colleagues identified (at least since 2008) the evolutionary trend and mutational characteristics of the "virus" which developed in 2014 into a regional disaster and international health crisis. This finding was further amplified in a report published on August 28, 2014, by the journal *Science*, detailing the results of a major surveillance study on "Ebola virus genomes" that involved 99 complete virus sequences. The report also stated that the West African Ebola strain was different from the strain that had circulated in Central Africa in the 1970s. The study was done by geneticists at the Broad Institute of MIT and Harvard University who sequenced the virus found in 78 patients treated at the Kenema Government Hospital in eastern Sierra Leone between May and June 2014. It confirmed that the virus that created the 2014 outbreak in West Africa had been present in the region since 2004, ten years before the outbreak.[13]

In 2004, US/European funded biodefense research operations were instituted in the dilapidated hospital grounds of the Kenema Government Hospital in eastern Sierra Leone. The differences of the viral strain that most likely caused the West African outbreak from other known "Ebola strains in other African regions" could also possibly mean that the viral haemorrhagic fever that caused the outbreak itself may be associated with Lassa fever, which carries the same signs and symptoms as Ebola and Dengue fever: profuse vomiting, diarrhea, followed by bleeding, renal failure, cardiac arrest, and then eventual death. Both Aniru Conteh, the Lassa fever doctor who died in 2004,[14] and Sheikh Umar Khan, who died in 2014, experienced the same signs and symptoms before their deaths. And, oddly enough, they were both infected through similar circumstances: treating infected pregnant women at the Lassa Fever Ward of the Kenema Government Hospital.

The problem with initially distinguishing the signs of the different haemorrhagic diseases became evident during the initial stages of the mass outbreak of the Ebola disease. The French medical charity, MSF, in its evaluation of the causes of the widespread explosion of the Ebola outbreak, singled out Metabiota for criticism, accusing its staff deployed in Sierra Leone of withholding critical information that would have assisted in the reversal of the casualties of the epidemic during the initial stages of the outbreak. MSF stated in a report released a year into the outbreak:

> From the onset of the epidemic, the US biotechnology company Metabiota and Tulane University, partners of Sierra Leone's Kenema hospital, had the lead in supporting Sierra Leone's Ministry of Health in investigating suspected cases. Their investigations came back Ebola-negative, while their ongoing surveillance activities seem to have missed the cases of Ebola that had emerged in the country.[15]

Metabiota, a member of the VHFC, had been a central player in the decade-old Western research operations in Kenema that followed the CDC's reclassification of the Lassa virus as a threat agent against Western security interests. Metabiota and Tulane University were on the ground and therefore instrumental in the transformation of eastern Sierra Leone (Kenema Government Hospital) into an outpost of the US war on terror through its Diagnostics for Biodefense project. While the reclassification of Lassa as a regional and international security threat attracted millions of dollars from biodefense coffers for research organizations and scientists, West Africa's public health concerns were never prioritized in the biodefense research operations of the VHFC. The fact that the Kenema–Kailahun axis, considered a major component of the Lassa belt and hub of the many Western funded biodefense research activities, became the initial site of the 2014 outbreak in Sierra Leone implicates the groups of organizations and scientists involved in the US and European funded biodefense research activities that were ongoing in the region. The contention that Western medical research activities in eastern Sierra Leone, supported by millions of biodefense dollars for research on pathogenesis and genomics, directly contributed to the 2014 health catastrophe in West Africa cannot be dismissed lightly.

The CDC's reclassification of Lassa as a potential bioweapon turned into a public health security risk for West Africa. But these security risks were embedded only within Western security concerns and these efforts did not prevent the occurrence of the kind of outbreak whose risk had laid the foundation for biodefense investments and research in West Africa a decade earlier. The money that went into Western laboratory research in Kenema did nothing to upgrade the health infrastructure in Sierra Leone, Liberia, and Guinea. The health situation in West Africa remained broken despite the influx of millions of biodefense funds into the region. There was no thermometer at the Lassa Ward in Kenema right up to the 2014 outbreak despite the presence of Western researchers and the fact that temperature readings are a key part of the case identification protocols for Lassa fever.

A study done on the Kenema Lassa Ward a year before the 2014 outbreak revealed the stark absence of basic protective equipment like gloves for health care workers handling Lassa cases. Nurses at the Lassa Ward reportedly re-used needles on patients, thereby increasing the risks of infection on health workers.[16] Local health units in remote villages in eastern Sierra Leone also complained of lack of equipment to diagnose and take samples from suspected Lassa cases for onward submission to the Lassa Laboratory in Kenema.[17] These conditions existed alongside the many Western biodefense research activities that occurred in Kenema from 2009 to 2014. These biodefense research operations in Kenema were carried out in a highly risky and mainly unprotected environment. This is in sharp contrast to safety procedures in the United States, where the Lassa virus studies are handled in biosafety *Level* 4 facilities. Researchers in such facilities are required to wear "space suits." These measures were never applied in Kenema.

The Kenema protective measures only included goggles, gloves, and masks, which were always in short supply. "Certainly we have less safety, less containment, but we do have the ability to do a lot more in the same amount of time," an American research scientist told the

Reuters News Agency three years ahead of the 2014 outbreak.[18] The absence of the required safety and containment measures needed to handle a CDC classified high-level threat pathogen in a dilapidated hospital facility posed severe risks to innocent health workers and the larger community. It was obvious that Western scientists and researchers working on Lassa at the Kenema Government Hospital made the larger eastern region communities of Sierra Leone, and by extension the entire sub-region, susceptible to the pathogenic risks that necessitated the millions of dollars in biodefense research operations in eastern Sierra Leone in the first place.

Could the 2014 West African outbreak have been the result of safety procedural violations that exposed both the health workers and the larger patient population to infectious risks at the Kenema Government Hospital, where a highly dangerous pathogen was being handled? Or could it have been a deliberate result of the experimentation of a *weaponized version* of the Lassa virus from the Kenema Lassa laboratory (Bah 2015)? These are crucial questions that could be answered by releasing all of the information and data associated with these facilities and the various kinds of research that were being conducted. The fact that the 2014 outbreak occurred within the same geographical space hosting some of the leading Western medical research institutions and major science groups from the United States and Europe renders suspect the zoonosis hypothesis in the 2014 outbreak by the German scientific team. To argue that the 2014 West African epidemic took the scientific world by surprise would be a deliberate effort to ignore the possible role of biodefense funding and Western medical research in the creation of the conditions for the epidemiological outbreak and failing to arrest its widespread transmission.

Without the release of information and transparency, it will be difficult to exonerate US and European funded biomedical research operations in eastern Sierra Leone, which defined Lassa as a potential bioweapon, from accusations of their complicity in triggering the 2014 health epidemic in West Africa. The efforts of Western scientists, the academic community, and Western media representatives to situate the 2014 West African outbreak in an obscure village in southern Guinea seems like deliberate attempts to divert public attention from seriously probing into the biomedical research projects at the Lassa Fever Laboratory of the Kenema Government Hospital in eastern Sierra Leone and their role in the outbreak.

This anomaly is captured squarely by MSF in its evaluation of the international response to the epidemic. The organization's report which criticized Metabiota, Tulane University, and government officials in Sierra Leone for hindering its operations was not a simple criticism of national and international response mechanisms to an outbreak, but it highlighted several issues which further challenges the truthfulness of the narrative, advanced by Leendertz, which now define the 2014 health tragedy in West Africa within Western society. According to MSF officials, Metabiota and health officials in Sierra Leone refused to release information relating to the contact lists of infected persons and kept all information about the outbreak in Sierra Leone to themselves. "When we set up operations in Kailahun, we realized we were already too late. There were cases everywhere," MSF stated.[19] Why had Metabiota, Tulane University, or any of the other members of the VHFC who were engaged in the years-long study of Lassa's bioweapon's potential in Kenema failed to report the outbreak of the epidemic when it first occurred? Why did they withhold relevant information that would have been instrumental in the battle against the outbreak?

These questions are central to understanding the timing, place of origin, and modes of transmission of the outbreak. Responding to questions on Metabiota's role in the outbreak response, Jean-Paul Gonzalez, a senior scientist with Metabiota stationed in Sierra Leone, told a PBS Frontline documentary crew that they initially felt the outbreak was not going to last more than two weeks. "We are not specialized in outbreak response. We know how to do it because we have some expertise in the domain, but we are a very small company," Gonzales told PBS Frontline.[20]

Corroborating the MSF charge against Metabiota, Amara Jambai, Sierra Leone's Director of Disease Prevention and Control, said government's initial reaction to the outbreak was based on advice from Metabiota. "We were advised by Metabiota that this is of a minor scale, but we never knew that it was going to be so big," he confirmed to PBS Frontline. At the initial stages of the outbreak, official records in Sierra Leone situated the origin of the epidemic in May 2014, attributing it to a traditional healer that had traveled to Guinea for a funeral, where it is claimed she was infected with the virus before returning to Sierra Leone in May. Recent evidence now confirms that the WHO and regional authorities in West Africa knew as early as February 2014 that infectious sick people in eastern Sierra Leone were migrating across the border into the southern region of Guinea – three months before the official narrative locates the virus in the country.

In particular, a patient named Sia Wanda Koniono from Kailahun had fallen sick and was said to have crossed into Guinea several times for medical treatment before she died (Sack et al. 2014). Individuals who were exposed to her in Guinea were later confirmed to have died of Ebola. An official report by a team of WHO experts and Guinean officials who had investigated the situation stated that authorities in Freetown and members of VHFC in Kenema had knowledge of Koniono's death from haemorrhagic fever, but they made no effort to trace the contacts that may have possibly been infected months ahead of the official declaration of the outbreak in Sierra Leone. MSF officials in Guinea disclosed that an e-mail attachment mentioning Koniono and other patients from Sierra Leone who were crossing into Guinea was sent to Dr. Sheikh Umarr Khan in late March 2014, several weeks before Sierra Leone officially acknowledged the presence of the virus in the country. It was alleged that neither Khan nor any of the VHFC members responded to the correspondences (Sack et al. 2014). MSF noted that "Ebola cases in Guinea were discovered that were reportedly coming from Sierra Leone." This is the opposite of the official narrative, based on Leendertz's account, which claimed the virus moved from Guinea into Sierra Leone and then into Liberia. This calls into question the official narrative, which claims that initial spread of the virus in Sierra Leone resulted from the funeral of an infected traditional healer.

Conclusion

Whether deliberate or not, it is difficult not to interpret "zoonotic origin of the West African Ebola epidemic" narrative advanced by Fabian Leendertz and his team as part of a cover-up or obfuscation of the actual chain of events that laid the foundation for the West African Ebola outbreak. By locating the origin of the 2014 West African Ebola epidemic within the realms of environmental concerns and African cultural behavior, the report of the German scientific team ignored the obvious historical exploitation and appropriation of the human and environmental resources of the region by multinationals and corporate entities for the purpose of medical research and experimentation. It provides an alibi as well as a larger discourse environment in which secretive biodefense research and questionable Western scientific practices are not accountable for being possibly involved in generating a disaster that has claimed thousands of innocent lives in West Africa and inflicted considerable damage to the region's socio-cultural fabric and its global image.

Notes

1 Even though Leendertz led the research, Saéz was listed first on the list of authors in the 2015 version of the report.

2 EMBO has its headquarters in Heidelberg, Germany. It is an organization of more than 1,700 leading researchers in the life sciences.

3 The literature on Ebola epidemiology in Africa since the 1970s linked the origins of all previous outbreaks to zoonotic factors associated with animal-to-human transmissions. See, for example Piot (2013); Quammen (2013).

4 There seems to be some confusion about the actual age of Emile in the Western media. The *New York Times* identified him as a one-year-old. See Kevin Sack, Sheri Fink, Pam Belluck, and Adam Nossiter, "How Ebola Roared Back," *New York Times*, December 13, 2014, http://www.nytimes.com/2014/12/30/health/how-ebola-roared-back.html?_r=0 (accessed September 16, 2016).

5 Interview with Etienne Ouamouno, father of Emile, in Meliandou, Guinea on December 28, 2014. For additional details see Bah (2015).

6 See, for example, "Autoimmune Technologies to Play a Key Role in $3.8 Million Biodefense Challenge Grant Research," a press release issued by Autoimmune Technologies LLC on November 9, 2009 in New Orleans. This press release clearly stated that the grant was awarded specifically for the development of diagnostic tools for bioterror threat agents as part of a project involving researchers from Tulane University's School of Medicine, the US Army Medical Research Institute of Infectious Diseases of Fort Detrick, Maryland (USAMRIID), Corgenix Medical Corporation of Denver in Colorado, and BioFactura Inc., of Rockville, Maryland.

7 Keith Brannon, "New $27.5 Million Tulane University Biosafety Lab Will Expand Research, Create Jobs," *Tulane University Media*, December 2008. Online July 6, 2016.

8 Ibid.

9 "Kenema Government Hospital," Viral Hemorrhagic Fever Consortium, 2011. Online July 6, 2016.

10 Simon Akam, "United States Anti-terror Outpost Tackles Rat-borne Virus," *Reuters*, February 2011.

11 Ibid.

12 "Inside the Ebola Wars," *The New Yorker*, October 2014.

13 See Gire et al. (2014). The researchers claimed that the viral variant of the of "Ebola" that created the West Africa outbreak "likely diverged from Central African lineages around 2004, (and) crossed from Guinea to Sierra Leone in May 2014 and exhibited sustained human-to-human transmission subsequently, with no evidence of additional zoonotic sources." It is important to note that this research work involved the participation of Sheikh Umarr Khan and four other Sierra Leonean healthcare workers attached to the Kenema Lassa Ward who all died

during the outbreak at least a month before this paper was published.

14 See, for more details, N. Mellor, "Aniru Conteh," *BMJ*, 328, 7447 (2004): 1078.

15 *Pushed to the Limit and Beyond: A Year into the Largest Ever Ebola Outbreak*, MSF Report, March 2015.

16 Annie Wilkinson, "Lassa Fever: The Politics of an Emerging Disease and the Scope for One Health," *STEPS Center*, 2015. Online July 6, 2016.

17 Ibid.

18 Akam, "United States Anti-terror Outpost."

19 Médecins Sans Frontières, *Pushed to the Limit and Beyond*, MSF Report, March 2015.

20 See the documentary *Outbreak* released on May 5, 2015 by PBS Frontline and produced by Dan Edge and Sasha Joelle Archili (excerpts located at 21:59–26:10 of the 55:55-minute documentary).

References

Andersen, K.G. et al. (2015). "Clinical Sequencing Uncovers Origins and Evolution of Lassa Virus," *Cell*, 162: 738–750.

Bah, Chernoh Alpha M. (2015). *The Ebola Outbreak in West Africa: Corporate Gangsters, Multinationals and Rogue Politicians*. Philadelphia, PA: Africanist Press.

Baker, Michael G. and Fidler, David P. (2006). "Global Public Health Surveillance Under New International Health Regulations," *Emerging Infectious Diseases*, 12, 7: 1058–1065.

Flatz, Lukas et al. (2010). "T Cell-Dependence of Lassa Fever Pathogenesis," *PLoS Pathogens* 6, 3: e1000836.

Garret, Laurie (2011). *I Heard the Sirens Scream: How Americans Responded to the 9/11 and Anthrax Attacks*. Amazon.com Kindle e-book.

Georges, A.J. et al. (1999). "Ebola Hemorrhagic Fever Outbreaks in Gabon, 1994–1997: Epidemiologic and Health Control Issues," *Journal of Infectious Diseases*, 179: S65–S75.

Gire, Stephen K. et al., (2014) "Genomic Surveillance Elucidates Ebola Virus Origin and Transmission During the 2014 Outbreak," *Science*, 345, 6202: 1369–1372. doi:10.1126/science.1259657.

Khan, A.S. et al. (1999). "The Reemergence of Ebola Hemorrhagic Fever, Democratic Republic of the Congo, 1995," *Journal of Infectious Diseases* 179: S76–S86.

Khan, Sheiku Humarr et al. (2008). "New Opportunities for Field Research on Pathogenesis and Treatment of Lassa," *Antiviral Research*, 78, 1: 103–115.

Leendertz, S.A., Gogarten, J.F., Düx, A., Calvignac-Spencer, S. and, Leendertz, F.H. (2016). "Assessing the Evidence Supporting Fruit Bats as the Primary Reservoirs for Ebola Viruses," *EcoHealth* 13, 1: 18–25.

Okeke, I.N. (2011). *Divining without Seeds: The Case for Strengthening Laboratory Medicine in Africa*. Ithaca, NY: Cornell University Press.

Olival, K.J. and Hayman, D.T. (2014). "Filoviruses in Bats: Current Knowledge and Future Directions." *Viruses*, 6: 1759–1788.

Park, D.J et al. (2015). "Ebola Virus Epidemiology, Transmission, and Evolution during Seven Months in Sierra Leone," *Cell*, 161: 1516–1526.

Pigott, David M. et al. (2016). "Updates to the Zoonotic Niche Map of Ebola Virus Disease in Africa," *eLife*. doi:10.7554/eLife.16412.

Piot, Peter (2013). *No Time to Lose: A Life in Pursuit of Deadly Viruses*. New York: W.W. Norton & Company.

Quammen, David (2013). *Spillover: Animal Infections and the Next Human Pandemic*. New York: W.W. Norton & Company.

Quammen, David (2014). *Ebola: The Natural and Human History of a Deadly Virus*. New York: W.W. Norton.

Russier, M., Pannetier, D., and Baize, S. (2012). "Immune Responses and Lassa Virus Infection," *Viruses*, 4: 2766–2785.

Sack, Kevin, Fink, Sheri, Belluck, Pam, and Nossiter, Adam (2014). "How Ebola Roared Back," *New York Times*, December 29.

Saéz, Almunda Mari et al. (2015). "Investigating the Zoonotic Origin of the West African Ebola Epidemic," *EMBO Molecular Medicine* 7, 1 (January): 17–23.

Walsh, Peter D. et al. (2003). "Catastrophic Ape Decline in Western Equatorial Africa," *Nature*, 422: 611–614.

Yozwiak, Nathan L. Schaffner, Stephen F., and Sabeti, Pardis C. (2015). "Make Outbreak Research Open Access," *Nature*, 518: 477–479.

Yun, N.E. and Walker, D.H. (2012). "Pathogenesis of Lassa Fever." *Viruses*, 4, 10: 2031–2048.

PART TWO

THE NEOLIBERAL AFFLICTION: DIFFERENT COUNTRIES, SIMILAR CONVULSIONS

3 | INTERPRETING THE HEALTH, SOCIAL, AND POLITICAL DIMENSIONS OF THE EBOLA CRISIS IN GUINEA

Alpha Amadou Bano Barry

Introduction

In late 2013 and early 2014, several eyewitness reports emerged from the forest region of the Republic of Guinea, describing an unknown infectious disease causing a sudden onset of fever accompanied by weakness and fatigue, muscle pain, headache, and sore throat. These symptoms were followed by diarrhea, vomiting, rash, and impaired liver and kidney function. External bleeding, and subsequent death by cardiorespiratory arrest occurred in 50 to 90 percent of cases. Without knowing it, Guineans were facing Ebola Virus Disease (EVD), one of the world's deadliest epidemics characterized by a high case fatality rate. Like other viral haemorrhagic diseases that have appeared over the last four decades in various parts of Africa (Lassa fever, the H1N1 and H5N1 strains of influenza, and the Nipah virus), Ebola is, in the main a zoonosis, caused by animal pathogens or originating in products of animal origin.

The factors responsible for epidemics and new infectious diseases are complex. A World Health Organization (WHO) report points out that "environmental exploitation and degradation and poor environmental management provide opportunities for viruses and their vectors to mutate into more infectious and virulent forms. Population displacement, urbanisation, poverty, overcrowding and weak health infrastructure provide ideal environments for infectious diseases to proliferate" (WHO 2012, vi). A glance at the map of the Guinean Forestiere region where the Ebola epidemic supposedly originated, confirms the link between the emergence of the disease and the exploitation and degradation of the forest environment.

Though unknown in the Mano River Union basin area of West Africa before 2013, Ebola is not a strange disease in parts of Eastern and Central Africa. Before reaching Guinea, Sierra Leone, and

Liberia, there have been close to 12 Ebola outbreaks in these parts of Africa from the mid-1970s onwards. The epidemic was first identified in 1976 in Nzara, South Sudan, and subsequently in Yambuku in then northern Zaire, in the Kikwit region of the former Zaire, in Côte d'Ivoire, in Gabon, and in Uganda in 2000.[1] All of these Ebola outbreaks, unlike the one that erupted in the MRU region between 2013 and 2016, were relatively limited in geographical scope, and numbers of fatalities, and were brought under control within a year.

In the case of Guinea, there are two competing views as to the source of the disease. The first is presented in an article published on October 24, 2014 in *Science*, which traces the start of the epidemic to the funeral of a healer in Sokoma village in the Kailahun District of Sierra Leone. The second version, published in the *New England Journal of Medicine* and reported by the French newspaper, *Le Figaro* in its issue of August 11, 2014, states that the first person infected was a two-year-old boy, who passed away in December 2013 in Meliandou, a village in Guéckédou prefecture in south eastern Guinea. The boy, Emile Ouamouno, supposedly contaminated the members of his family who, in turn, contaminated health care workers in Guéckédou. In any event, it was not until March 22, 2014 that the Ebola virus was formally and officially[2] identified, after epidemiological investigations were undertaken and blood samples were sent to Lyon, France and Hamburg, Germany.[3]

Despite the scientific confirmation of the presence of EVD in Guinea, there were popular denials of the very existence of the disease, and repeated attacks were directed against health care facilities, health care administrative staff, and fieldwork and awareness teams. In Womey, a town in the Nzérékoré prefecture, eight members of an awareness team were killed by the inhabitants, after rumors circulated that they were contaminating people.[4] What explains this situation? We conducted a series of studies between October and December 2014 in areas where violent resistance by communities was most prevalent, including: Matoto in Conakry; Coyah, Forécariah, and Kindia in Lower Guinea; Faranah, Kankan, and Siguiri in Upper Guinea; and Guéckédou, Macenta, and N'Zérékoré in Guinea Forestiere.[5] In this chapter, I discuss how illness and death are managed within Guinean families, and how this influenced their attitudes toward the Ebola epidemic. These attitudes are situated both with the framework of Guinean health care policies and Guinean politics.

Managing illness and death in Guinean families

Although there is a diversity of ethnic groups and cultural practices linked to death in Guinea, our study reveals broad and consistent indications of how Guineans deal with sickness. When an illness occurs within a family in Guinea, the cost of care is covered by the head of the family. However, this does not preclude the participation of the other active members of the family, such as the wife or wives and children. The decision to utilize treatment in a health care facility seems to be linked to the social status and level of education of the head of the household. Group interviews showed that people who are younger, more educated, and hold a salaried position are more likely than others to take their children or other dependent household members to health care facilities when they are ill.

Caring for the sick in Guinea is highly gendered, and it is almost the exclusive responsibility of women. Women act as nurses and personal care attendants, attending to bodily hygiene as well as other health care support responsibilities. Within this gendered caring responsibility, however, there is a clearly structured division of labor: "If it is a child, it is the mother, if it is the father, it is his wife, if it is the wife, it is the husband, and if it is a protégé, it is the mother. If there is vomiting, then the women or older children clean it up."[6] Women do not play a major role in ritual purification of the deceased. However, women seem to be on the front lines when it comes to care and social protection within families, which makes them more vulnerable than other family members to the chain of contagion in an epidemic.

The preparation and purification of the dead for burial is largely the domain of males. Ritual washing of dead bodies and the prayer for the deceased are usually performed by men – specifically members of the mosque council, older men, and those who have learned the Koran: "The prayer is said by the imams, the Koranic teacher of the deceased, or a person chosen by the deceased during his lifetime."[7] Women are only involved in ritual bathing of the deceased under very specific circumstances. They must be over the age of 60, and the deceased must be their own husband, one of their children, or another woman; "if it is a girl, then the women wash the body," according to participants in focus groups conducted at Mamou. The participants also revealed that the wife of the deceased plays an important role in washing the body when both parties are in their advanced years. In such cases, the wife provides the initial care before the members of the mosque council and the elders take over.

When the body is being washed, the members of the mosque council are often accompanied by representatives from the family "to bear witness to the customary properness and conformity of the acts performed."[8] There are strict rules regarding the ritual purification of the deceased in order to help them to overcome obstacles on the journey to the beyond. Among the Pulaar in Guinea, to ritually purify a body is *few nu ghol*, literally meaning to "straighten." Focus group discussion (FGD) and individual interviews also revealed that people of a certain age and social status could appoint a person or persons during their lifetime to ritually wash their body and even conduct the funeral prayer. They could also select their burial sites, more often than not next to their father, mother, and/or grandparents. Survivors regard the wishes expressed by such people during their lifetimes as a sacred duty, even at the risk of their own lives.

Popular views and attitudes on Ebola in Guinea

The data from our fieldwork suggest that there were three phases of response to EVD among the Guinean people: incomprehension, rejection, and fear. In the first phase, between the emergence of the disease and its spread throughout the country toward June 2014, there was much ignorance about the true nature the disease and how it should be treated. This was unsurprising due to "the fact that Ebola symptoms were similar to ordinary illnesses (fever, headache, fatigue, malaria, vomiting, and bleeding) [which] convinced some that the illness they were suffering from was not Ebola."[9]

During the first year of the epidemic, the quest to better understand the disease was combined with palpable fear. Like HIV/AIDS, which is known as the "monster" in certain Guinean dialects, Ebola became known in certain areas of the country as *Fimba* or *Fèmba*, meaning the "very dark" or "big thing." *Fimba* refers to the dark spots that appear on the bodies of people with Ebola. Yet, these dark spots are not only physical manifestations of a deadly disease, they are also signs of an unfathomable social affliction: they are dark marks that affect the whole family. The analogy between the color, black, and the darkness of the disease was mostly made by the inhabitants of Laya Sando in the Faranah prefecture, an area hit hard by the epidemic. *Fèmba*, on the other hand, refers to the unspeakable, namely a great misfortune, a major catastrophe or a monster. It is also a code word deployed by people who do not want "others" or "outsiders" to know what they are talking about. This way of framing the epidemic could also be a way of expressing real contempt for the disease or the extreme fear it arouses. This version of the term was used in Marel, a sub-prefecture of Faranah, from the time of the popular revolt against the authority of the sub-prefect.

In the eyes of the majority of Guineans, Guinea was a long way from Congo, and they could not see how a disease from the equatorial forest could come to their country. This disbelief in the presence of Ebola in their midst was influenced by the fact that the term "Ebola" was first invoked in Guinea by "foreigners," namely staff of Doctors Without Borders (Médecins Sans Frontières – MSF). MSF were the first to care for patients in the countryside far from the capital city, whereof the inhabitants had only seen "white men" in books, films, or on television. Furthermore, the death of nearly all the EVD patients treated by these white people in hazmat suits had a devastating impact on public acceptance and treatment procedures. The statement that there was no medication and that the fatality rate was 90 percent discredited health centers and helped position marabouts and charlatans. However, it has been proven that when care is provided early on, the chances of recovery are significantly increased.

Furthermore, it did not help that the doctors focused their initial public discourse on two aspects of the epidemic: the origin of the disease (consumption of monkeys and bats) and the high fatality rate because, they claimed, the health care system had no vaccine or treatment for the disease. Because of the alleged link to the consumption of monkey and bat meat, people in the Forestiere region felt stigmatized and reacted negatively. They pointed out they had consumed such meat from time immemorial without catching EVD, so they did not see how they could suddenly contract the disease in 2014. Jean Marie Dore, a politician hailing from the Forestiere Region of Guinea and an incomparable orator, pointed out that there were no monkeys left in his region. He contended that if the disease came from monkeys, they should look to Middle Guinea, since the monkeys consumed came from that region. This public pronouncement was damaging to the explanation provided by the doctors, since it was true there were virtually no monkeys left in the Forestiere Region.

The Guinean government, for its part, was doubtful initially about the presence of EVD within its territory. In the absence of national expertise capable of confirming or denying the existence of the epidemic, the government focused its energies on attracting investors after the signing and ratification of its contract with Rio Tinto and on the visit to Guinea by the king of Morocco in March. Contradictory statements from the highest authorities of the nation in the early days of the epidemic created doubts about the existence of the disease. Too many ministers came out with contradictory and often knee-jerk reactions.[10] In April 2014, the president, Alpha Conde, indicated the outbreak was under control.[11] He also traveled to Guéckédou to shake hands with the population, a gesture designed to demonstrate the futility of the precautions dictated for the containment of the disease. This only served to confuse the issue further and intensify levels of denial among the general population. Never having heard a convincing explanation for its emergence in Guinea and surprised by its mode of transmission, Guineans found their own explanations for the sudden appearance of the disease. These explanations were usually in accordance with their political sensibilities, their ethnic and/or religious ties. They also reflected their mistrust of the Guinean political class and territorial administrators.

Rejection, and the deflection of responsibility for the disease to others, was the second phase in the evolution of response by the Guinean population. Supporters of the government adopted the doubts of the authorities and asserted, in the cafés of Conakry, that the disease had been introduced by Beny Steinmetz, a French-Israeli billionaire. Steinmetz was involved in a legal mining dispute with the government that is pending in a US court.[12] Others suspected the authorities, maintaining that the president had imported the disease to disrupt elections in 2015. The elites of the Forestiere region community theorized that the disease had been imported by the authorities in order to decimate their community and seize their land to facilitate the exploitation of the iron mines. They speculated that these lands would be placed in the hands of members of the Malinké community, who were perceived as supporters and beneficiaries of the Alpha Conde government. Some supporters of the Union des Forces Démocratiques de Guinée (UFDG), the chief opposition party, with a strong following in the Pulaar community, held that the epidemic was a divine punishment meted out to a community and a region where hundreds of heads of cattle were massacred by locals following recurring disputes between herders and farmers. While opposition supporters saw an ethno-political dimension to the disease, African-style Marxists amongst Guineans analyzed with broad strokes, asserting: "Ebola is not a natural disease but a political disease, because all of the victims of Ebola are among the poor."

If some Guineans saw devious politico-economic calculations behind the disease, others sought explanations in the eschatological. For them, this latest disease was none other than "a divine punishment for the deviant behaviors of humanity." In a region with deep Islamic roots and history, it is not surprising that a religious official from Télimélé that was interviewed maintained that it was predicted in the Koran that "you will be tested with things like sickness, fear, hunger, death and natural disasters." The belief that EVD was an instrument of mass decimation of Guineans also had currency with conspiracy theorists. Some of the Guineans who participated in the focus groups organized for this study were convinced that Ebola was "a means for the coordinators [of sensitization campaigns] to get rich," while others thought that "white people use this disease to reduce the number of black people." Health centers "have become centers for inoculating people with Ebola" and people hired to promote awareness and/or monitor contacts "are just locals paid on a pro rata basis according to the number of people they bring to health centers to be inoculated with the Ebola virus" was the narrative.

The misinformation spread by politicians and their supporters in the early stages of the epidemic is symptomatic of the excessive politicization of Guinean national life and it became one of the biggest obstacles in the fight against the epidemic. This politicization was evident in the fact that the health discourse lost its neutrality and its scientific basis; it became partisan and subjective. Guineans accepted, rejected, or contested explanations and public health messages about Ebola on grounds of opposition or allegiance to the ruling regime. In a country divided and excessively ethnicized, and where there were "multiple presidents," the political opposition was, initially, neither asked to participate nor included in the public awareness campaign. It probably did not seek to participate, since many opposition supporters saw Ebola as proof of the "bad luck of the ruling government" and something that would definitively discredit the government in the eyes of the population.

From July 2014, in the light of the scale and geographical reach of the EVD epidemic, the government discourse changed. It sought more assistance from WHO, ECOWAS, AU, and later the UN to combat the disease. However, the government's change of perspective and the additional responses to the disease did not put much of a dent in popular denial. Belated, it did not stop the spread of the epidemic or even less restore the faith of the people in the measures proposed to wipe out the disease. Ebola Treatment Centers (ETCs) and safe and dignified burials by the staff of the International Federation of Red Cross and Red Crescent Societies (IFRC) came to be viewed as very problematic. Guineans found it difficult to accept the prohibition on returning the bodies of the deceased to their home villages, even when they did not die of Ebola. The ETCs were viewed by the population as places where people go to die; you enter walking and you leave feet first in a black plastic bag. In an ETC, you cannot visit your son, your father, or your mother. You do not see doctors examining people or giving them medicine. In these "camps," which followed a model developed by MSF, Guineans found themselves with a new and terrifying form of medical care: "those who enter either leave dead or frightened, because nobody knows why him and not the others," according to one interviewee.

While the prohibition of the transportation of the remains of persons who died of Ebola or any other disease from one area to another was certainly understandable for protecting public health, it was still difficult for families and communities to accept. All of the participants in the focus groups for this study confirmed their desire to be able to bring the remains of their kin back to their native villages, and to bury them according to local customs. Indeed, the most difficult thing for the people to accept was allowing staff or volunteers from IFRC to wash and bury their dead. This difficulty was significantly complicated by the age of local Red Cross staff, and their knowledge (or lack thereof) of the Koran and of customary usages and practices. After the decision had been made to hand over the task of ensuring safe burials to them, certain IFRC staff members displayed a lack of tact and even intelligence in their handling of human remains that exacerbated rather than reduced social hostilities.

Using more experienced IFRC employees and volunteers and including members of the mosque councils as well as providing training and protective equipment much earlier on would have assuaged social tensions. The places where the IFRC hired the "right people" or placed them in the forefront of the burial process had the fewest issues with public disaffection with the handling of human remains during the EVD outbreak. These included Pita prefecture, where it seems that the local IFRC used people who were usually in charge of handling dead bodies as an interface. One interlocutor in the study pointed out that in certain more active areas of the Ebola epidemic, "The prayer for the dead was carried out by the community after the bodies were washed or disinfected in the case of Ebola by a few Red Cross staff members."[13]

Failures and inadequacies

If the Ebola epidemic generated incredible, and certain counterproductive speculations, it also became a vehicle for seeking self-aggrandizement in Guinea. Following the announcement that international aid would ensue to support various aspects of the response to the outbreak, awareness-raising in the field became a flocking point for idle civil servants from Conakry and the interior as well as unemployed people disguised as stakeholders in non-governmental organizations. Dr. Sakoba Keita, the national coordinator of the Ebola response, stated:

> I received text messages from strangers threatening me with bodily harm if I did not give them enough money for conducting awareness activities. They said I took too long to process their applications. That is why the security services assigned two gendarmes to my protection. The money does not belong to me; it belongs to the state. I refuse to support NGOs that want to twist my arm to give them two billion for awareness in Conakry. (Quoted by Bah 2014, my translation)

At the height of the emergency situation, too many people in Guinea were engaged in awareness campaigns with dubious efficacy. Every town or village had resource persons with real power, whose word was respected, and these people were initially not leading these campaigns. It also did not help that these awareness campaigns were conducted by non-natives of the targeted towns or villages, in a highly administrative manner by political staffers who openly displayed their party affiliations. This contributed significantly to the negative reactions that were observed in the field.

In an environment heavily laden with suspicion between the government and the governed, the autocratic and intimidating behavior of territorial administrators interfered with the effectiveness of the awareness messages. For example, certain territorial administrators made threats such as: "if you don't come out we'll gas you." In addition to giving the impression that spraying houses with chlorine to disinfect them was a punishment, such statements reminded the people of the harsh colonial practices of the French that were marked by abuses and harassment of all kinds. There was also a failure to teach and lead by example: local authorities should have started with the disinfection of their own homes to reassure the population of the safety of the procedure.

The response to the Ebola epidemic in Guinea also revealed the lack of a rigorous system of surveillance and monitoring of the movements of the populations, within the country and between Guinea, Sierra Leone, Liberia, and later Mali, all of which became part of the Ebola epidemic zone. The data very clearly indicates that EVD was spread by the movements of people. This is readily apparent if we look at the chain of contagion in certain prefectures:

> In Kindia, it was brought by infected individuals from Coyah; in Pita, it came from a cola nut vendor from Sierra Leone followed by other members of the family who had contact with him; in Faranah, from people who came from Macenta; in Télémélé, from an individual who came from Sierra Leone; and in Dabola, from a body that was brought home and through a traditional healer who claimed he could cure Ebola. (Summary of five interviews in Kindia, Pita, Faranah, and Télimélé prefectures)

For well over a year after Ebola appeared, no mechanism was in place to control population movements to prevent "free movement of the disease." Such a mechanism would have targeted bus stations linked with the "active" zones of the epidemic so that records could be kept of travelers. Similarly, there should have been serious monitoring of the Guinean borders to the south with Sierra Leone and Liberia, with checkpoints having temperature checks and record sheets, such as those utilized at the Conakry airport. Because of the nature of the disease, and its process of transmission, even a prefecture with no cases or that had managed to wipe out all cases of Ebola were still under threat due to population movements. Disease centers considered "quiet," "extinct," or "virgin" may become "active" as people moved around – particularly because there is a very strong tradition in Guinean communities that it is preferable to grow old, convalesce, or pass away in one's place of birth. This was demonstrated much later in 2014 and 2015, with the flaring up of new EVD outbreaks in areas which were considered clear of the disease.

The large-scale EVD infections and deaths of several health care personnel and the almost total lack of implementation of security or preventive measures, revealed the failings of the Guinean health care system.[14] In addition to discrediting the system, the infections of health care personnel showed their lack of preparedness for epidemics, the absence of screening centers to detect new diseases, and the lack of suitable equipment to deal with such outbreaks. The EVD epidemic contributed to disorganization with the Guinean health care system, and loss of faith in health care facilities and staff. It was not just Ebola that was killing Guineans, but other diseases as well, because they could no longer be managed and treated efficiently.

The ability of the Guinean health system to respond to diseases has not always been parlous and inefficient. Prior to 1984, and before the liberal reforms initiated and supported by the Bretton Woods institutions, Guinea had set up epidemic prevention and response teams within a streamlined, mobile health care system staffed with highly trained professionals that the population referred to as "Tripano."[15] By 1985, Guinea had changed its health care system, placing more focus on primary health care (PHC) and essential drugs. While this reform allowed the country to successfully deal with maternal, child, and newborn health, it let epidemic prevention and response fall by the wayside.

Compounding the shift in emphasis in public health care was the problem of renewal and expansion of health care personnel and budget allocations to the sector. In 2003, forecasts indicated that in 2014, nearly 25 percent of health care personnel in Guinea would have retired. Most of the retirees would be public health technicians (73 percent), midwives (52 percent), and radiology technicians, lab technicians, and pharmacy technicians (50 percent) (Ministère de la Santé publique 2004, 12). These disciplines, which are key in responding to epidemics, were already understaffed in the system and professional training institutions, are few and far between in Guinea. Furthermore, the share of the health care operating budget in the national budget has been in the region of 3 per cent for more than 30 years, whereas the Community of West African States (ECOWAS/CEDEAO), the African Union (AU), and WHO recommend spending 10 percent of the national budget on the sector. In Guinea, 90 percent of the health care budget is earmarked for the salaries of health care personnel. The remainder goes to administrative overhead, especially the ministry and health care centers (Ministère de la Santé et de l'Hygiène publique and Institut de Recherché en Sciences de la Santé du Burkina Faso 2011, 45).

Aside from the weaknesses of the health care system, the biggest error in the Ebola epidemic response in Guinea was the government's failure to carry out serious behavioral analysis to support its communication strategy. And yet, it has long been common known that: "Evidence, experience and common sense dictate that social mobilization strategies designed in collaboration with the target audience will be more effective than those imposed without consultation or opportunities for meaningful dialogue" (WHO 2012, 97). Studies conducted in different contexts have shown that African people faced with disease respond with family health production, meaning that extended family networks are usually actively involved in medical decision making, health care advice, and even treatment. Patients turn to family or friends first and only subsequently see a healer or health care professional once they have pondered, assessed, and possibly even decided on a diagnosis or a course of treatment. When care cannot be obtained in health care centers, or when it is said that there is no medicine, then family, healers, and marabouts became the next recourse.

Research conducted on therapeutic strategy in Guinea over the past two decades has shown that a majority of patients either begin or end their health care with traditional medicine. When certain symptoms appear (such as jaundice, for instance), patients are never taken to a modern health care center, unless they are in the terminal stages. This approach is demonstrative of the importance attached to traditional medicine by Guineans and the impact of various cultural beliefs on their chosen therapeutic options (Ministère de la santé publique 2004, 9).

Effects of EVD on social cohesion

The denial of the disease witnessed in the early months of the epidemic, when many people had never seen a person who was ill with or had died of Ebola, was replaced by fear and anxiety. These feelings increasingly affected social ties within families and between Ebola survivors and others. Indeed, in societies where physical contact is a part of life and people are constantly touching, as in Guinea, where people shake hands all day, share meals, and are in close contact at endless social ceremonies such as marriages, baptisms, and funerals, a viral disease spread by physical contact was a terrifying proposition, because it severely interrupted rituals that initiated, affirmed, and reinforced social ties.

In Guinean societies, illness and death are not events that weaken these ties; in fact, they reinforced them even more. The sick are cared for by their families, who accompany them in the process of healing or death. Even in hospitals, it is not uncommon to find a relative sleeping on the floor beside a patient's bed. People are duty-bound to visit the sick, to sit with them and chat, and wish them a speedy recovery. With Ebola, these social interactions became impossible. It is not without reason that Benjamin Hale (2014, 5), in a renowned article entitled "The Most Terrifying Thing about Ebola," wrote: "This virus preys on care and love, piggybacking on the deepest, most distinctively human virtues" and added, "In short, Ebola parasitizes our humanity." When an infected person was sent to an Ebola treatment center, they left their family with a sense that they will probably die. For fathers, mothers, sisters, and brothers, seeing a loved one disappear into a dehumanized medical space, with no opportunity to enter into physical or visual contact, caused anxiety that laid the foundation for interpretations that were sometimes quite fanciful.

EVD also left visible, and indelible socials scars on individual Guineans, health professionals, and their communities (Sow et al. 2016). Infected people suffered from two kinds of discrimination. First, the epidemic forced them to leave their families, who could no longer touch them or their personal items. Second, within the family, and between family members, their neighbors and their relations, they were ostracized once again. These different restrictions were traumatic and, in communities weakened by several years of ethnic and political tensions, they aroused feelings of suspicion and undermined progress made in achieving social cohesion. This situation altered social relationships within affected family units, communities, and regions. Suspicion and stigmatization did not only apply to families that had experienced cases of Ebola, but also affected people who had recovered from the disease. The latter suffered not only from problems of acceptance by their neighbors and colleagues, but also in their relations with certain members of their own families.

Conclusion

Long after the deadline imprint of EVD became unavoidable or undeniable in Guinea and the MRU sub-region, many Guineans continued to deny the existence of the disease and to attack anyone who discussed it in their vicinity. Many factors accounted for this seeming irrational behavior. First, the similarity of Ebola symptoms with other commonplace diseases in the country made any suggestions that it was something radically new implausible. The newness and sudden emergence of the disease and the general ignorance of its nature provided fertile ground for popular rejection. Unfortunately, rather than dispelling ignorance, official communication about the disease, which focused on its origin and fatality rate, negatively interfered with popular receptiveness of messages about prophylaxis.

Against a backdrop of ignorance, negative reception, and excessive politicization grounded in the pre-independence years, the Ebola response policy developed by the organizations in charge was unsound. The awareness campaign that was conducted was not grounded in serious social or behavioral analysis of target communities. It was rife with multiple discourses, which sometimes contradicted local common sense, and ultimately undermined efforts to educate, promote understanding, and assuage fears. An awareness campaign conducted by card-carrying, demagogic, partisan administrators, NGOs made up of the unemployed disguised as humanitarians, and foreigners with very little knowledge of local customs, in a sociopolitical environment steeped in suspicion and tribalism produced doubt rather than clarity in the minds of Guineans. Between those who talk about Ebola (UNICEF), go door to door looking for the sick (the WHO), wear hazmat suits, like cosmonauts, to care for the sick (MSF), feed isolated and stigmatized families (World Food Programme), and take away bodies in black plastic bags and bury them without a purifying ritual (IFRC), Guineans felt trapped in all kinds of gigantic, hidden plots.

EVD had hit a country weakened by years of poor governance and wide-scale predation, with an economy subsidized by a handful of bilateral and multilateral donors. Recurring outbreaks of cholera and meningitis in Guinea had already shown the limits of the country's health care system. The epidemic had degraded and disorganized what was left of it, fueling popular disaffection about the value of health care facilities. Ebola was not the only disease that killed Guineans on a large scale between 2013 and 2016; many died from other diseases because of lack of competent care and infrastructural support.

The Ebola epidemic ruptured, hopefully only temporarily, social bonds by reducing people's presence at social ceremonies (weddings, baptisms, funerals) and, above all, by the suspicion it engendered within and between families. Suspicion, loss of trust, and a refusal to share the same spaces (beds, meals, transportation, work spaces, etc.) and even to buy products sold by people from active Ebola zones were realities that were difficult to evade. This breakdown of social bonds, if they are not quickly repaired, would be highly problematic for a society with a significant social economy.

Notes

1 "Outbreaks Chronology: Ebola Virus Outbreaks," Center for Disease Control and Prevention, http://www.cdc.gov/vhf/ebola/outbreaks/history/chronology.html (last accessed October 16, 2016).

2 According to reliable and confidential sources, it seems that prior to March 2014 (toward the end of November 2013 to be exact), samples drawn from a few patients were sent to France by international organizations operating in Guinea that had identified the Ebola virus.

3 Médecins Sans Frontières, *Pushed to the Limit and Beyond: A Year into the Largest Ever Ebola Outbreak*, MSF Report, March 2015, 5.

4 "Outbreak: Guinea Health Team Killed," *BBC News*, September 19, 2014, http://www.bbc.co.uk/news/world-africa-29256443 (last accessed October 12, 2016).

5 See UNMEER External Situation Report, November 12, 2014; UNMEER External Situation Report, November 18, 2014. See also ACAPS, "Ebola in West Africa: Guinea: Resistance to the Ebola Response," file:///Users/home/Downloads/h_guinea_resistance_to_the_ebola_response_24_april_2015.pdf (last accessed October 16, 2016).

6 Interview with a 62-year-old man in Mamou.

7 Interview with an Imam from Télimélé.

8 Interview with a customary chief from Pita, a locality of Moyenne Guinée.

9 Interview with a 43-year-old man from Dabalo.

10 Certain ministers, such as Tata Vieux Condé, claimed on two separate occasions (in June 2014 and January 2015) in Faranah prefecture (Layasando and Tiro) that there was no Ebola in Guinea.

11 Beth Balen, "Ebola Under Control per Guinean President," *Liberty Voice*, May 1, 2014, http://guardianlv.com/2014/05/ebola-outbreak-under-control-per-guinea-president/ (last accessed October 16, 2016).

12 For the exploits of this controversial businessman in Guinea, see Tom Burgis, *The Looting Machine: Warlords, Oligarchs, Corporations, Smugglers, and the Theft of Africa's Wealth* (New York: Public Affairs, 2015).

13 Interview with interlocutor, December 14, 2014, Pita prefecture.

14 See Annex of Guinea Response Plan in WHO: WHO Ebola Response Roadmap, August 28, 2014.

15 "Tripano" is short for trypanosomiasis or sleeping sickness. It was the first disease the epidemiological prevention and response team dealt with.

References

Bah, B.L. (2014). "Insécurité en Guinée: La vie du coordinateur national de lutte contre Ebola menacée?" http://www.Africaguinee.com/articles/2014/09/21/insecuriteenguineelaviedu coordinateurnational deluttecontreebola (accessed February 28, 2015).

Hale, B. (2014). "The Most Terrifying Thing about Ebola: The Disease Threatens Humanity by Preying on Humanity," September 19. http://www.slate.com/articles/health_and_science/medical_examiner/2014/09/why_ebola_is_terrifying_and_dangerous_it_preys_on_family_caregiving_and.html (accessed October 18, 2016).

Ministère de la Santé et de l'Hygiène Publique (Guinée) and Institut de Recherche en Sciences de la Santé du Burkina Faso (2011). "De l'analyse de la situation de la planification familiale en Guinée," Conakry, Guinea.

Ministère de la santé publique (2004). "Plan stratégique de développement sanitaire, 2003–2012," Conakry, Guinea.

Sow, S., Desclaux, A., Taverne, B., and Groupe D'Etudes PostEboGui (2016). "Ebola en Guinée: formes de la stigmatisation des acteurs de santé survivants," *Bulletin de la Societe de Pathologie exotique*, 1–5.

World Health Organization (WHO) (ed.) (2012). "Communication for Behavioural Impact (COMBI): A Toolkit for Behavioural and Social Communication in Outbreak Response." http://www.who.int/ihr/publications/combi_toolkit_outbreaks/en/ (accessed February 28, 2015).

4 | THE POLITICAL ECONOMY OF THE EBOLA EPIDEMIC IN LIBERIA

George Klay Kieh, Jr.

Introduction

The Ebola Virus Disease (EVD) epidemic in Liberia and its aftermath have witnessed the emergence of scholarly interest in the examination of the domestic, economic, political, and social contexts that shaped the phenomenon. The emergent literature can tentatively be subsumed under three major frameworks: governance, socio-economic development, and infrastructural change (physical). The centerpiece of the governance explanation is that the Ebola epidemic exposed the underbelly of poor governance in the country (Dempsey 2014; Ryan 2014; Curson 2015). That is, weak institutional capacity, the lack of a regime for addressing epidemics, and rampant corruption, among others, hamstrung the government's capacity to respond to the crisis adequately.

The socio-economic model is premised on the argument that human well-being in the country is in a sordid state (Hartman 2014; Nsoedo 2014; Ryan 2014; Obilade 2015; Sanders et al. 2015). This is reflected in, for example, abject mass poverty, high unemployment, especially among the youth, underemployment, and food insecurity. Importantly, the drivers of the country's socio-economic malaise include an inadequate health care infrastructure characterized by the dearth of trained medical personnel, facilities, equipment, and supplies, and the lack of investment in food production. These conditions militated against the country's capacity to contain and defeat the virus.

As for the infrastructural explanation, it is anchored on the woeful state and inadequacy of the country's physical infrastructure – roads, bridges, clean drinking water, medical equipment, sanitation, and the lack of electricity (Ryan 2014; van de Pas and Belle 2015). There were two major resulting implications for addressing the epidemic. It was extremely difficult to travel through the country, and this made it very difficult to deliver various supplies, including health-related and food. The other lacuna was that the inadequacy of clean drinking water and sanitation provided an enabling environment for the spread of the Ebola virus, thereby adversely affecting the containment efforts.

Against this background, while the various explanations focus on particular sets of factors as the axles that conditioned and shaped the Ebola epidemic in Liberia, this chapter will focus on the peripheral capitalist Liberian state. This is because it is the state that is the generator of the factors that conditioned and shaped the epidemic. Accordingly, an examination of the portrait of the state – nature, character, mission, structure and power relations, and policies, among others – would help us understand the context or crucible within which the epidemic occurred, and the resulting impact. The central question that the chapter seeks to address is how did the peripheral capitalist Liberian state impact the Ebola epidemic? To address this question, the chapter is divided into four sections. The first section examines the portrait of the peripheral capitalist Liberian state, and the resulting governance and development trajectories. Second, the nature of governance and development in Liberia are examined both historically, and specifically during the regime of Ellen Johnson Sirleaf. Third, the chapter interrogates the nature and dynamics of the Ebola epidemic and the response of the Sirleaf regime. Fourth, the prospects for the post-Ebola era are examined, with a focus on the possibility of the much needed systemic and structural transformation in the future.

Theorizing the peripheral capitalist state

The peripheral capitalist state is essentially a social formation that has a capitalist materialist base as its mode of production. Central to it is the private ownership and control of the major means of production (Ziemann and Lanzendorfer 1977). Importantly, ownership and control of the major means of production are mainly in the hands of the owners of the metropolitan-based multinational corporations, who have a collaborative (but patron–client) relationship with the state managers in the peripheral state (Prado 1966).

In terms of the broader relations of production, there are two major clusters of classes: the ruling and subaltern classes. The former has two major wings: the internal one comprises state managers and local businesspeople. The external wing consists of the owners of foreign-based multinational corporations and other businesses. Importantly, the internal wing, especially its bureaucratic element (state managers), creates propitious conditions for the external wing to amass wealth through predatory accumulation (surplus through profits). As for the members of the internal wing, especially the state managers, they accumulate wealth through the use of their respective positions by engaging in various corrupt practices, including stealing public funds, extortion, the receipt of bribes, and fraudulent procurement schemes. The subaltern classes are made up of the workers, farmers, and the unemployed, among others. Significantly, the members of the ruling class use the state to benefit them materially, while visiting mass poverty and social malaise on the subalterns.

Another major element is that the lifeblood of the economy is supplied by the production of raw materials for the industrial and manufacturing complexes of the developed states (Emmanuel 1972). In turn, the peripheral formation relies on the developed states for manufactured goods. Significantly, the prices for both raw materials and manufactured goods are set by the developed capitalist states as part of the unjust "system of unequal exchange" (Emmanuel 1972).

Further, the portrait of the state consists principally of its nature (the historical roots or foundation), character (orientation or behavior), mission, and policies. Its nature is the by-product of colonialism, neocolonialism, and imperialism. The character is multidimensional: it has been described variously as "exploitative," "criminalized," and "negligent" (Agbese 2007). Its purpose is to create an enabling environment in which the members of the ruling class can accumulate wealth through predatory means, while neglecting the basic human needs of the members of the subaltern classes. Also, the state's various policies are designed to promote the general interests of the ruling class as a whole.

The related element is that the structure of the state's political economy has two major dimensions: the political and economic structures. The former consists of the public institutions that are lodged in the legislative, executive, and judicial branches. These are managed by those Prado (1966) refers to as the "bureaucratic bourgeoisie." The latter comprises the domestic and global economies. The former is an appendage of the latter (Ziemann and Lanzendorfer 1977; Frank 1978).

Moreover, the peripheral capitalist state performs several major functions. One of them is the reproduction of the social, political, and economic structures of ruling-class dominance (Fatton 1988). Also, the state provides "law and order" (Graff 1994), so as to ensure that enabling conditions are created for the members of the ruling class to exploit the subalterns, and to accumulate wealth through various predatory means. In addition, the state, as has been discussed, serves the general interests of the ruling class. In so doing, it mediates conflicts between the various factions and fractions of the class (Miliband 1973). Furthermore, in the case of conflicts between the ruling and the subaltern classes, the state always intervenes on behalf of the former. At the external level, as an appendage of the world capital system, the peripheral capitalist state functions as a handmaid of the advanced capitalist states within the context of dependency and subservience (Frank 1969; Amin 1974).

The crucible: the Liberian state The examination of the portrait – nature, character, mission, structure and power relations, and policies – of the peripheral capitalist Liberian state is the *sine qua non* for understanding the economic, political, social, and other factors that shaped and conditioned the Ebola epidemic in the country. The rationale is that as the arena of struggle (Glasberg and Shannon 2011), the Liberian state sets the parameters for the various developments that take place within it. Generally, the Liberian state is either a facilitator or an inhibitor.

At the vortex of the portrait of the peripheral capitalist Liberian state is its unrepresentative and non-inclusive nature. That is, the Liberian state is not representative of the historical and cultural experiences of its various ethnic groups and stocks (Sawyer 1992; Kieh 2008; Kieh 2012a). Instead, it represents only the historical and cultural experiences of the manumitted Africans, who were repatriated to Liberia, beginning in 1820 (Liebenow 1969; Wreh 1976; Sawyer 1992; Kieh 2008; Kieh 2012a). The repatriation project and the resulting formation of the Liberian state were ostensibly designed to help solve the American "race problem" (Smith 1972). In other words, these Africans were repatriated to Liberia (first to Sierra Leone) as the result of the initial disintegration of the system of slavery in the United States. Fearful of a large unemployed pool of blacks, the American ruling class and its government made the determination that the solution to the emergent "black problem" was to repatriate the freed Africans to Africa, the land of their ancestry (Smith 1972). Unfortunately, conditioned by what Brown (1941, 10) aptly refers to as a "slave psychology," the repatriated Africans went to Liberia with hubris: since they had lived in the United States, although as slaves, they were therefore superior to their African kin, who they met on the Grain Coast (now Liberia) (Kieh 2008; Kieh 2012a). Hence, they embarked on a so-called "civilizing and Christianizing mission" (Liebenow 1969; Liebenow 1987; Wreh 1976; Beyan 1991; Sawyer 1992; Kieh 2008; Kieh 2012a). At the heart of this parody of the colonial "*mission civilisatrice*," was the demonization and desecration of the cultures of the various indigenous groups that they met on the Grain Coast. The emergent independent Liberian state was a settler one that privileged the descendants of the repatriated Africans in every sphere (Sawyer 1992: Kieh 2008; Kieh 2012a). Even with the finalization of Liberia's incorporation into the world capitalist system in 1926, and the ascendance of class as the pivot of the power relations, the communal current and its accent on privileging the descendants of the repatriated Africans remained ensconced in the country's political economy until the 1980 military coup (Kieh 2008; Kieh 2012a). Ultimately, the nature of the state created a dialectical tension between the privileging of the members of the local wing of the Liberian ruling class (state managers, local economically well-off business people, and others) and their relations with the subalterns. This in turn shaped the formulation and implementation of public policies – from health care to job creation.

In terms of its character, the Liberian state has been described variously as "criminalized," "exploitative," "negligent," and "predatory" (Agbese 2007; Kieh 2008; Kieh 2012a). As Agbese (2007, 45–46), aptly observes in the general case of the African state, "The African state [is] a composite of an oppressor, terrorist, a criminalized entity, a criminal enterprise, and a beggar or client of a foreign power. Which of these tendencies is more dominant at any given time is a function of several factors." Hence, the state and its government have had no interest in serving the interest of the Liberian people, including providing for their basic needs such as jobs, health care, education, food security, clean drinking water, and sanitation. Importantly, this orientation has not changed. The people, especially the subalterns are vulnerable to hunger, malnutrition, undernourishment, and diseases.

Clearly, the mission of the Liberian state vividly reflects its "Janus-faced" complexion: on the one hand, the state provides propitious conditions for the members of the local ruling class and their relations to live fulfilled lives by serving as a vehicle for the provision of their basic human needs. But, on the other hand, the state visits mass abject poverty, unemployment, food insecurity, and vulnerability to diseases as the result of inadequate health care on the subalterns. The resulting *raison d'être* of the state is twofold. First, it creates an enabling environment in which metropolitan-based multinational corporations and other businesses engage in the predatory accumulation of capital (Kieh 2008; Kieh 2012a). Second, the faction or fraction of the local wing of the Liberian ruling class that controls state power at particular historical junctures uses it as an agency for engagement in the primitive accumulation of capital through sundry illegal and immoral means such as the insistence on the receiving of bribes, extortion, the stealing of public funds, and procurement fraud (Kieh 2012b). Nzongola-Ntalaja's (1992, 14) poignant summation of the prebendalization of the African state by the ruling class is apropos to the Liberian case: "The state has been likened to a warehouse where each member of the [ruling] class collects his or her loot. Corruption together with the adoption of misguided policies, have seen the country's economy deteriorating to a moribund one." Thus, the Liberian state has, and continues to be presided over by a local ruling class, whose primary interest is not the delivery of public goods such as jobs, education, health care, and food security, but the primitive accumulation of wealth through the agency of the state. Hence, the subalterns lack the requisite socio-economic "safety net" that would prepare and enable them to withstand the vagaries of epidemics.

Significantly, power relations are lodged in two major spheres. At the societal level (the meta-level) power relations are anchored on a class system (Mason and Sawyer 1979; Kappel et al. 1986; Kieh 2008; Kieh 2012a) that comprises three major clusters: ruling, *petit bourgeois*, and subaltern. The ruling class, which consists of two wings – internal (state managers and local business people and others, who are relatively well-off economically) and external (the owners of metropolitan-based multinational corporations and other businesses) – owns and controls the major means of production and the state. The *petit bourgeois* class consists of intellectuals and entertainers. The subaltern classes comprise the workers, farmers, the unemployed, and the *hoi polloi*. At the governmental level, there is an asymmetrical relationship between the presidency, the hegemonic institution, on the one hand, and the legislative and judicial branches, on the other. Under this arrangement, the presidency dominates the political landscape of the country with very limited checks from the legislative and judicial branches (Wreh 1976; Sawyer 1992; Kieh 2008; Kieh 2012a).

The motor force for public policy formulation and implementation is the creation of an enabling environment for predatory accumulation by both metropolitan-based corporations and other businesses and the faction of the local wing of the ruling class that is manning state power at particular moments. Hence, issues such as health care, food security, clean drinking water, and sanitation that are critical to the health and overall material well-being of the subaltern are neglected.

Significantly, the peripheral capitalist Liberian state generated multidimensional crises of underdevelopment. Among them are political, economic, and social fissures that became ensconced in the country's landscape. At the political level, the crisis found expression in several key areas. A major one was the emergence of an authoritarian governance system in which the human rights of the people were violated by the state and its functionaries (Freedom House 2017). For example, the state and its various regimes frowned upon the expression of views that were contrary to the policies of the government. In several cases, critics of the government were harassed, imprisoned, tortured, forced into exile, and even murdered (Wreh 1976). S. David Coleman, an opposition leader, was murdered during President William Tubman's regime (Watkins 2007). In the case of the Tolbert regime, after the April 14, 1979 mass demonstration against the excesses of the ruling class and its government, it arrested, charged with treason, and imprisoned the leaders of the various pro-democracy movements that organized the action (Cordor 1979). Under the Doe regime, opposition leaders and pro-democracy activists, including student leaders, were routinely harassed, arrested, and imprisoned (Sawyer 1992; Kieh 2008; Kieh 2012a). The Taylor regime continued the practice of muzzling the freedom of speech, and of the press by, among other things, arresting and imprisoning pro-democracy activists and journalists, and closing down media organizations for criticizing his regime (Kieh 2012a; Freedom House 2017).

Another major dimension of the political crisis was the issue of weak public institutions, as the result of the emergence of the "hegemonic presidency" during the Arthur Barclay regime in 1904 (Sawyer 1992; Kieh 2008; Kieh 2012a; Kieh 2012b). In essence, the legislative and executive branches were subordinated to the executive. As Wreh (1976, ix) laments, "Under Tubman's rule, there was no countervailing power from the people or from the constitutionally created National Legislature … [an institution] which should provide the checks and balances to the executive branch … Unchallenged and unfettered, Tubman had everything to himself and ruled as he pleased." Also, the political culture nurtured the lack of accountability and transparency in the conduct of the affairs of the state, as well as the absence of the "rule of law." One of the resultant effects was the emergence of a culture of impunity, under which the members of the ruling class and their relations were above the law. Hence, they could violate the law without being held accountable for their actions.

The economic crisis was captured by several major indicators. For example, by the end of the Doe regime and the beginning of the first civil war, unemployment stood at about 36.2 percent. During the same period, there was a skewed distribution of wealth and income. In the case of the former, the ruling class accounting for about 6 percent of the population, cornered about 70 percent of the national wealth (Kieh 1997). As for the latter, the ruling class accounted for about 68 percent of the national income (Ministry of Planning and Economic Affairs 1989). The inequitable distribution of income was reflected in the country's Gini Coefficient of 0.53 (Peters and Shapouri 1997, 45). By the end of the Taylor regime in 2003, the rate of unemployment burgeoned to 85 percent (United Nations Development Programme 2006). During the same period, the rate of poverty (below the poverty line: people living on less than US$1 per day) stood at an alarming 76.2 percent (United Nations Development Programme 2006). Amid mass abject poverty, the members of the bureaucratic wing of the ruling class (state managers) and their relations engaged in the criminalization of the state through sundry corrupt means. For example, using their respective public offices as the agencies, state managers, including the president, plundered and pillaged the public coffers through thievery. During his tenure as head of state, President Doe and his faction of the local wing of the ruling class accumulated over $300 million through predatory means (Ballah 2003). Similarly, during the Taylor regime, rampant corruption continued through the use of various illegal means, including the receipt of bribes, extortion, procurement fraud, and the stealing of public funds.

As for the social crisis, it was manifested in various ways. For example, at the end of President Taylor's tenure in 2003, the adult mortality rate was an astronomical 537 per 1,000 persons (United Nations Development Programme 2006). Clearly, the scourge of undernourishment contributed to this high mortality rate – about 50 percent of the population was malnourished (United Nations Development Programme 2010). In addition, only 26 percent of the population had access to safe drinking water (United Nations Development Programme 2006), and 45 percent to acceptable sanitation (United Nations Development Programme 2006).

Not unexpectedly, the multidimensional crises of underdevelopment that were generated by the authoritarian peripheral capitalist state led to civil unrest and armed conflict. The latter metamorphosed into two civil wars from 1989 to 1997 (first civil war), and 1999 to 2003 (second civil war). Among other things, the two wars destroyed the country's already underdeveloped physical infrastructure – roads, bridges, electrical grid, water, and sanitation systems – and led to "brain drain," including doctors, nurses, and other health care professionals, who fled the country for safety.

After the termination of the first civil war in 1997, the international community initiated a liberal post-conflict peace-building project. However, the Taylor regime rejected the project, and instead opted to establish a "garrison state" in a militarized environment. For example, the Taylor regime retained the *ancien* authoritarian governance system, and the anti-people and anti-development peripheral capitalist economy. Consequently, the confluence of authoritarianism and socio-economic malaise created the propitious conditions for the outbreak of the second civil war in 1999.

When the second civil war ended in 2003, again, the international community led by the United States and the United Nations re-imposed the liberal peace-building template on Liberia. Importantly, the model's thrust is neoliberal state reconstitution. Operationally, this entails the establishment of formal liberal democratic rules and processes – what Yidana (2009, 1) perceptively refers to as "form driven democracy – and a peripheral capitalist economy that is controlled by multinational corporations and other businesses mainly from the "Global North." Importantly, these structural modalities set Liberia on the course to another "false start." This is because these frameworks are incapable of addressing the country's perennial multidimensional crisis of underdevelopment. Hence, by adopting them, the country commenced another phase in its seemingly unending cycle of underdevelopment.

Governance and development under the Sirleaf regime

Background President Ellen Johnson Sirleaf was elected President in 2006, amid high hopes among Liberians that she would provide the requisite stewardship in building a new democratic and prosperous country for all Liberians. And the sense of expectancy was increased in two major ways. At the global level, various major actors, especially the United States under the Bush administration, heaped various accolades on President Sirleaf, hailing her as the country's "savior." President Sirleaf promised in her two inaugural addresses (she is currently in her second term of office) to tackle the vexatious issues of undemocratic governance and the socio-economic crises of underdevelopment (Johnson Sirleaf 2006; Johnson Sirleaf 2012).

As the pathways, the Sirleaf regime embraced the liberal peacebuilding project that was imposed by the international community under the leadership of the United Nations and the United States. Specifically, the Sirleaf regime adopted the hybrid governance system and the neoliberal *Weltanschauung*. The former is a mixture of authoritarianism and democracy (Freedom House 2015). Specifically, Liberians do freely exercise their political and civil rights. However, at various times, when the regime determines that its grip on power is being threatened, it could curtail the exercise of civil liberties in the name of national security (Kieh 2015). The latter is a development model that, among other things, minimizes the role of the state, and places primary control of a country's economy in the hand of so-called "market forces" such as multinational corporations and other businesses (Saad-Fiho 2008). Both the implicit and explicit postulate is that the "market" would serve as the engine of national development (Saad-Fiho 2008).

This section of the chapter examines the travail of governance and development during the Sirleaf regime. In the case of the former, focus will be on the state of democratization, the functioning of public institutions, and the pedigree of institutional capacity, including the existence of protocols and processes for managing the affairs of the state. As for the latter, the emphasis will be on human well-being. The rationale is that this should be the *raison d'être* of development.

Governance

Political democracy

Compared to its predecessors – Tubman, Tolbert, Doe, and Taylor – the Sirleaf regime has made appreciable strides in seeking to liberalize the Liberian polity. In comparative terms, Liberians are able to exercise their constitutionally guaranteed political rights and civil liberties with fewer constraints than in the past. A major case in point is that Liberians can openly criticize the Sirleaf regime without facing reprisals; and this is evident on the various radio talk shows in the country (Liberia Data Project 2015). In addition, elections are comparatively freer and fairer than in the past, when electoral fraud was the norm (Liberia Data Project 2015). One of the resulting effects is that several incumbent members of the National Legislature of Liberia – both representatives and senators – have lost their re-election bids. For example, during the 2014 Senate by-election, all but two of the incumbents, who sought re-election, lost their bid (National Election Commission of Liberia 2014).

However, despite the progress in the area of political democracy, the authoritarian reflex is ever present. That is, the Sirleaf regime has resorted to the use of repressive methods, when its hold on state power has been threatened. During the 2011 presidential election, when the incumbent President Sirleaf sought a second term, the regime closed down media organizations that gave favorable coverage to the Congress for Democratic Change (CDC), the main opposition party. King FM and Clar TV, Love FM and TV, and Shiata Power and TV were shut down by armed police (Committee for the Protection of Journalists 2011). Similarly, during the same period, President Sirleaf "suspended and replaced the Liberian Broadcasting System (LBS) Director-General Ambrose Nmah … due to the broadcast of a press conference in which the leaders of [the] main opposition party were critical of the president" (Freedom House 2012). Clearly, President Sirleaf's action was in violation of Article 15, section d of the Liberian Constitution, which guarantees equal access to the state's media outlets by all political parties.

Overall, under the Sirleaf regime, Liberia has become a hybrid state in terms of its democratic status (Freedom House 2017). The status reflects the fact that political democracy and authoritarianism are co-existing in a contradictory manner: the gains that are being made in the process of political democratization are being undermined by the persistence of authoritarian tendencies.

The functioning of public institutions

As in the past, public institutions remain weak and ineffective. One of the major contributing factors to this phenomenon is persistence of the "hegemonic presidency." Essentially, this entails the subordination of public institutions, including the legislature and the judiciary, to presidential suzerainty (Kieh 2012b). Three major cases are quite instructive. In September 2006, President Sirleaf requested the legislature to grant her the authority to appoint city mayors (Kennedy 2006; Kieh 2012b). While the request was pending, the Supreme Court of Liberia, based on a lawsuit that was filed by two Liberian opposition political parties challenging the constitutionality of President Sirleaf's request for the expansion of presidential appointive powers, issued a stunning ruling on the matter: the country's highest court ruled that Article 54 of Liberia's Constitution gives the president the authority to appoint mayors (Boweh 2008; Kieh 2012b). With the ruling, for the first time in the country's history, the president acquired the power to "appoint virtually every official in the executive and judicial branches" (Kieh 2012b, 23). Even during the heyday of authoritarianism in the country, city mayors were elected.

Similarly, in 2007, President Sirleaf appointed herself Chair ex-officio of the Board of Governors of the Booker Washington Institute – a technical high school (Government of Liberia 2007). This action was unprecedented, because no president of the country has ever been a member of the Board of Governors of any public educational institute (Kieh 2012b). In addition, President Sirleaf followed the precedent set by her predecessor in appointing the principal of the high school. A year later, President Sirleaf dismissed the president of the University of Liberia, the country's flagship public tertiary institution (Press Office, Executive Mansion 2008). This action continued the practice of the politicization of the administration of public educational institutions in the country. This no doubt undermined the autonomy of academic institutions as public spaces for free and unencumbered debates, and the search for solutions to the major challenges facing the country.

Furthermore, President Sirleaf also tampered with the independence of the judiciary when she interfered with the assignment of Judge Charles Williams of the First Judicial Circuit Court of Montserrado County. Specifically, President Sirleaf ensured that Judge Williams was transferred to another circuit court. The reason was that Judge Williams allegedly incurred the consternation of President Sirleaf when he refused to issue a guilty ruling in the trial involving Charles Julu (now deceased) and others, who were accused of plotting to overthrow the Sirleaf regime (Borteh 2008).

The lack of protocols for managing national crises

One of the glaring manifestations of the lack of institutional capacity under the Sirleaf regime is the lack of protocols for conducting the affairs of the state. For example, there are no protocols for managing health crises such as epidemics. In other words, the Sirleaf regime has failed to develop the modalities that would serve as guides for addressing health and other crises that pose major threats to the country's national security (Liberia Data Project 2015). In addition, there is the lack of an inter-ministerial and inter-agency organizational architecture for addressing national emergencies such as health epidemics.

Importantly, the Ebola epidemic exposed the lack of the aforementioned modalities. Particularly, this was reflected in the Sirleaf regime's ad hoc and uncoordinated approach to addressing the epidemic. For example, President Sirleaf appointed a taskforce for addressing the epidemic. However, the absence of protocols for addressing health and other crises required the taskforce to invest an enormous amount of time in trying to formulate strategies for addressing the epidemic. Undoubtedly, if the Sirleaf regime had an established institutional mechanism and protocols for addressing crises such as the Ebola epidemic, they would have greatly enhanced the efforts to contain the spread of the virus.

Patronage

The Sirleaf regime has made patronage a major cornerstone of its governance trajectory. Two major cases are quite instructive. Like her predecessors, President Sirleaf has appointed several of her relatives to key positions in her regime. For example, Estrada Bernard, the president's brother-in-law, is the Adviser to the President on Legal and National Security Affairs; A.B. Johnson, the president's cousin, served as the First Minister of Internal Affairs, until he was forced to resign under public pressure, for allegedly embezzling money from the county development fund; Fumbah Sirleaf, the president's son, is the Director-General of the National Security Agency, the country's principal intelligence unit; and Charles Sirleaf, the president's son, is Deputy Governor of the Central Bank (Liberia Data Project 2015).

The other major case of neo-patrimony was the directive President Sirleaf issued to cabinet ministers and the heads of various government agencies in February 2010 "to employ at least two members each of the ruling Unity Party" (Clarke and Wenyu 2010, 1). In a strong rebuke of President Sirleaf's promotion of patronage, Jefferson Elliott, the President of the Civil Servants Association of Liberia, exclaimed: "[This] is a return to the 'spoils system,' and an attempt to politicize the civil service and to give it a partisan picture, and violates section three of the Civil Service Standing Order" (Clarke and Wenyu 2010, 1).

Corruption

Corruption has become a pervasive feature of public administration during the Sirleaf regime. Even the US State Department (2009, 1) was forced to admit, "Corruption and impunity are endemic through all levels of [the Liberian] government." Against this backdrop, there have been many cases of corruption since the inception of the Sirleaf regime in 2006. For example, in 2008, the late Willis Knuckles, then Minister of State for Presidential Affairs (President Sirleaf's Chief of Staff) and a confidante of the president, was accused of engaging in influence peddling, and the resultant illegal accumulation of wealth through the process. In response to the public outcry, President Sirleaf appointed a commission to investigate the matter. But, after spending about a $1 million on the investigation, President Sirleaf refused to make the commission's report public, and to act on it.

Again, in 2013, the Managing Director of the Roberts International

Airport, was accused of embezzling over $350,000. But, in a stunning development, the accused indicated that she had tape recordings that could reveal President Sirleaf's personal involvement in various corrupt acts. This revelation is consistent with similar claims that have been made by others. For example, Zaza (2009, 1) asserted, barely four years into President Sirleaf's first term of office, that "President Sirleaf and her cronies are seizing businesses ranging from banks to mining gold, mining diamonds, logging, consulting, and importing rice." Corruption under the Sirleaf regime reached a crescendo in 2013, as reflected in Liberia being ranked the most corrupt country in the world by Transparency International (2013). Specifically, the results of the survey revealed, "the vast majority of Liberians surveyed said they believe the country (Liberia) is run largely or entirely by few entities acting in their own selfish interests (Hess and Sauter 2013, 1). In addition, 96 percent of the Liberians surveyed rated the country's legislature as very corrupt (Hess and Sauter 2013, 1).

Critically, the lack of political will on the part of President Sirleaf to bring to justice government officials who are accused of corruption has led to the further institutionalization of the culture of impunity. That is, government officials, who are accused of corruption, very rarely face trial. In fact, some of them are rewarded with appointments to major positions in the government (Sungbeh 2013). As Frances Johnson Morris, the then Chair of the Liberia Anti-Corruption Commission, asserts, "the Executive Branch of government, which is charged with the responsibility of enforcing laws and mustering the political will in this fight [against corruption], is found wanting with respect to transparency and accountability in matters of financial management" (Sieh 2009, 1).

Development As has been discussed, neoliberalism is the development strategy being pursued by the Sirleaf regime. Accordingly, the Sirleaf regime has taken various steps to create propitious conditions for multinational corporations and other foreign-based businesses to invest in the Liberian economy. For example, Sime Darby, a Malaysia-based multinational corporation, was given a 63-year lease for 220,000 acres of land to produce palm oil (Ford 2012). Similarly, Golden Veloreum, an American and Indonesian palm oil corporation, was given a 65-year lease for 865,000 acres of land (Baron 2012). In some cases, the Sirleaf regime forced farmers from their land (Ford 2012). Consequently, there have been protests by farmers and others, whose lands were taken and given to the owners of foreign capital. Overall, during its first term of office (2006–2012), the Sirleaf regime mortgaged about 33 percent of Liberia's total land mass to foreign-based multinational corporations and other businesses for so-called investment projects primarily in the agricultural, logging, oil, and mining sectors (Siakor and Knight 2012). One of the major resulting consequences of mortgaging the country's land is the growing and dangerous problem of food insecurity. Characteristically, President Sirleaf has responded to the critics of her land-mortgaging scheme by asserting, "When your government and the representatives sign any paper with a foreign country, the communities can't change it … You are trying to undermine your own government. You can't do that" (Johnson Sirleaf 2011).

Another major step taken by the Sirleaf regime is the allocation of oil wells to foreign-based corporations, especially from the "Global North," including the US-based Chevron-US (Global Witness 2011). As usual, the oil well allocation process has been fraught with characteristic corruption. At the core is the receipt of bribes by various Liberian government officials, including legislators, as the *quid pro quo* for privileging certain corporations (Global Witness 2011). The regime has created an enabling environment for foreign-based corporations to exploit the country's vast forest resources (Global Witness 2011). For example, corporations such as Forest Ventures, Nature Oriented and Timber, Atlantic Resources, and Southeastern Resources are plundering and pillaging vast expanses of forests throughout the country. In turn, the exploitation of the country's vast forest resources is contributing to various ecological problems, including deforestation.

By 2011, the total foreign direct investment in Liberia stood at about $19 billion (United States Department of State 2011). However, this has not contributed to improvement in the material conditions of ordinary Liberians. In 2014, the unemployment rate stood at an astronomical 85 percent (Bertelsmann Stiftung 2014, 15). Similarly, 84 percent of the population lived on less than US$1.25 per day (Bertelsmann Stiftung 2014, 15). Furthermore, 14 percent of the population was severely food insecure (Food and Agricultural Organization 2014, 1). To make matters worse, the

Sirleaf regime has not made human needs top priorities. This is clearly reflected in the allocation of public resources. For example, in the country's 2014–2015 national budget, only a paltry 10.6 percent and 16.5 percent respectively were allotted for education and health care respectively (Ministry of Finance and Development Planning 2014). Consequently, the overall state of human development during the Sirleaf regime has been poor. While the country's Human Development Index (HDI) has increased from 0.350 in 2006 to 0.412 in 2013 (United Nations Development Programme 2014) Liberia has consistently retained its low ranking of 175 out of a total of 187 countries, and remained in the lowest tier of the HDI (United Nations Development Programme 2014).

The crisis of legitimacy The overall poor performance of the Sirleaf regime in the areas of governance and development has led to the erosion of the public's trust in the government (Liberia Data Project 2015). Consequently, the regime is engulfed in a crisis of legitimacy. Specifically, in spite of the appreciable progress that has been made in the area of political democratization, the Sirleaf regime has failed to cage the authoritarian demon, strengthen public institutions by, among other things, ending the excesses of the "hegemonic presidency," develop the requisite modalities for addressing national emergencies, including health crises, and improve the material conditions and well-being of ordinary Liberians. To make matters worse, corruption is spinning out of control, aided by an entrenched culture of impunity. In short, the dialectical tension between the advancement of the material well-being of the members of the ruling class and their relations, and the neglect of the human needs of the subalterns has reached a crisis point. A major manifestation is the continual deterioration in the standard of living of ordinary Liberians.

Essentially, the crisis of legitimacy has found expression in two major areas. A key one is that the vast majority of Liberians do not trust the Sirleaf regime (Liberia Data Project 2015). In fact, the regime is derisively viewed as a marauding band that uses the state as an instrument for the predatory accumulation of wealth through the engagement in various corrupt acts (Liberia Data Project 2015). Concomitantly, there is the overwhelming belief that the regime does not have any interest in the welfare of ordinary Liberians. In fact, the talk shows on the various radio stations, especially in the capital city region, are inundated on a daily basis by the recurrent expression of the mass belief that the Sirleaf regime is woefully negligent (Liberia Data Project 2015). The other major area is the emerging perception from below that the Sirleaf regime is an irritant that needs to be avoided at all cost, challenged, and even cheated (Liberia Data Project 2015).

How the peripheral capitalist state made Ebola a possibility

The Ebola virus first hit Liberia in March 2014. Initially, both the number of people that were infected with the virus and the geographic expanse were small. However, the disengaged attitude of the Sirleaf regime, and its resulting failure to take quick action to contain the spread of the virus, ultimately led to its spread. According to the World Health Organization (2015, 1), "Liberia's first two cases of Ebola, in the Foya District of Lofa County near the border with Guinea, were confirmed on March 30, 2014."

Clearly, the lack of a response by the Sirleaf regime coupled with the poor state of the country's health care infrastructure and the related critical issue of poor sanitation provided an enabling environment for the spread of the virus. So, by June 2014, the virus had engulfed various regions of the country. Consequently, a state of fear gripped the country, as the virus infected hundreds of people, and the overwhelming majority of them died. So, how did the country's peripheral capitalist state make the spread of the Ebola virus possible? First, the Janus-faced complexion of the peripheral capitalist state in Liberia has led to the situation in which the construct creates propitious conditions for the members of the ruling class and their relations to have all of the comforts of life, such as health care, on the one hand. But, on the other hand, the same state visits mass deprivation and malaise on the subaltern classes that constitute the majority of the society. The Liberian state has failed to invest in the health care infrastructure that is indispensable to containing the spread of diseases such as EVD. For example, at the onset of the EVD epidemic, the country had only 10,052 health care workers – doctors, nurses, physician assistants, among others (Ministry of Health, Liberia 2015, 24). Also, there were a total of 656 health care facilities in the country. Of this number, 404 were public, and the remaining 252 private (Ministry of Health 2015). Among the health care facilities were a total of 36 hospitals in the entire country (17 public and 19 private) (Ministry of Health 2015). There were also 48 health care centers and two referral hospitals (Ministry of Health 2015). Further, in a classical demonstration of the internal core–periphery chasm, 240 of the 656 health care facilities were located in Monrovia, the capital city and its environs (Ministry of Health 2015).

To make matters worse, 26 percent of the public health care facilities were not structurally sound; about 45 percent lacked primary power sources for electricity; about 13 percent lacked access to safe drinking water; and about 43 percent lacked functioning incinerators to dispose of waste (Ministry of Health 2015, 8). Furthermore, about 29 percent of the population lacked access to health care facilities that were within an hour's walking distance of their homes (Ministry of Health 2015, 8).

The failure of the peripheral capitalist Liberian state to invest in health care was vividly demonstrated by donor dependence. For example, due to the negligence of the peripheral capitalist state, metropolitan-based non-governmental organizations (NGOs) provided more than 90 percent of health care delivery service in the country (Ministry of Health 2015, 8). More broadly, the peripheral capitalist Liberian state relies preponderantly on the United States, the European Union, and other states to annually fund its health care system (Ministry of Health 2015).

Similarly, the peripheral capitalist Liberian state failed to invest in the physical infrastructure, thereby making it difficult to contain the spread of the Ebola virus. For example, only about 25 percent of the population had access to clean drinking water (Front Page Africa 2016, 1). This meant that about 75 percent of the population relied on unsafe sources of water such as polluted streams. This made them vulnerable to the Ebola virus. Similarly, only about 10 percent and 20 percent of the population respectively had access to acceptable sanitation and decent toilet facilities (WaterAid 2016, 1). This increased their vulnerability to the Ebola virus.

The failure of the peripheral capitalist Liberian state to invest in agriculture in order to ensure food production contributed to food insecurity, and the resulting adverse effects on the health of Liberians. This helped to make them vulnerable to the Ebola virus. For example, about 33 percent of the population was classified as undernourished (International Food Policy Research Institute 2015).

In terms of food insecurity, about 16 percent of the population was food insecure (World Food Programme 2016). In addition, about 18 percent of households relied on begging as the major means for providing for their food needs (World Food Programme 2016).

The primacy of predatory and primitive accumulation of wealth has led to the diversion of capital away from health care and other critical national development areas to the enrichment of the foreign owners of capital and the local compradors who serve as their handmaids. In the case of predatory accumulation, the various factions of the compradors or the local wing of the Liberian ruling class that have managed the state have focused on creating an enabling environment in which multinational corporations like Firestone can reap huge profits at the expense of human needs such as health care, and the development of the physical infrastructure such as roads. Similarly, the faction of the local ruling class that runs the state at a particular historical juncture uses state power as an instrument for the primitive accumulation of capital through various non-productive means such as extortion, embezzlement, and procurement fraud. Thus, the financial resources that are required for making investment in health care and the physical infrastructure, so that they can position the country to deal effectively with epidemics such as the Ebola virus, are diverted to self-enrichment.

Another major issue is that the peripheral capitalist state in Liberia has created a culture of insensitivity among the members of the local wing of the ruling class. That is, the members of the local wing of the Liberian ruling class have a contemptuous attitude toward the subalterns. Based on this mindset, which is anchored on pathological hubris, the compradors view the subalterns as marginal and unimportant. Hence, the thrust of policy making and implementation is not the making of public investments in health care and the other basic human needs of the members of the subaltern classes. Instead, the emphasis is on using the agency of the various state positions to make themselves rich. Interestingly, the compradors measure their ill-gotten wealth by the scope and destitution of the subalterns. So, building hospitals and other health facilities, and the training of health care professionals, as well as the development of the physical infrastructure are not priorities for the state.

The related point is that the insensitivity among the ruling class toward the members of the subaltern class has also found expression in the former's lack of vision in terms of planning for national emergencies such as epidemics. Therefore, it was no surprise that when the Ebola epidemic broke-out, the state did not have in place the protocols for dealing with it precisely because there were no policies in place for dealing with such an emergency/epidemic. Similarly, there were no institutional mechanisms in place for dealing with an epidemic. Hence, the government had to scramble to formulate and implement protocols for addressing the Ebola epidemic in an ad hoc and very disorganized manner. Importantly, the lack of protocols to address the epidemic led the Liberian government to abdicate its responsibility for caring for the well-being of its citizens, and to subsequently rely on the United States, other countries, and non-governmental organizations to contain and address the epidemic.

The Sirleaf regime's response to the EVD epidemic The Sirleaf regime responded to the epidemic in two major ways: apathy and indifference, and "doing too little too late." As has been discussed, the first response was characterized by indifference and disengagement. In fact, President Sirleaf dismissively indicated that she had a pending trip to Equatorial Guinea; and that she would make the trip, in spite of the epidemic (Liberian Association of Metropolitan Atlanta 2014). In addition, she asserted that those who had the responsibility for health matters would address the epidemic (Liberian Association of Metropolitan Atlanta 2014). The attitude demonstrated by President Sirleaf raises the important issue whether the health and well-being of the people are not the top priorities of the President of Liberia (Kieh 2015). Basically, the nonchalant attitude of the Sirleaf regime, and its lack of protocols and institutional mechanisms to address health epidemics made the containment of the virus difficult.

The second response of the Sirleaf regime was framed by the avalanche of domestic and international criticisms and pressure to act. But, handicapped by the lack of institutional modalities to address health epidemics, the Sirleaf regime became rudderless, as evidenced by its inability to develop effective strategies for addressing the growing epidemic. However, by the time the Sirleaf regime was able to take some steps to address the epidemic, including the declaration of a "state of emergency" for 90 days, and the closure of all government offices and schools, the virus had virtually engulfed the entire country. In short, the Sirleaf regime's actions were tantamount to "too little too late." Frank (2014, 1) provides a poignant summation of the Sirleaf regime's handling of the Ebola epidemic:

> Liberians are experiencing the worst public health safety crisis in living memory. And possibly, since the country declared independence in 1847. After almost eight years in office, Ebola has rudely unmasked the Johnson Sirleaf administration's failure to build working institutions to cope with extraordinary circumstances and national disasters, as well as provide overall good governance and stability for Liberia.

Amid the poor handling of the Ebola crisis by the Sirleaf regime, various actors in the international system, including the United States and China, had to intervene to help address the epidemic. For example, the United States sent a contingent of military personnel to the country to help battle the deadly epidemic. However, the combination of poor governance, a poor physical infrastructure, inadequate health services, the lack of clean drinking water, and the poor sanitary conditions, major dimensions of the country's crises of underdevelopment, impeded the international relief efforts. Furthermore, the crisis of legitimacy adversely affected the efforts to address the epidemic. That is, based on their distrust of the Sirleaf regime, the overwhelming majority of Liberians did not believe the regime's public awareness efforts about the virus (Blair et al. 2016). Instead, it was widely believed that the Sirleaf regime had concocted the claim about the Ebola virus as part of its characteristic efforts to swindle the international community of money.

Conclusion

Clearly, the Ebola virus exposed the underbelly of the multidimensional crises of underdevelopment that have been generated by the peripheral capitalist Liberian state for almost nine decades. Essentially, the crises of underdevelopment provided propitious conditions for the Ebola virus to spread. For example, the lack of clean drinking water and the horrendous sanitary conditions provided fertile grounds for the entry and subsequent spread of the virus. In addition, the poor physical infrastructure militated against efforts to contain the virus. Accordingly, although the continuing health-related efforts to contain and prevent the re-occurrence of the epidemic are important, they need to be transcended. The broader focus needs to be on the structural transformation of Liberia covering all spheres, including economic, political, and social. The success of the transformation would position the country well to be able to address emergencies and crises, including health-related ones, in the future.

However, since the World Health Organization (WHO) declared Liberia Ebola free in September 2015, the Sirleaf regime has yet to begin the much-needed process of democratically reconstituting the peripheral capitalist Liberian state, including its portrait. Unless this is done, Liberia will not be able to deal with any national emergency – health or otherwise. Essentially, the democratic reconstitution of the Liberian state would require several major steps. First, the current peripheral capitalist state and its hybrid governance architecture need to be deconstructed. Second, the state needs to be rethought. Third, a new state construct, preferably a social democratic developmental one with "social citizenship" at its core" (Marshall 1950, 149), needs to be designed.

The major derivative will be the development of a new portrait for the emergent social democratic developmental state. In terms of its nature, the state would need to represent the historical and cultural experiences of all of the major ethnic stocks that constitute Liberia. The primary mission of the state would be to promote the cultural, economic, political, religious, security and social rights of all Liberians, including the advancement of material well-being and the restructuring of power relations, so that the people can have what Ake (2001, 130) aptly calls "real decision-making power." In addition, public policies would be designed primarily to promote human-centered democracy and development, including the protection of the political rights and civil liberties, and massive state investments in health care, education, public housing, clean drinking water, sanitation, food security, and the physical infrastructure. As well, public institutions would be strengthened, and the modalities would be developed for addressing emergencies and crises, including epidemics.

However, if Liberia maintains its peripheral capitalist state, its hybrid governance system, and neoliberal development strategy, it will not be able to address the underlying multidimensional crises of underdevelopment that provided the crucible in which the Ebola virus thrived. Thus, the country will remain vulnerable to other epidemics.

References

Agbese, Pita Ogaba (2007). "The Political Economy of the African State," in George Klay Kieh, Jr. (ed.) *Beyond State Failure and Collapse: Making the State Relevant in Africa*. Lanham, MD: Lexington Books, 33–48.

Ake, Claude (2001). *Democracy and Development in Africa*. Washington, DC: The Brookings Institution Press.

Amin, Samir (1974). *Accumulation on a World Scale: A Critique of the Theory of Underdevelopment*. New York: Monthly Review Press.

Ballah, Henrietta (2003). *Ethnicity, Politics and Social Conflict: The Quest for Peace in Liberia*. University Park, PA: McNair Program of Penn State University.

Baron, Ethan (2012). "Palm Oil Industry Accused of Land Grabs in Liberia," *Global Post Rights*, December 27, 1–2.

Bertselsmenn Stiftung (2014). *Liberia Country Report*. Gutersloh: Bertelsmann Stiftung.

Beyan, Amos (1991). *The American Colonization Society and the Creation of the Liberian State*. Lanham, MD: University Press of America.

Blair, Robert, Morse, Ben, and Tsai, Lily (2016). "Public Health and Public Trust: Evidence from the Ebola Virus Disease Epidemic in Liberia." www.ssrn.com/abstract=2864029 (accessed February 5, 2017).

Borteh, George (2008). "Julu, Dorbor Retrial Begins Today," *Analyst*, February 14, 1.

Boweh, Bruce (2008). "No Municipal Elections: Supreme Court Recognizes President Sirleaf's Appointment of Mayors," *Star Radio*, January.

Brown, George (1941). *The Economic History of Liberia*. Washington, DC: Associated Publishers.

Clarke, Robert and Wenyu, Moses (2010). "President Sirleaf Wants Ministers to Create Employment for UP Partisans," *Star Radio*, February 8.

Committee for the Protection of Journalists (2011). "Liberian Government Silences Three Broadcasters," *Alerts/Liberia*, November 8, 1.

Constitution of Liberia (1986). Monrovia.

Cordor, S. Henry (1979). *The April 14 Crisis in Liberia*. Occasional Paper. Monrovia.

Curson, Peter (2015). "The Ebola Crisis and the Failure of Governance," *Geodate*, 28, 3: 2–4.

Dempsey, Thomas (2014). "Ebola, Security and Governance in West Africa: Why a Limited Problem Needs a Global Response," *Georgetown Journal of International Affairs*, August 11, 1–3.

Emmanuel, Arghiri (1972). *Unequal Exchange: A Study of the Imperialism of Trade*. New York: Monthly Review Press.

Fatton, Robert (1988). "Bringing the Ruling Class Back In: Class, State and Hegemony in Africa," *Comparative Politics*, 20, 3: 253–264.

Food and Agricultural Organization (2014). "FAO/WFP Crop and Food Security Assessment Liberia," *FAO in Emergencies*, December 17.

Ford, Tamasian (2012). "Liberia Land Deal with Foreign Firms 'Could Sow

Seeds of Conflict'," *The Guardian*, February 29.

Frank, Andre Gunder (1969). *Capitalism and Underdevelopment in Latin America*. New York: Penguin Books.

Frank, Andre Gunder (1978). *Dependent Accumulation and Underdevelopment*. London: Macmillan.

Frank, Cecil (2014). "Understanding Governance in Liberia through Ebola," *Front Page Africa*, October 6, 1–2.

Freedom House (2012). "Liberia." *Freedom of the Press*. Washington, DC: Freedom House.

Freedom House (2015). "Liberia." *Freedom of the Press*. https://freedomhouse.org/report/freedom-press/2015/liberia.

Freedom House (2017). *Freedom in the World: World Historical and Comparative Data, 1972–2016*. Washington, DC: Freedom House.

Front Page Africa (2016). "25 Percent of Liberia's Population Access Clean Drinking Water," April, 1.

Glasberg, David and Shannon, Deric (2011). *Political Sociology: Oppression, Resistance and the State*. Thousand Oaks, CA: Sage.

Global Witness (2011). *Curse or Cure? How Oil Can Boost or Break Liberia's Post-War Recovery*. London: Global Witness.

Government of Liberia (2007). "BWI Board, Inter-Ministerial Forestry Concessions Committee Constituted," Press Release, December 20, 1.

Graff, William (1994). "The State in the Third World," Paper Presented at the Conference of the British International Studies Association, York, December.

Hartman, Sophie (2014). "Ebola and the Politics of a Global Health Crisis," *E-International Relations*, 1: 1–2.

Hess, Alexander and Sauter, Michael (2013). "The Most Corrupt Countries in the World," *USA Today*, July 14. www.usatoday.com (accessed October 4, 2015).

International Food Policy Research Institute (2015). *Global Hunger Index 2015. Liberia: Health System Assessment*. Monrovia: Ministry of Health.

Johnson Sirleaf, Ellen (2006). *First Inaugural Address*. Monrovia: Government Printing Office.

Johnson Sirleaf, Ellen (2011). *Remarks Delivered to Rural Community Members Affected by the Operations of Sime Darby, a Multinational Oil Producer*, December 6.

Johnson Sirleaf, Ellen (2012). *Second Inaugural Address*. Monrovia: Government Printing Office.

Kappel, Robert, Korte, Werner, and Maschler, R. Friedegund (1986). *Liberia: Underdevelopment and Political Rule in a Peripheral Society*. Bremen: Institute of African Studies.

Kennedy, Joey (2006). "President Sirleaf Writes Senate, Wants to Appoint City Mayors," *Star Radio*, September 12.

Kieh, George Klay (1997). "The Crisis of Democracy in Liberia," *Liberian Studies Journal*, 22, 1: 23–29.

Kieh, George Klay (2008). *The First Liberian Civil War: The Crises of Underdevelopment*. New York: Peter Lang.

Kieh, George Klay (2012a) *Liberia's State Failure, Collapse and Reconstitution*. Cherry Hill, NJ: Africana Homestead Legacy Publishers.

Kieh, George Klay (2012b). "The Hegemonic Presidency and Post-Conflict Peacebuilding in Liberia," *Africa Peace and Conflict Journal*, 5, 2: 14–26.

Kieh, George Klay (2015). "Political Developments in Liberia," in

Ndongo Sylla (ed.) *Recent Political Developments in West Africa*. Dakar: Rosa Luxemburg Foundation, 75–99.

Liberia Data Project (2015). Multi-Sectoral Data on Liberia. Douglasville, GA.

Liberian Association of Metropolitan Atlanta (2014). "Statement on the Ebola Crisis and the Governance and Human Development Deficits in Liberia," Lilburn, GA, August 24.

Liebenow, J. Gus (1969). *Liberia: The Evolution of Privilege*. Ithaca, NY: Cornell University Press.

Liebenow, J. Gus (1987). *The Quest for Democracy in Liberia*. Bloomington, IN: Indiana University Press.

Marshall, T.H. (1950). *Citizenship and Social Class and Other Essays*. Cambridge: Cambridge University Press.

Mason, Dew Tuan-Wleh and Sawyer, Amos (1979). "Labor in Liberia," *Review of African Political Economy*, 6, 14: 3–15.

Miliband, Ralph (1973). "Poulantzas and the Capitalist State," *New Left Review*, 82, 1: 83–93.

Ministry of Finance and Development Planning, Liberia (2014). *National Budget of Liberia, 2014/2015*. Monrovia: Ministry of Finance and Development Planning.

Ministry of Health, Liberia (2015). *Liberia: Health System Assessment*. Monrovia: Ministry of Health.

Ministry of Planning and Economic Affairs, Liberia (1989). *Economic Survey of Liberia*. Monrovia: Government Printing Office.

National Election Commission of Liberia (2014). *The Results of the Senatorial Elections*. Monrovia: NEC.

Nsoedo, Ezeakukwu (2014). "The Ebola Crisis in the West African Region: Should It Have Been So Severe?" *Open Journal of Social Sciences*, 2, 1: 98–104.

Nzongola-Ntalaja, Georges (1992). *The African Crisis: The Way Out. Seminar Paper No. 1*. Harare: SAPES.

Obilade, Titilola (2015). "The Political Economy of Ebola Virus Disease in West African Countries," *International Archives of Medicine*, 8, 40: 1–10.

Peters, May Mercado and Shapouri, Shahla (1997). "Income Inequality and Food Security," *Economic Research Service*, 9: 44–47.

Prado, Caio (1966). *The Political Evolution of Brazil*. Sao Paulo: Editora Brasiliense.

Press Office, Executive Mansion, Liberia (2008). "President Sirleaf Removes U.L. President Dr. Conteh," Press Release, April 14, 1.

Ryan, Jordan (2014). "Can a Post-Crisis Country Survive in the Time of Ebola? Issues Arising with Liberia's Post-War Recovery," *Harvard International Review*, 36, 2: 25.

Saad-Fiho, Alfredo (2008). "Marxian and Keynesian Critique of Neo-Liberalism," *Socialist Register*. 44, 10: 337–345.

Sanders, David, Sengupta, Amit, and Scott, Vera (2015). "Ebola Epidemic Exposes the Pathology of the Global Economic and Political Systems," *International Journal of Health Services*, 45, 4: 643–656.

Sawyer, Amos (1992). *The Emergence of Autocracy in Liberia: Tragedy and Challenge*. San Francisco, CA: Institute for Intercultural Studies.

Siakor, Silas and Knight, Rachel (2012). "A Nobel Laureate's Problem at Home," *The New York Times*, January 12. www.nytimes.com (accessed September 25, 2012).

Sieh, Rodney D. (2009). "Ellen Writes Hilary: No Lack of Political Will on Corruption," *Front Page Africa*, July 7, 1.

Smith, Robert (1972). *The American Policy in Liberia, 1822–1971*. Monrovia: Providence Publications.

Sungbeh, Tewroh Wehtoe (2013). "RIA Saga Reinforces Sirleaf Administration's Image as Corrupt," *Liberian Dialogue*, March 17, 1.

Transparency International (2013). *Corruption Perception Index*. Berlin: TI.

United Nations Development Programme (2006). *Liberia National Development Report*. New York: Oxford University Press.

United Nations Development Programme (2010). *Liberia National Development Report*. New York: Oxford University Press.

United Nations Development Programme (2014). *Human Development Report*, 1990–2013. New York: Oxford University Press.

United States (US) Department of State (2009). *Human Rights Report: Liberia*. Washington, DC: US State Department.

United States (US) Department of State (2011). "2011 Investment Climate Statement – Liberia," March. www.state.gov/e/eb/rls/othr/ics/2011/157311.htm (accessed September 30, 2015).

Van de Pas, Remco and van Belle, Sara (2015). "Ebola the Epidemic That Should Never Have Happened," *Global Affairs*, 1, 1: 95–100.

WaterAid (2016). Liberia. www.wateraid.org/us/where-we-work/page/liberia.

Watkins, Samuel R. (2007). *Liberia Communication*. London: Authorhouse.

World Food Programme (2016). *Liberia*. www.wfp.org/countries/liberia (accessed September 24, 2016).

World Health Organization (2015). "Liberia: A County – and Its Capital – Are Overwhelmed with Ebola Cases," January, 1.

Wreh, Tuan (1976). *The Love of Liberty Brought Us Here: The Rule of Williams V.S. Tubman in Liberia, 1944–1971*. London: C. Hurst.

Yidana, Richard (2009). "Discussion Notes on the State and the Political Economy of Africa." Grand Rapids, MI.

Zaza, Yanquoi (2009). "Liberian President's Corruption Tree," *Liberian Forum*, November 22, 1–2.

Ziemann, W. and Lanzendorfer, M. (1977). "The State in Peripheral Societies," *Socialist Register*, 14, 3: 145–177.

5 | CONFRONTING EBOLA WITH BARE HANDS: SIERRA LEONE'S HEALTH SECTOR ON THE EVE OF THE EBOLA EPIDEMIC

Ibrahim Abdullah and Abou Bakarr Kamara

Introduction

Three countries in the Mano River Union (Guinea, Liberia, and Sierra Leone) were recently hit by the worst health crisis in the recorded history of the sub-region. The first case of Ebola Viral Disease (EVD) in the Mano River Union (MRU) basin was reported in the Gecko prefecture, Guinea and supposedly began with the illness of a two-year-old child, who died at the end of December 2013 (Ryan Fall 2014\Winter 2015). From Guinea, EVD allegedly spread over into Sierra Leone in May 2014 and quickly enveloped the three chiefdoms along the eastern border district of Kailahun. The porous nature of the border as well as the common ethnic and cultural identities shared by the people on both sides of the national boundaries partly facilitated the spread of the disease.[1] What initially appeared as an isolated and localized case of viral infection quickly spread and engulfed the three nations resulting in total of 28,599 cases of infections and a death toll of 11,299 or about 40 percent case fatality rate (CFR).[2] By November 7, 2015, when the World Health Organization (WHO) declared the end of EVD transmission in Sierra Leone, the country's Ministry of Health and Sanitation (MoHS) had recorded 8,704 confirmed cases, 3,589 deaths, 4,051 treated, survived, and discharged from the disease.[3] The World Health Organization (WHO) provides much higher figures for the same period, recording 14,122 cases of infection (about 50 percent of the total cases for the three countries) and 3,955 deaths for a CFR of around 28 percent.[4] The discrepancy between WHO and Government of Sierra Leone figures is due to the fact WHO factored in their calculations all confirmed, probable, and suspected cases while the government of Sierra Leone only recorded confirmed cases.

Prior to the outbreak, the Sierra Leone economy was supposedly on an upward swing – and lauded in official circles as the fastest growing economy in the world. This dubious claim based on the short-lived iron ore boom, translated into double-digit real GDP growth in two consecutive years, 15.2 percent in 2012 and 20.1 percent in 2013 (Ministry of Finance and Economic Development 2014). Sierra Leone recorded significant improvement in macroeconomic stability with marked reduction in its external current account and fiscal deficits. This stability was evident in single-digit inflation, declining interest, and relatively stable exchange rates. Despite these positive indicators, Sierra Leone was ranked 183 in the 2013 United Nations Development Programme (UNDP) Human Development Index (HDI) with a score of 0.374, far less than the regional average of sub-Saharan African (SSA) countries of 0.502. With very high infant and under-five mortality rates, high maternal mortality rates and morbidity rates, and low life expectancy averaging 49 years, Sierra Leone is regarded as one of the worst countries in the world to live.[5] In an effort to improve these horrendous health statistics, the Sierra Leone government introduced several health programs with funding from internal and external sources. These included free HIV/AIDS/TB/malaria diagnosis and treatment, and the Free Health Care Initiative in April, 2010.[6] Even though some improvements have been recorded, these programs remain fragmented and without clear government ownership, focus, and leadership. This has hindered their overall quality and sustainability.

The EVD outbreak in the MRU region was unprecedented in its geographical scale, epidemiological complexity, morbidity, and efforts to control it. It is the first occurrence of the disease that was transnational as well transcontinental. Infected people from the region surfaced in seven other countries: Italy, Mali, Senegal, Nigeria, Spain, United Kingdom, and the United States. Unlike previous outbreaks, EVD in the three MRU countries quickly spread from its rural abode to urban areas where those infected with the virus thronged to seek medical attention. The outbreak generated widespread fear and panic, and by late 2014 it had overwhelmed the fragile health systems of Guinea, Liberia, and Sierra Leone, effectively ensuring the diversion of focus on other diseases and national health care needs. By the time EVD was contained in late 2015, about 28,601 people had been infected.[7] The emergency measures adopted by the governments of

Guinea, Liberia, and Sierra Leone between mid-2014 and early 2015 to control the disease also created hardships for citizens and residents: schools and colleges were closed in Liberia and Sierra Leone, places of leisure and entertainment shuttered, communities quarantined, and population movement severely restricted. Paid employment in many government and private institutions and commercial activities almost ground to a halt. Contact with the external world was put on hold with few foreign airlines willing to fly to Liberia and Sierra Leone, and many ships avoided berthing at their ports.[8] The suspension of airline and shipping operations, which effectively isolated the three countries from the rest of the world, mirrored the quarantine of Ebola patients as a strategy to contain the disease.

The extant literature, which the EVD has spawned, or more appropriately, the Ebola library – from academic think pieces to blogs to newspaper articles and policy briefs – remains heavily loaded with analysis and descriptions of the economic dimension of the disease. Relatively very little has been done – mapping out and analyzing the medical and health infrastructure of the three most affected MRU countries on the eve of Ebola. Comprehending the rudimentary nature of broken medical and health infrastructure is central to understanding how and why EVD could claim so many lives in so short a time. This chapter attempts to offer insights on this crucial question by providing an overview of the Sierra Leone medical and health infrastructure on the eve of the EVD outbreak. It focuses especially on the serious challenges being experienced with the human resource capacity, financing, and adequate maintenance of the logistics, health care information, and disease surveillance systems of this infrastructure around 2013 and 2014.

The chapter is divided into four sections: the first section presents the human resource capacity with a detailed analysis on the quality, quantity, and distribution of the workforce. The second section discusses financing wellness with emphasis on the quantum of funds allocated to the health sector and reliance on out-of-pocket/private expenditure to finance health service delivery. The infrastructure, logistics, health information, and surveillance system are discussed in the third section; while the Kenema Government Hospital, the treatment center that dealt with the first cases of EVD, is presented as a case study highlighting the ills confronting the health sector on the eve of the outbreak.

Human resources: quality, quantity, and distribution

The quality of any health service largely depends on staff size, capacity, and availability as well as an enabling environment with the appropriate infrastructure, equipment, and logistics to function as a health service unit. In Sierra Leone, there is a dearth of skilled personnel to adequately provide services especially at public facilities. With a population of 7,075,641 people, the country had less than 200 medical doctors (specialists and medical officers combined), 6,147 nurses[9] (with Maternal and Child Health Aides (MCHA) and Nursing Aides accounting for about 45 percent of the nursing population) prior to the EVD outbreak.

A little over a decade ago WHO estimated that a critical threshold of 23 skilled health providers, including doctors, nurses, and midwives, per 10,000 persons is needed for the provision of minimal levels of basic health care for pregnant women and children (Chen, Evans, et al. 2004). Currently the Sierra Leone health system has only two skilled providers per 10,000 population, making delivery of basic services extremely challenging. The country is ranked fourth from the bottom on a list of 49 priority low-and-middle-income countries for health worker-to-population ratio. The ratio of physician per 10,000 population is 0.2 compared to one for neighboring Guinea and 2.6 for the rest of Africa.[10] It is also worth mentioning that more than 70 percent of the Sierra Leone medical doctors are medical officers or general clinicians. Before the EVD outbreak Sierra Leone could only boast of 16 specialists: three obstetricians and gynecologists; one pediatrician; three internal medicine; one family medicine; three surgeons; one radiologist; one ophthalmologist; two dental surgeons; and one anesthetist. In all, there were about 145 medical officers as full time staff on the government pay roll.[11]

The Sierra Leone health care system is facing a serious problem with the maintenance and expansion of its cohort of highly trained doctors. Over 65 percent of the country's specialists are above 50 years of age – getting closer to retirement with no mechanism for recruitment to replace retired staff. The deployment of medical personnel, especially medical doctors, is largely skewed towards urban areas or affluent districts of Sierra Leone. As Table 5.1 shows, Freetown, the capital city and the economic nerve center of the country, has almost 70 percent of medical doctors and about 90 percent of all specialists. This lopsided concentration in medical

TABLE 5.1 Gap analysis and distribution of specialist doctors in Sierra Leone

Area of Specialization	Number in Post	Required Number	Present Location
Obs/Gynecologists	3	54	Freetown
Pediatrician	1	54	Freetown
Internal medicine Family medicine	3 1	54 32	Freetown Freetown
Surgeons	3	54	Freetown, Kenema, and Makeni
Radiologists	1	25	Freetown
Ophthalmologists	1	17	Freetown
Dental surgeon	2	17	Freetown
Anesthetist Pathologist	1 0	25 5	Freetown

Source: Ministry of Health and Sanitation Report on Human Resource Status (2014)

personnel in the capital city begins to explain why people with serious and debilitating diseases often go to Freetown to seek medical attention. The situation is so dire that, as at the time of writing this chapter, there were no government employed specialist doctors in any of the government-owned hospitals outside the Western Area, Bo, and Kenema districts.

The chronic lack of qualified medical personnel and their overwhelming deployment in the Freetown area is worsened by their concentration in lucrative donor-funded projects as administrators. These personnel, mostly medical doctors and senior nurses, are bunched in public health projects where their expertise is really not needed – mainly performing administrative tasks that could be competently handled by non-health specialists. There are about 50 trained medical doctors and a similar number of senior nurses involved in such projects, depriving the nation of their life-saving skills and services in the name of making money. To make matters worse, the available evidence seems to suggest that it is the best performing doctors and nurses that are withdrawn from medical practice and deployed as administrators to work in these donor-funded projects at the national level. There is also evidence of a high attrition rate – primarily qualified practitioners voting with their feet for greener pastures.[12]

To compound the situation, the existing educational infrastructure cannot produce the medical and health human resource capacity to meet the needs of the country. The College of Medicine and Allied Health Sciences (COMAHS), the principal training institution for medical sciences in the country, does not have the resources, staffing, or infrastructure to train sufficient numbers of qualified medical personnel. Education at the college is largely at the undergraduate level as the school lacks the required expertise and resources to administer graduate programs or train specialists. A revised Education Act, allowing the Ministry of Education to supervise educational institutions offering training in the field of medicine, has not produced the desired result. A Polytechnic Act (2002) allowed the academic boards of the accredited polytechnic institutions to design and implement nursing and other similar health care training programs using certain minimum standards. But this rather laissez faire approach to the training of nurses and other health care professionals has opened a Pandora's box: there has been a proliferation of nursing programs, especially for State Enrolled Community Health Nurses (SECHN), offered by unsupervised private institutions which mushroomed in the wake of the 2002 Act. The result is the mass production of nurses, whose training and understanding of the profession barely meets the minimum standards agreed in the Act. Furthermore, a large number of these nurses trained by different institutions cannot be immediately absorbed into government service for several reasons, including financial constraints. Those that are eventually absorbed into government or private practice receive very little continuous education in the form of in-service training.

There is a serious geographical imbalance, mirroring the case of medical doctors, in the distribution of nurses and similar health care workers across Sierra Leone. Over 70 percent of the trained nurses, particularly SRN, SECHN, and midwives, are concentrated in urban areas, leaving the less qualified Community Health Assistants (CHAs), Maternal and Child Health Aides (MCHAs), Nursing Aides, and volunteers to staff rural and remote areas. There are a number of facilities, particularly Maternal and Child Health Post (MCHP), with only one staff on the government payroll. Attempts to address the dearth of qualified staff in the rural areas, especially at the primary care level, led to the formalization/harmonization of the services of community health workers, mostly volunteers. Consequently, a National Community Health Worker (CHW) Policy and Strategic Plan were unveiled in 2012. Partners have trained and supported about 15,000 CHWs to provide a range of services including integrated community case management (ICCM), growth monitoring and nutritional counseling, and the distribution of family planning commodities, primarily on a voluntary basis. However, this intervention is largely fragmented, uncoordinated, with varied duration, and inconsistent approaches on training and duties of the community health workers. There are also issues of rivalry between the CHWs and the MCHAs as they are yet to fully accept them as a complementary health work force.

The World Bank-funded decentralization project has also affected performance in the health sector. Primary and secondary health services were devolved to local councils to administer as part of their governance functions. But as was usually the case with most of the post-conflict legislations in Sierra Leone, they were hardly examined or debated at the local level where it really mattered. The result has been a grinding overlap with other legislations, which has made things difficult in the health sector to function the way they should. The 2004 Local Government Act, which ushered in the decentralization of power to local institutions, was amended in 2008.[13] Two others legislations, the Hospital Board Act (2007) and Health Service Commission Act (2011), were also promulgated to improve service delivery in the health sector. Inter-ministerial rivalry and power politics has meant that the Ministries of Health and Sanitation and that of Local Government became locked in mortal combat for control of institutions and resources emanating from these acts. Conflicting roles and overlapping responsibilities have hampered the smooth functioning of various institutions empowered by the different legislations. Thus while the delivery of primary and secondary health services has been devolved to local councils, the Ministry of Health and Sanitation still retains its primary function of policy formulation, supervision, monitoring, and evaluation. However, health officials at the district level remain loyal to national authorities at the center as recruitment, posting, and promotion remain the responsibility of the Health Service Commission and by extension ministry officials.

Financing wellness: how much money is available and who pays?

Adequate financing of health care delivery has been identified as a prerequisite for a resilient health delivery, including attaining and maintaining universal health coverage. Access to needed health services – prevention, promotion, treatment, and rehabilitation – should be available, without causing financial ruin for users because they have to pay excessively for them (WHO 2010). The centrality of finance in providing quality health care has been the subject of two World Health Assembly (WHA) Resolutions – WHA 58.33 and WHA 64.9. With respect to Sierra Leone, financing the health sector remains a major and daunting challenge. Funding, particularly from government to the health sector, is not only inadequate and untimely but also unreliable, thereby impeding planning and implementation. WHO has estimated that a country needs to spend a minimum of US$44 per year on health per person to enable the provision of basic life-saving services (WHO 2012). In Sierra Leone, government is spending less than US$10 per year on health per person (Ministry of Health and Sanitation 2013).

The major sources of funding for the health sector are budgetary appropriations from the government, external donors and NGO support, and private out-of-pocket expenditure.

TABLE 5.2 Total health expenditure, 2013

Financing Source	Amount (US$)	Percentage of Total Health Expenditure
Government of Sierra Leone	40,142,638.00	6.8
Donors	143,610,224.00	24.4
Non-Governmental Organizations	42,229,458.00	7.2
Out-of-Pocket (OOP)	362,660,015.00	61.6

Source: Ministry of Health and Sanitation – National Health Accounts (2013)

For 2013 the global average total health care expenditure was about 9.8 percent of average global GDP while it was 3.7 percent of GDP in Africa. Sierra Leone's expenditure of 2.1 percent was not only far below the global average but also 45 percent less than the African average. As shown in Table 5.2, the government's $40.1 million contribution, however, represented a mere 6.8 percent of overall total health expenditure or around 2 percent of the country's GDP that year. This overall government contribution was well within the African Region average of 3.7 percent.[14]

TABLE 5.3 Government allocation to the health sector as a percentage of GDP and total government expenditure

Year	Health Expenditure as a Percentage of GDP	Health Expenditure as a Percentage of Total Government Expenditure
2008	N/A	8.2
2009	2.9	10.4
2010	2.8	8.2
2011	2.8	8.4
2012	2.5	8.5
2013	2.1	11.2

Source: Ministry of Health and Sanitation – National Health Accounts (2013)

Despite being below WHO recommended levels, Sierra Leone government expenditure on the health sector had increased from 8.2 percent in 2008 to 11.2 percent in 2013.[15] While 2009 and 2013 witnessed small spikes of over 2 percent from the previous year, the average annual increase over a five-year period has been less than 1 percent. The very low growth rate in government health expenditures lagged significantly behind the country's projected population growth rate of about 3 percent.

Absolute figures on health expenditure can be misleading. The 11.6 percent of GDP or US$584 million (a US$96 per capita health expenditure) Sierra Leone expended on health care was relatively high compared to other Mano River Union (MRU) countries. In Guinea, it was 5 percent and in Liberia, 9 percent in 2013. However, as demonstrated in Table 5.2, 61.6 percent of the Sierra Leone amount came from private individuals (out-of-pocket) (Ministry of Health and Sanitation 2013). Out-of-pocket payments have been identified as a major barrier for the poor households trying to access medical goods and services. The percentage of out-of-pocket payments has dropped significantly from 2009, when it was 80 percent of total health expenditure, and Sierra Leone was rated as the second country in the world with the highest out-of-pocket health expenditure as a proportion to total health expenditure. Furthermore, government contribution to total health expenditure is the lowest amongst the MRU countries. Since 1995, the Sierra Leone government's expenditure on health per capita has hovered around US$10 to US$15. In Guinea, where the proportion of private out-of-pocket contribution (88 percent) is equally as high as Sierra Leone, the government per capita expenditure is $29 and in Liberia $42. Donor contribution as a percentage of Sierra Leone's total health expenditure remains high, even though it has more than halved from 27 percent in 2010 to 13 percent in 2012. The trend suggests possible donor fatigue or a degree of disengagement as the Sierra Leone government increases its contribution.

The high out-of-pocket expenditure shows that the government's flagship project, the Free Health Care Initiative, introduced in April 2010 is not having its envisaged impact. A major justification for this popular initiative, among others, was to remove financial barriers and minimize costs associated with accessing health care particularly for pregnant women, lactating mothers, and children under five. After almost six years of implementation, the data and public experience suggests the opposite (Maxen 2013; M'Cormack-Hale and M'Cormack McGough 2016). Costs and private payment for health services is increasing rather than decreasing. The free health care initiative, despite the fanfare that accompanied its launching, is really not free. This requires special attention and detailed analysis that may proffer alternate or complementing financing strategy.

Additionally, an analysis of the out-of-pocket expenditure suggests that 60 percent of that money goes to public facilities, of which 20 percent is allocated to peripheral health units (PHU). By its nature, out-of-pocket expenditure is primarily a means to incentivize health workers, and services at the PHUs are largely for the beneficiaries of the free health care initiative. Thus, payment for services at that level shows the inadequacy of the government's free health care initiative. Prior to the introduction of the free health care initiative, government increased health workers' salaries by more than 100 percent and introduced remote location allowance for staff in hard-to-reach areas as an incentive to get staff to underserved rural communities. It also instituted a performance-based financing (PBF) scheme to improve service delivery in key maternal and child health indicators. These measures were geared towards incentivizing staff to improve on the delivery of services and to prevent request for payment particularly from people within the free health care target population. A significant proportion of out-of-pocket expenditure purported to be spent on PHUs requires a rethink – appropriate measures could be adopted to save the government's flagship project.

A review of the report of the Audit Service for the past five years suggests leakages and financial impropriety within the health sector.[16] The recent Ebola Audit Report revealed the built-in malfeasance prevalent in the health ministry. The issues and challenges identified include, among others, procurement irregularities, mismanagement of fixed assets, payments without supporting or adequate documentation, and absence of regular bank reconciliation. This speaks to the capacity issues in managing financial resources allocated to the sector.

Broken health infrastructure, information system, and inadequate logistics: a perennial malaise

The nature of the Sierra Leone health service delivery system with government, while open and offering a variety of choices for users, was not robust, well structured or well regulated before the EVD outbreak. It was a pluralistic system consisting of faith-based organizations, non-governmental organizations, and the private sector (private for profit and private not for profit providing different kinds of medical and health services).[17] There are also traditional healers, mostly herbalists, who have a large and arguably expanding clientele. The latter were unarguably the most popular first choice for a majority of people in the rural areas.[18] And, it is not surprising that they were the most vulnerable health care workers during the Ebola holocaust.

The country's network of 1,184 peripheral health units (PHUs) and 40 hospitals (public and private) was grossly inadequate for its population of around six million in 2013 or projected demographic increases in the ensuing years.[19] The state-run health services, which are the largest within the formal system, account for approximately 80 percent of public health service utilization. The formal private sector, which is relatively small and mainly concentrated in major cities like Freetown and Bo, caters predominantly to the rich; those who can afford to pay the huge medical bills for their services. The state-run health delivery system is organized in the form of a triad:

1. primary health care, delivered by peripheral health units consisting of Maternal and Child Health Posts,[20] Community Health Post,[21] and Community Health Centers;[22]
2. secondary care, delivered by district hospitals; and
3. tertiary care, delivered by regional/national hospitals.

TABLE 5.4 Distribution of hospital beds and peripheral health units by district and region

District/Province	Hospital Bed Capacity	Number of PHUs	Projected Population for 2014
Eastern Province	474	278	1,443,064
Kailahun	80	74	465,048
Kenema	220	119	653,013
Kono	174	85	325,003
Northern Province	949	449	2,164,215
Bombali	250	102	494,139
Kambia	85	68	341,690
Koinadugu	150	71	335,471
Port Loko	224	106	557,978
Tonkolili	240	102	434,937
Southern Province	569	351	1,436,564
Bo	300	121	654,142
Bonthe	50	55	168,729
Moyamba	150	99	278,119
Pujehun	69	76	335,574
Western Area	1,214	106	1,304,507
Freetown	1,214	106	1,304,507
Sierra Leone	3,206	1,184	6,348,350

Source: Statistics Sierra Leone Population Projection Monograph and Ministry of Health and Sanitation's Basic Package of Essential Health Services (2015)

People encountered serious challenges with accessing health facilities particularly in the remote and hard-to-reach areas like Koinadugu in the north and Bonthe district on the Atlantic Ocean – particularly the island. Clinics were far apart, and the rugged terrain was difficult to ply especially during the rains. The choice, in the absence of adequate resources, seemed to be between constructing additional facilities with compromised standards for the country's burgeoning population or improving existing infrastructure to guarantee the provision of quality services.

Quality of care is also very critical in health service delivery and remains a major and persistent challenge for Sierra Leone. Over 90 percent of health facilities in the country provide maternal and child health services (MCH). However, the quality of the services provided on the eve of the EVD outbreak was largely sub-optimal. More than 10 percent of PHUs did not have access to water supply, less than 40 percent have functional incinerators, and 88 percent used unprotected pits to burn medical waste, whilst 59 percent did not have at least two toilets as specified in the Primary Healthcare Handbook. Additionally, over 60 percent of the PHUs did not have access to electricity. Power supply was notoriously erratic; and the substitute generator, even with fuel, hardly ran for 24 hours. The chronic lack of power supply to keep refrigerators working made it impossible to store delicate medical supplies like blood and immunization material.[23]

The condition of state-run health care facilities seems to be declining rather than improving over time. Following the introduction of the Free Health Care Initiative, the Ministry of Health and Sanitation set up a Facility Improvement Team (FIT) to regularly assess the readiness of facilities to implement the Free Health Care Policy with a view to improving maternal and newborn health services based on set criteria/enablers.[24] Prior to the commencement of the assessment, 65 Community Health Centers (CHCs) – five from each of the 13 districts, were identified nationwide to be upgraded to provide Basic Emergency Obstetric Neo-natal Care (BEmONC), while 13 hospitals (all the district hospitals and the Princess Christian Maternity Hospital (PCMH) – the principal maternity hospital in the country – were to be upgraded to provide Comprehensive Emergency Obstetric Neo-natal Care (CEmONC) services. Significant investments were made by both government and donors to upgrade these facilities before the free health care was rolled out. The objective of the exercise was to assess the facilities and recommend areas that require support. While few facilities met the set minimum criteria in July 2013,[25] the report for July 2014 came out with a stunning but unexpected finding: none of the facilities nationwide could pass the test!

The 2014 FIT Report revealed the following:[26]

1. About 85 percent of the facilities did not meet the criteria set for water and sanitation. This was largely attributed to faulty machines to pump water, no pipe connection, and poor waste management (inadequate incinerators).
2. About 80 percent of facilities had non-functional laboratories with no reagents and lack of trained personnel.

3. Eighty percent of the facilities lacked the required equipment to function qua hospital – Personal Protective Equipment (PPE), delivery bed, elbow gloves to provide Emergency Obstetric Neonatal Care (EmONC).
4. Stock out of tracer drugs was a major issue as 85 percent of the facilities reported stock out.
5. Almost 88 percent of the facilities did not have the required staff.

The FIT findings were consistent with earlier findings, most notably the Health Facility Assessment Report.[27] And it is general knowledge that the hospitals throughout the country lacked the wherewithal to function as hospitals. Why nothing was done to beef up these facilities remains an unanswered question – could it be lack of planning, lack of finance, or both? To make matters worse the assessment by officials from the Ministry of Health and Sanitation were never presented to the local councils that had been empowered under the Local Government Act for the provision of primary and secondary health care. Instead they were presented to donors to access funding that was not geared to improving conditions in the hospitals. Without knowledge of the needs in these facilities the local councils could not include such items in their budget.

Before the EVD outbreak, medical protocol governing infection, prevention, and control measures were not routinely distributed, practiced, and observed at public health facilities. Most health workers in public facilities seemed to have operated on norms prescribed by dint of the circumstances in which they found themselves. It was never a case of adhering to the rigorous protocols of the profession; there was in fact no professionalism. Staff routinely flouts medical protocols. They do not adhere to these protocols in part because of inadequate refresher training, absence of requisite technology, or – in some cases – inadequacy or lack of personal protective equipment (PPEs). Consequently, patient diagnosis, examinations, and treatment were largely done with bare hands, with doctors and nurses seemingly oblivious to the inherent risks.

Laboratory infrastructure and capacity were largely inadequate prior to the Ebola outbreak. This impeded real time contribution to diagnosis and patient management, disease surveillance, or outbreak investigation. Appropriate equipment and supplies were generally lacking, and bio-safety and bio-security practices virtually non-existent, thereby presenting a serious risk to the staff and the environment. It is hardly surprising that only one adequately equipped and functional laboratory was available in the whole country when Ebola struck in 2014 (Ministry of Health and Sanitation 2011)!

The palpable lack of equipment, facilities, and trained personnel were exacerbated by the almost non-existent information and surveillance system. Reliable, adequate, and timely information is the centerpiece for informed decision making. But this is fraught with debilitating challenges in health care delivery in Sierra Leone. There are several stand-alone information databases managed at the ministry by different units and/or programs. The four major information databases are: District Health Information System (DHIS), Integrated Disease Surveillance Information System (IDSI), Integrated Human Resource Information System (IHRIS), and CHANNEL for logistic management. Each of these data units seems to exist independent of the others. Prior to the EVD outbreak in 2014 only the DHIS and CHANNEL were fully operational with up-to-date data.

The DHIS is the national system for data management and analysis for health program planning, monitoring, and evaluation. Data is collected at the facility level in paper form submitted to the District Health Management Team where it is inputted into the software. District health workers collect data from health facilities on a monthly basis on services provided and utilization of drugs and supplies. The quality of the returns is, however, contingent on several factors ranging from when they are sent in to when they are recorded. However, primary data fed into the DHIS was not only incomprehensive as hospital and private facilities were not captured, but also untimely and not reliable. There is evidence of inconsistencies between what is inputted in the registers (the first source) and what eventually goes into the system – frequent breakdown of server and data validation continues to hamper its smooth operation. These grave shortcomings impede the ministry's ability to provide relevant national or district-level data on demand, which subsequently compromise the reliability of the data for any serious planning.

The IHRIS was rolled out to capture staff data (attendance, qualification/training, age, etc.). This was intended to be used for the cleaning of the payroll and update staff records, among others. Prior to the EVD outbreak, payroll cleaning was a major problem for government. A huge number of staff are on the payroll but not at their designated facilities, leading to significant financial burden to government. The system, which was intended to resolve this anomaly, though installed, remained confined to the Western Area. Appropriate structures, including adequate capacity to support the system, were not established. Consultants were recruited to design and roll out the system without adequate participation of ministry officials, especially at the district level. Accordingly, once the consultants' contract expired, the system collapsed.

The IDSI, another non-functional database, was most important in the area of disease surveillance, and outbreak. The system was intended to capture disease surveillance data and provide feedback. However, even at the central level the system was not fully functional and there was inadequate staff at the district level for surveillance activities. This led to the irregular updating of the system, which therefore made effective surveillance impossible. The grim health situation in Sierra Leone could be gleaned from the conditions that existed in one of the major hospitals in the country located in the initial epicenter of the dangerous Ebola Virus Disease.

The Kenema Government Hospital: the initial treatment center of the Ebola epidemic

The deadly cocktail of insufficient medical personnel, inadequately trained health care workers, lack of basic health facilities, and scarce equipment proved fatal when Ebola struck in May 2014. The Kenema Government Hospital – the original treatment center for the Ebola epidemic – typifies the general conditions prevailing in the country on the eve of the outbreak (Senga et al. 2016). As the main referral hospital, equipped with 280 beds, in the eastern part of the country, it was virtually impossible, even in normal times, to provide the needed medical care to about a third of the population. When Ebola struck in May, the Kenema hospital became flooded with patients from Kailahun, an adjacent district; and the two became the points from where the deadly virus spread to eventually envelope the whole country. The Kenema Government Hospital is a metaphor for all the ills that characterized the health sector in Sierra Leone: confronting Ebola with bare hands!

Consisting of ten wards and about 220 beds for a population of roughly 700,000, it would be swamped with patients, literally bursting at the seams when Ebola struck. On the eve of the EVD outbreak the hospital could only boast of five medical doctors – two of these would be consumed by the epidemic – Dr. Khan, the only virologist in the country, and Dr. Rogers, a retiree. Of the 42 nurses stationed at the hospital, the majority were nursing aides and volunteers. At a time when patients were coming from all over the region, the hospital only had one functional ambulance attached to the maternity ward – a donation from the International Rescue Committee (IRC). The shortage of health care workers and ambulances was compounded by erratic power supply and inadequate provision of water – key supplies in normal and emergency periods. There were only three stretchers to carry the sick and the dying, which were shared by all the patients irrespective of their ailments. The drugs in stock were only 30 percent of what the hospital needed; and even then, the storage facilities were inadequate.[28]

The above inventory of the conditions in Kenema was published in September 2014 – four months after the outbreak of the deadly virus. During that four-month period there was a 34-day "moratorium on movements"; but the lack of equipment and personnel made it impossible to control the spread of the disease. Consequently, Kenema district moved from zero infection in May to "becoming the second epicenter with about 395 infections" in September 2014.[29] What, then, was the problem?

As the only referral hospital in the region, Kenema was completely swamped with patients from all over the region and beyond, yet without the resources to cater for the increasing numbers. Much more important is the history of the hospital and its organic linkages with infectious disease. The Kenema Government Hospital had been the site of a massive research outfit funded by WHO, CDC, and Merlin, the British medical relief organization, since the early 1970s when Lassa fever ravaged the nearby towns of Tongo and Panguma, in the Kenema district. Initially located at the Nixon Memorial Hospital in Segbwema, a Sierra Leonean virologist, Dr. Aniru Conteh, was hired to head the Lassa fever program. When the CDC, the principal funding agency, abandoned the project after war broke out, Dr. Conteh shifted base to the Kenema hospital where a Lassa ward was established.

In spite of the chronic lack of funding during the war years, and the continued spike in the rate of infection, Dr. Conteh soldiered on. Even when no support was forthcoming from a government at war, he continued his own one-man war against the deadly Lassa haemorrhagic fever. He subsequently succumbed to the deadly virus after an accident in April 2004. It was only after his demise that the program got a new lease of life with massive funding from external sources, principally the US. A task force was quickly assembled by the United States Agency for International Development (USAID) to address the Lassa scourge in the region. It included representatives from the three countries of the MRU that were ravaged by the Ebola virus disease, the WHO, the European Union, and other NGOs. Funding was to come from the US government, channeled to the WHO for the setting up of a Lassa Fever Laboratory at the Kenema Government Hospital.

A coordinating body was also proposed, the Mano River Union Lassa Fever Network (MRU-LFN), to strengthen scientific cooperation, patient management, outbreak surveillance, and laboratory capacity (Bah 2015). A Lassa laboratory would be constructed in Kenema to serve as an "international medical research center" linked to other laboratories in the region as part of the MRU-LFN research network. An EU-funded Lassa Isolation Ward at Kenema Government Hospital would complete the new multilateral funding to the revived Lassa fever research project. But these high-profile interests and extra funding for research on a deadly infectious disease in the region did not, however, translate into any meaningful improvement in the facilities or equipment available at the hospital. Even with the massive funding that came in after Lassa fever was reclassified by the CDC as a possible Category A pathogen and the establishment of the Viral Hemorrhagic Fever Consortium (VHFC), the hospital remained unchanged – a veritable contrast to the research money made available for Lassa fever (Bah 2015). Sierra Leone's only virologist, whose death marked a turning point in the war against Ebola, Dr. Umar Khan, is on record to have complained about the conditions in the hospital. "I'm afraid for my life. I must say I cherish my life, and if you are afraid of it you will take the maximum precautions,"[30] he is reported to have told a journalist. The original Lassa fever ward, now the Ebola treatment center, would eventually consume Dr. Khan as he struggled single-handedly to contain the deadly virus.

The appalling conditions in Kenema even extended to the Lassa fever ward right up to the outbreak of the deadly Ebola

Virus Disease. And the basics in infectious disease protocol were not even observed. There were reportedly no thermometers in the ward and safety precautions were hardly ever observed as routine practice. A study conducted on the eve of the outbreak revealed the "absence of basic protective equipment like gloves for health care workers handling Lassa cases" (Bah 2015). There was lack of diagnostic equipment to collect specimen; needles were routinely reused; while health workers went about without protective gear. These working conditions not only endangered the lives of health workers but also patients whose ailments where not contagious. In a situation where water and power supply were erratic, ambulance service virtually non-existent, and the few available stretchers were used by all irrespective of their clinical conditions, the possibility of spreading a deadly infection became a frightening proposition for all – patients as well as health workers.

It is therefore not surprising that two weeks after Dr. Khan perished amidst deteriorating conditions in the overcrowded Kenema Government Hospital, the president had to publicly express his disappointment with the lack of external support for what his government should have provided in the first place:

> I am disappointed at the international community in their delay in responding (sic) towards the fight against the deadly Ebola virus in Sierra Leone. We have not been provided with enough equipment, resources, qualified health officers, and we have lost the only expert we had in the country to the disease amidst the declaration of the international health emergency on Ebola.[31]

This volte-face in trying to shift the blame to outsiders was as unhelpful as it was disingenuous. The problem with the war against Ebola was not only about lack of equipment and personnel; it was also about governance or its absence.

The story of the Kenema Government Hospital as a reflection of the whole national health system cannot be complete without an assessment of the role-played by the District Health Management Team (DHMT) – the body statutorily entrusted with the running of health services at the local level. Consisting of 16 chiefdoms, at the center of which is Nongowa chiefdom, where Kenema city, the site of the hospital, is located, the district shares a border with Kailahun district – the original epicenter of the deadly disease. As early as June 2014, when the disease was ravaging Kailahun, the local council allegedly designed a "response plan covering case management, surveillance and social mobilization" in collaboration with the DHMT. This was long before officials from above discovered social mobilization as an effective strategy to counter the deadly disease. The Ministry of Health and Sanitation only confirmed the disbursement of funds totaling 7,969,200,015 Leones to the 13 DHMT on August 11, 2014. By then many local councils were allegedly compelled to raise funds on their own. The two local councils in Nongowa raised a total of Le50 million to fund a management health center for 30 patients. This project was undertaken under the guidance of Dr. Khan, the only virologist in country.[32]

This seeming self-help from below simply meant that institutions statutorily tasked with carrying out specific duties were not allowed to function precisely because of the extreme centralization of power in Freetown – far away from the epicenter of the raging disease. There is evidence to suggest that even by September 2014, when Nongowa recorded 92 percent of all infection in Kenema district, health officials in Freetown refused to budge, preferring to channel resources through the DHMT as opposed to the local councils. The apparent disconnect between local councils and the DHMT would hamper any robust attempt to tackle the raging disease. Before the spike in infection rate in Kenema, Le542 million was disbursed by ministry officials to the DHMT; while close to Le700 million was made available to parliamentarians from Kenema, plus another Le2 billion to Freetown-based civil society and NGOs specifically earmarked for Kenema. What would later become a national scandal – appropriating Ebola funds for personal use – seems to have started with the Kenema situation. Ironically, the popular response from below would be the pathway to salvation as the nation stumbled from one ineffectual strategy to another in the on-going war against the Ebola Virus Disease.[33]

Conclusion: the limits of fighting Ebola with bare hands

With its still unclear origins, stealthy attacks, and frequently fatal impact on the body, an EVD outbreak can generate panic and quickly wreak havoc on local health systems. Yet, in four decades since it first appeared in the Democratic Republic of Congo (DRC), and then Gabon, Uganda, and South Sudan, national governments with the support of WHO, CDC, and other organizations have devised strategies to contain localized outbreaks and quickly get the situation under control. The lack of familiarity with the disease could be blamed for the initial poor response to its outbreak and spread. Once the presence of EVD in Guinea had been definitely confirmed by April 2014, the failure for stopping it from mutating into a sub-regional epidemic lay with global organizations like WHO, tasked with containing infectious diseases, and the inadequate national health systems in the three MRU countries. While there are slight national variations, the health systems of the three most affected MRU countries mirror each other and contain the same fundamental weaknesses in financing, medical personnel, logistics, medical data, and disease surveillance that made containing the virus and stopping its transmission from person to person and place to place immensely difficult. Senegal, Mali, and Nigeria, with their more robust and responsive medical systems, were able to marshal the necessary resources to limit the spread of EVD within their borders.

In Sierra Leone, the increase in government health expenditure, the extensive foreign donor contributions, and high out-of-pocket payments, coupled with a raft of health care legislation and high-profile Free Health Policy could not quickly reverse the havoc created by decades of decline in the health sector, and the decade long civil war. The inputs into the systems could not effectively rectify the disparities and imbalances in the system, which limited access of Sierra Leoneans in rural areas and marginal urban areas to timely, affordable, and reliable medical and health care. The tussles between state officials regarding control over health care resources, the ineffective communication between governance institutions at different levels, and recurrent financial malfeasance did not inspire public trust or confidence in the system. At the very extreme, Ebola could be read as the terrifying magnification of a deficient health care system that had struggled to reduce the incidence of familiar and endemic infections like typhoid, malaria, and cholera.

The large-scale intervention of UN agencies, under the leadership of UNMEER, the AU, ECOWAS, and several foreign medical teams provided the necessary finance, personnel, and infrastructure within a short timeframe to contain and eventually help stop the outbreak. Most of these inputs were temporary and could not be repurposed or converted into long-term contributions to the Sierra Leone health system. With the subsidence of the outbreak, there have been many discussions of the lessons learned and post-Ebola health sector recovery plans have been crafted by the Sierra Leone government in concert with various international agencies, donor countries, and NGOs. Whether or not lessons have been truly learned and the truly transformative ideas in these plans will be translated into reality remains to be seen. The National Ebola Recovery Strategy unveiled last year has partially delivered on its first primary objectives: restoring basic access to health care, getting children back to school, and rolling out social protection.[34] This was to cover the first six months. The long term objective of "building a resilient health system" – which includes the formulation and implementation of a stand-alone Public Health Master Plan, a graduate program in medical and health related professions, the establishment of a center for the control of infectious diseases, and the setting up of a well-capacitated Directorate for Environmental Sanitation and Hygiene – will have to wait until the economy recovers from the "twin crisis" that allegedly sent it to recession.[35] An austerity regime proclaimed at the beginning of October will be in force until the first half of 2017.[36]

While acknowledging that the "rapid spread of the disease was due to major shortcomings in governance, social cohesion, and missed opportunities in exploiting the benefits of sub-regional collaboration, such as MRU," things have seemingly slipped back to "business as usual." A recent survey of the health facilities in the over-crowded Freetown area – where the majority of the nation's inhabitants are to be found – has unearthed serious lapses in health service delivery, poor accountability, corruption at all levels, and deteriorating conditions across all the public health facilities in the area.[37] While the role of international agencies and donor countries cannot be ignored, the responsibility for creating a truly robust, responsive, trustworthy, and accessible health care system rests solely with the government and people of Sierra Leone, and the larger sub-region within which they reside.

Notes

1 Sierra Leone Government, Ministry of Finance and Economic Development, "Preliminary Assessment of the Impact of the Outbreak of the Ebola Viral Disease on the Sierra Leone Economy," September 2014.

2 These numbers are based on "suspected, probable and confirmed" cases rather than just confirmed cases. See http://www.cdc.gov/vhf/ebola/outbreaks/2014-west-africa/case-counts.html.

3 National Ebola Response Center (NERC) daily updates/reports, http://www.nerc.sl/ (accessed September 16, 2016).

4 WHO Ebola Situation Report, November 11, 2015, http://apps.who.int/iris/bitstream/10665/194050/1/ebolasitrep_11Nov2015_eng.pdf?ua=1&ua=1 (accessed September 16, 2016).

5 Infant mortality rate was 127/1,000 in 2008 and 92/1,000 in 2013, and the under-five mortality rate was 194/1,000 in 2008 and 156/1,000 in 2013. Maternal rate was 857/100,000 in 2008 and 1,165/100,000 in 2013. See Sierra Leone Demographic and Health Survey (2013).

6 The Free Health Initiative is the government flagship project, which allows free treatment for pregnant women, lactating mothers, and children under five years in all government-owned health facilities.

7 WHO Ebola Situation Reports, December 30, 2015, http://apps.who.int/ebola/sites/default/files/atoms/files//who_ebola_situation_report_30-12-2015.pdf?ua=1&ua=1 (accessed September 25, 2016).

8 See UN Security S/2014/669: Letter dated September 15 from the Secretary-General address to the President of the Security Council. It contains a letter from Ernest Bai Koroma, President of the Republic of Sierra Leone, Ellen Johnson Sirleaf, President of the Republic of Liberia, and Alpha Condé, President of the Republic of Guinea, detailing the impact of EVD on their countries.

9 Sierra Leone Government, Ministry of Health and Sanitation Report (2014).

10 See WHO, "Sierra Leone Health Profile, 2012."

11 Sierra Leone Government, Ministry of Health and Sanitation, Report on Human Resource Status (2014).

12 An OECD policy brief produced four years before the onset of the epidemic lists Sierra Leone as one of five African countries, which include Mozambique, Liberia, Angola, and Tanzania, as parts of world which have 50 percent rates of expatriation of its doctors. See OECD Policy Brief, February 2010, "International Migration of Health Workers: Improving International Co-operation to Address the Global Health Workforce Crisis," http://www.who.int/hrh/resources/oecd-who_policy_brief_en.pdf (accessed September 29, 2016).

13 See p. 64 of the Supplement to the *Sierra Leone Gazette Extraordinary*, 135, 14 (March 1, 2004): The Local Government Act, 2004.

14 See WHO, "Global Health Expenditure," http://data.worldbank.org/indicator/SH.XPD.TOTL.ZS?end=2014&start=2013&year_high_desc=true (accessed September 28, 2016).

15 This is less than the 15 percent target agreed to in Abuja, Nigeria in April 2001.

16 See Auditor General's Annual Reports (2009, 2010, 2011, 2012, and 2013), http://www.auditservice.gov.sl/reports-2-annual-reports.html (accessed September 16, 2016).

17 Government of Sierra Leone and Ministry of Health and Sanitation, National Health Sector Strategic Plan (2010–2015), November 2009, http://www.internationalhealthpartnership.net/fileadmin/uploads/ihp/Documents/Country_Pages/Sierra_Leone/NationalHealthSectorStrategicPlan_2010-15.pdf (accessed September 25, 2016).

18 This chapter does not deal with traditional healers.

19 Sierra Leone Health Sector Recovery Plan (2015–2020).

20 The MCHPs are designed to serve between 500 to 5,000 people within a three-mile radius and provide antenatal care, delivery, and postnatal care services.

21 The CHPs are designed to serve between 5,000 to 10,000 people within a five-mile radius and provide all MCHPs services plus basic curative services.

22 The CHCs are designed to serve between 10,000 to 30,000 people within a five-to-ten-mile radius and provide all CHPs services plus inpatient care and laboratory services. Additionally, they also supervise the CHPs and MCHPs.

23 Government of Sierra Leone, Ministry of Health and Sanitation, "Facility Improvement Team Report" (2015).

24 The enablers assessed are: water and sanitation, electricity, referral, equipment, blood and laboratory, staff, and drugs and supplies.

25 Only eight of the 65 CHCs (12 percent) BEmONC and three of the 13 hospitals (23 percent) met the minimum criteria.

26 Government of Sierra Leone, Ministry of Health and Sanitation, Reproductive and Child Health Directorate, "Making Health Facilities Safe in an Ebola Outbreak: Facility Improvement Team Assessment Report" (2014).

27 Sierra Leone Health Facility Survey, December 3, 2014, http://www.unicef.org/emergencies/ebola/files/SL_Health_Facility_Survey_2014Dec3.pdf (accessed September 16, 2016).

28 Institute for Governance Reform, "Making the 3-Day National Lockdown Meaningful: Lessons from the Governance of Ebola in Kenema District, 14 September 2014," http://awoko.org/2014/09/22/sierra-leone-news-making-the-3-day-national-lockdown-meaningful/ (accessed September 25, 2016).

29 Ibid.

30 "Profile: Leading Ebola Doctor Sheikh Umar," *BBC News*, July 30, 2014, www.bbc.com/news/world-africa-28560507.

31 Umaru Fofana, "Blaming WHO, Blaming Sierra Leone President," *Politico SL*, August 21, 2014, http://politicosl.com/articles/blaming-who-blaming-sierra-leone-president (accessed September 16, 2016).

32 Institute for Governance Reform, "Making the 3-Day National Lockdown Meaningful."

33 A coherent and robust strategy to tackle the Ebola virus only emerged when UNMEER was set-up at the end of 2014. Conversation with Mr. Amadu Kamara, UNMEER official, November 2014.

34 Government of Sierra Leone, "National Ebola Recovery Strategy for Sierra Leone, 2015–2017" (July 2015).

35 Ibid., 41.

36 Government of Sierra Leone, Press Release: State House, Freetown, October 3, 2016.

37 Campaign for Human Rights and Development International (CHRDI), Press Release, Devastating Impact of Service Failure across the Health Care Sector in Freetown, October 3, 2016.

References

Bah, C.A. (2015). *The Ebola Outbreak in West Africa: Corporate Gangsters, Multinationals and Rogue Politicians*. Philadelphia, PA: Africanists Press.

Chen, L., Evans, T. et al (2004). "Human Resources for Health: Overcoming the Crisis," *Lancet*, 364: 1984–1990.

M'Cormack-Hale, Fredline A.O. and M'Cormack McGough, Fredanna (2016). "Promises and Pitfalls of the Free Health Care Initiative in Sierra Leone: An Early Analysis," in Mustapha, Marda and Bangura, Joseph (eds) *Democratization and Human Security in Postwar Sierra Leone*. New York: Palgrave, 199–216.

Maxen, Amy (2013). "Sierra Leone Free Health Care Initiative: Work in Progress," *The Lancet*, 381, 9862 (January): 191–192.

Ministry of Finance and Economic Development (2014). "Preliminary Assessment of the Impact of the Outbreak of the Ebola Viral Disease on the Sierra Leone Economy," September.

Ministry of Health and Sanitation (2011). "National Laboratory Strategic Plan 2011–2015."

Ministry of Health and Sanitation (2012, 2013 and 2014). "Facility Improvement Team Report," various issues.

Ministry of Health and Sanitation (2013). "National Health Account Report."

Ryan, Jordan (Fall 2014/Winter 2015). "Can a Post-crisis Country Survive in the Time of Ebola? Issues Arising with Liberia's Post-war Recovery," *Harvard International Review*, 36, 2: 25.

Senga, Mikko et al. (2016) "Factors Underlying Ebola Virus Infection among Health Workers, Kenema, Sierra Leone, 2014–2015," *Clinical Infectious Diseases*, 63, 4 (August 15): 454–459. doi:10.1093/cid/ciw327.

Sierra Leone Auditor General's report (2009, 2010, 2011, 2012, and 2013).

Sierra Leone Demographic and Health Survey (2013).

Sierra Leone Health Facility Assessment Report (March 2015).

Sierra Leone Health Sector Recovery Plan (2015–2020).

Sierra Leone National Ebola Response Center Daily Ebola Updates/Reports.

Sierra Leone National Health Sector Strategic Plan (2010–2015).

World Health Organization (2010). *Health Systems Financing: The Path to Universal Coverage*. Geneva: WHO. http://www.who.int/whr/2010/en/index.html.

World Health Organization (2012). *Global Health Expenditure Atlas*.

PART THREE

DEVELOPMENT, GENDER, AND ITS DISCONTENTS

6 | STRUCTURAL VIOLENCE, PUBLIC HEALTH, AND THE MILITARIZATION OF ASSISTANCE

Julia Amos

Introduction

Sierra Leone's under-resourced and dysfunctional health system was as unprepared for the humanitarian emergency of the Ebola Virus Disease (EVD) outbreak in 2014 as the army had been for the rebel invasion in 1991 that started the country's long civil war. As with the war, the disease entered from the south-east, in a rural hinterland where the presence of the state is weak and the primary sources of governance are the traditional authorities.[1] The southeast is also considered a stronghold of the Sierra Leone People's Party (SLPP), the main opposition party, a factor that has been blamed locally for the initial slow intervention and little trust in the central government. The distance between the national elite based in the capital Freetown and the poor rural districts on the border with Liberia and Guinea has historically been great, their relationship characterized by suspicion and neglect.

Deadly though the virus is to those infected, previous outbreaks elsewhere in Africa have been effectively contained (there had been no known outbreak in Sierra Leone, Guinea, or Liberia). It is now clear the Mano River Union (MRU) outbreak would not have grown into the epidemic without the combination of political, economic, and social factors affecting the country. At the same time, the responses of the government and the international community to the situation – characterized by militarized practices and language – had an impact on the social and political environment that will outlast and is ultimately likely to outweigh the immediate health consequences. As with the war (Keen 2005) there will be no way to understand the political economy of Sierra Leone without taking into account the changes wrought by the epidemic. These impacts, which this chapter explores, include the loss of human capital resulting from the death of medical staff and health care workers, and the closure of schools and universities. It also includes the social capital, trust, and government legitimacy that were forfeited with the revelation of the dismal state of the health system, and the banning of touching and public gatherings. Finally, the situation also raises important questions about relations between developed and developing countries and the nature of development support, especially in a post-conflict setting when there is a risk of over-prioritizing national security at the expense of individual wellbeing.

Development theory and practice: structural violence or expanding capabilities?

It should not come as a surprise that a major disease outbreak would require a humanitarian response, or indeed that such a response would not be immediately successful, given that Sierra Leone's health system was not advanced enough to weather such a shock. Duffield characterizes relations between developed and developing countries, and development assistance, as the containment and localization of poor, uninsured populations. He raises the concern that relief and development aid may be essentially circular when developmental self-reliance is sought at a level where the precarity of uninsured populations risks collapsing into humanitarian disaster (Duffield 2007; Duffield 2008). The debate over the response to Ebola essentially parallels earlier debates within development about the political economy of famine (Sen 1981; Drèze and Sen 1991; Keen 1994). Sen (1981; Drèze and Sen 1991) famously argued that occurrences of famines were not simply due to natural disasters and food shortfalls, but as the result of an "entitlement failure" unlikely to take place in a democratic country. Entitlement in Sen's usage covers the relations that govern the bundle of commodities that an individual or family can legitimately acquire within a particular socio-economic setting. The entitlement to adequate life-supporting health facilities failed in Sierra Leone; the inadequacy of state and non-state provisions were shown up by the Ebola epidemic.

Paul Farmer, a medical doctor and infectious disease specialist and the most famous theorist of global health inequalities as structural violence, has recently applied his work to Sierra Leone and Liberia. He pointed out how Ebola mortality rates could have been dramatically reduced through basic treatments that were initially unavailable to vulnerable patients because of a lack of basic equipment (Farmer

2014). Such equipment includes intraosseous needles, which might have been especially useful in the treatment of dehydration in children, who initially almost all succumbed to the disease when infected. Farmer argues that the poor state of health facilities in Sierra Leone is the product of an abusive historical legacy and can therefore be described as structural violence. Galtung developed this concept of structural violence in 1969 to show how institutionalized attitudes may prevent the achievement of fundamental human needs by different categories of people. It was then used by Farmer (2004) in a public health setting to show how the legacy of slavery and racism affects the risks to Haitians of succumbing to diseases such as AIDS and tuberculosis.

However, intentionality and the agency of a perpetrator, as well as physical pain, is central to our taken-for-granted conceptualizations of violence, meaning that definitions that de-emphasize these aspects may back-fire, inviting ridicule and rejection. Suspicions of definitions of terms propagated by academics and other educated elites that radically transform their meaning and uses should not be written off as reactionary "jitters" stemming from the guilty conscience of "everyone who belongs to a certain [violent] social order … still geared to pinning praise or blame on individual actors" (Farmer 2004, 307). The recognition of inequitable historical legacies, practices, and systems is not the *same* as participating in naming practices that oppose them: this is a separate political project, the case for which has to be made explicitly. There are good grounds for not using labeling in this way: support for a political project centered on conceptual redefinition is likely to be correlated with education and socio-economic background, or class, and thus exclude a wide social strata of Sierra Leoneans. Moreover, such practices may serve to disguise the considerable opposition that such a project would encounter from those wealthier countries portrayed as obligated to help (more on which below). Finally, conceptual clarity is necessary to enable a debate about how to (re-)build trust in the failed Sierra Leonean health system. As Moran and Hoffman write (2014): "[i]n the current epidemic, as in the violence that preceded it and in the long uncertain period to come, intervention and understanding are not separate. One is not possible without the other."

On the one hand, we are faced with the stark reality of very low levels of development, including public health provisions, in an historical context that has been shaped by exploitative international relations including the transatlantic slave trade and British colonialism (Shaw 2002; Ferme 2001). On the other hand, the entitlements and resources that any nation's citizens can draw upon within the current global political system are delineated by national boundaries, and it is practically and politically very hard to make claims on resources outside of this framework, however compelling the moral arguments. Ferguson (2006) draws attention to the lack of entitlements available to the population of Lesotho compared to those living in the so-called homelands created in apartheid South Africa: the resources we are able to draw on for sustenance are literally circumscribed by such arbitrary national borders.

Although health expenditure in Sierra Leone makes up a comparatively high proportion of the country's GDP, at over 10 percent (a larger share than in the UK, for example), the absolute numbers involved are tiny. Per capita spending on health before the EVD outbreak was less than $100/year, with government spending accounting for less than 15 percent of that sum[2] (compared with nearly $3,600 in the UK and over $9,000 in the US). Out-of-pocket expenditure[3] by citizens accounts for over 60 percent of total expenditure on health, and external resources (NGOs etc.) make up over 30 percent. The majority of health expenditure is made up of direct purchases by citizens from non-state providers, including unregulated and traditional health workers, and with a large NGO health sector as an additional provider. Persistent problems of insufficient understanding of diseases, patchy coordination, poor coverage, and weak oversight of the health sector have proved devastating in the context of the Ebola epidemic.

Those that describe the legacy of historical injustice as a form of structural violence against poor, uninsured populations, argue for a transfer of resources from developed to developing countries as a form of restitutional justice. However, since there is no international legal framework where such claims can be put forward they tend to rely on the goodwill of envisaged payees, in this case the United States and Latin American countries that benefitted from the extractive practices of the slave trade, and the UK, the former colonial power. Within our current political framework these countries are only directly responsible to their own electorates, which given the controversy in the United States about providing basic medical insurance to its own citizens, and the recent dramatic UK welfare cuts, are unlikely to be supportive of such commitments.

How do academic development studies attempt to square the transatlantic triangle of historical exploitation, to address current shortfalls in a way both just and practical? Sen's argument overcomes this difficulty by offering a localized political economy version of the systemic global critiques of Duffield, Ferguson, and Farmer: centering on the responsibilities of individual national democracies towards their citizens. As such it is a popular lens in development studies; however, it is a lens that is capable of showing up the discipline's own weaknesses in terms of struggling to effect sustainable solutions that require political change, rather than short-term or minor inputs of materials or policy suggestions – especially as those seeking to effect such changes are often operating in a foreign country. Sen elaborated his approach into what is known in development studies as the capabilities approach (see also Nussbaum 2000).[4] Crucially, this approach, when transplanted into the public health domain, offers developed countries the opportunity to participate (as technical support partners and donors) in the project of ensuring that all have the capability of being healthy and pursuing a life plan, by making this the goal, rather than fair and equal access to the same health provisions globally (Venkatapuram 2011).

Such an approach does not have to be as reactionary and unambitious as it sounds. It may be more successful in securing the necessary funds to improve the Sierra Leonean health system from external donors, and by making the national state and its relationship with its citizens the primary focus it can potentially enable the pursuit of more pro-poor and locally appropriate health care solutions than would be the case if a global consensus had first to be sought. One of the most remarkable features of the Ebola crisis has been the South-to-South assistance missions by countries including China[5], Cuba,[6] and Kenya:[7] these make the possibility of fitting the outbreak within the narrative of developing country solidarity movements an attractive possibility. Sierra Leone has a rich educational and intellectual history, Fourah Bay College was founded in 1827 and affiliated with Durham University, making it the first Western-style university in the region and earning the colony its epithet "the Athens of West Africa" (Paracka 2003). It also has a strong political tradition of Pan-African discourse, animating youth constituencies especially (as in the case of the National Provisional Ruling Council (NPRC) coup, see Opala 1994).

While other countries initially pledged mainly monetary support, Cuba sent a large early contingent of medical doctors. This in part exemplifies Cuba's foreign relations strategy of providing this sort of humanitarian aid, but it is also reflective of its national approach to health care provision. The Cuban approach may hold important lessons for Sierra Leone compared to the very expensive approaches of developed countries such as the United States – which relies on high levels of private medical provision and nevertheless failed to prevent nosocomial (within hospital) EVD transmission. Cuba views universal health care as a human right, a belief enshrined in its 1976 constitution. The aftermath of the EVD epidemic provides opportunities for South-to-South knowledge exchange and cooperation in terms of suitable models for the provision of affordable and robust primary health care. One such proposed model is pooled investment to scale up national community health worker coverage.[8] However, to ensure that such a system is sustainable it needs to be properly resourced, which requires long-term financial commitment from donors as well as difficult political choices for governments to prioritize health care over other spending.

Ebola in context: Sierra Leone's political economy

The Sierra Leone civil war started at a point of popular disillusionment with a process aimed to transition the country from a post-independence history dominated by one-party rule by the All Peoples Congress (APC). The external interventions in the war, and the reconstruction models that they deployed, sought to rebuild the political system according to a liberal democratic model. The goal was to create a stable state, governed by elected politicians and protected by security forces, which were subject to civilian oversight. The UK, various UN programs and the international financial institutions invested in Security Sector Reform (SSR) programs to reshape the army and the police and an economic agenda of liberalization and measures intended to benefit the poorest (through Poverty Reduction Strategy Papers that looked remarkably similar to those of other developing countries). Despite declarations about the importance of local or national ownership such cookie-cutter policies were in fact pre-conditions for external aid, investment, and expertise.

Elections were held during the war in 1996 and 2002, both were won by the Sierra Leone People's Party (SLPP). The first of these elections sought to replace the military regime of the NPRC, but the resulting government was overthrown in 1997 by another junta, the Armed Forces Redemption Council (AFRC), leading to the continuation of conflict. This reinforced the placement of national security and SSR at the top of the development agenda, seeking to protect the country from armed actors both external and internal. However, it was complaints about ethnically based corruption and discrimination, and popular impatience with the slow pace of progress in improving the standard of living for average Sierra Leoneans that led to the first shift in government after the war, which I witnessed for myself during the 2007 elections. Sierra Leone's two largest ethnic groups (both with approximately 30 percent of the population),[9] the Mende and Temne, are associated with the two contending political traditions, the SLPP and the APC respectively. These politicized ethnic cleavages were not the cause of the country's conflict but were exacerbated by the nature of external interventions aimed at ending the conflict and (re-)launching an electoral democracy. With low average educational levels and comparatively strong ethnically delineated neo-traditional forms of local governance the resulting political system favored ethnic mobilization, as well as the incumbent party, leading to recruitment of young people into acts of intimidation and fueling distrust in the state.

In 2007 enthusiasm for the new APC government was high, and I observed it being re-kindled by re-election in 2012. The country had started exporting iron ore in 2011 and was one of the fastest growing economies in the world.[10] However, the mining boom ended with a collapse in the international price of iron ore from $190 in 2011 to $60 in 2014,[11] just before the Ebola epidemic. Around the same time, complaints about the lack of progress for non-elites were already being voiced once more. Faith that development would provide a minimum international standard of living for Sierra Leoneans was disrupted by the economic crisis accompanying the epidemic, and this has had real local political consequences in terms of stability and faith in the government.

Sierra Leone is now in a very different place to the 2012 elections, when macro-economic indicators were stabilizing, inflation was finally contained to single figures, and consistent double-digit economic growth predicted.[12] The World Bank (WB) has adjusted its growth figure for 2014 from 14 percent to 4 percent[13] and the International Monetary Fund (IMF) is projecting negative growth for 2015 of -21.5 percent.[14] The production of iron ore, the biggest export earner (IMF 2015, 4) has stopped and it is unclear if and when it will be resumed.[15] The twin crises of EVD and the economy have been rapidly politicized and the murmurs on the streets of Freetown are echoed in the academic press, in statements such as that of Fodei Batty (2014) about the "stubborn correlations between the presence of the APC party in power and major national and regional calamities." How the Ebola outbreak was and is handled is both a reflection of, and major future influence on, state legitimacy and national identity.

Popular rumors styled EVD as a manufactured crisis, a source of funding for elites and foreign interests. Some Sierra Leoneans cast the disease as an evil too powerful for its originators to control, exemplified in rumors circulated by text messages in the Northern Province describing the sudden spates of deaths being caused by witches crashing their night-airplanes into residential neighborhoods (Bolten 2014). Although many of the claims made may seem outlandish, the reasons for such suspicions are not. As Keen (1994) showed in the famine response in Sudan, complex humanitarian emergencies have powerful beneficiaries, including political elites and traders within the affected nation, and shortcomings that affect responses may in part be caused by the organizational modes of practice of the responders. Similar weaknesses have affected the Ebola response, where the massive external resources invested have been controlled by foreign NGOs and national elites, leaving survivors unsupported to cope with after-effects such as ocular impairments (Bausch 2015b) on their own amongst persistent allegations of financial mismanagement.[16]

The government reacted to the EVD outbreak by putting into place stringent emergency legislation. In one incident on October 21, 2014 in Koidu Town, the regional center of the diamond mining area, Kono, with a strong tradition of youth mobilization, a female youth leader protested the removal of her grandmother who was suspected of having Ebola. Two participants in the ensuing unrest were shot dead[17] with others arrested and detained for six months without charge under the emergency laws. These laws circumscribed the right to expression and peaceful protest and suspended the right to assembly in the interest of disease control. They were also used to effect the arrest of opposition and dissenting government officials and to control critical journalists.[18] Throughout the outbreak public health and political interventions shaded into each other. Curfews and a hastily prepared three-day Ebola lockdown at the end of March 2015 followed on the heels of the removal of the vice-president, Sam Sumana, from office amidst rumors about his intention to start a break-away party using his Kono support base. In other words, donor-funded security sector reform in Sierra Leone contributed to a militarized Ebola response with ambiguous political and human consequences. To paraphrase the old saying, when donor policy focuses on the handing out of hammers then people may worry that they look like nails (see also McGovern 2014).

The implicit theory of Sierra Leone's international partners in both aid and trade as to how to best support good governance has also been misguided. It hinged on the other two foci of attention and investment apart from security sector reform – support for electoral democracy and local NGO, or so-called third sector, partners.[19] As late as February 13, 2014, these remained the priorities of the UK Department for International Development (DfID) as outlined at the meeting with its "delivery partners" (about 50 NGOs, INGOs, and contractors funded directly by DfID). The main focus, apart from continued security cooperation, was economic, on job creation and growth, and the response to a direct question about the need for more of a focus on cross-border issues was that London dealt with regional issues. However, London is even farther from the rural border region areas than the home of the national governmental and NGO elites in Freetown. In the month that followed, EVD crossed from Guinea into Sierra Leone, and by May 26, 2014 the first Sierra Leonean fatality of the outbreak was officially confirmed, and the dangers of the weak national governance and heath infrastructure combined with cross-border health risks were painfully realized.

Ebola changes everything?

While on the one hand "Ebola changes everything," the crisis precipitated by the outbreak was at least partly the result of systemic weaknesses that are still not being adequately addressed. My previous research has highlighted how NGO provisioning of basic social services can lead to social capital accruing to civil society actors rather than the state, undermining the government's ability to mount a credible conflict resolution initiative (Amos 2009a; Amos 2009b; Amos 2011; and Amos forthcoming). There are parallels here with the weaknesses affecting the efforts to counter and contain EVD which spread from areas where government clinics were not the primary providers of health care. The population instead relied on a patchwork of NGO provisions and traditional healers with limited or no understanding of the transmission of the EVD and disease in general that proved devastating (Ferme 2014; Richards and Mokuwa 2014; Richards et al. 2015). We have seen why in the aftermath of Sierra Leone's long civil war security sector reform was top of the donor agenda, arguably to the detriment of more holistic conceptions of security that include individual wellbeing and health, such as human security (Gbla 2007). This may be a general weakness of recent post-conflict reconstruction models and a general lesson to take away from the Ebola epidemic.

At the end of the war in 2002 the International Military Assistance Training Team (IMATT) of 115 UK armed forces personnel was established to assist the transformation of the Sierra Leone Army into a modern army (Amos 2011). The Office of National Security (ONS) was created under the Office of the President, on the model of the UK government's crisis management facility (often known as COBRA).[20] Yet, the state emergency management capacity that donors (led by the UK) sought to create in the war's aftermath did not materialize. The EVD response was instead initially directed by the Ministry of Health and Sanitation (MoHS), which received much criticism for its approach: underplaying the outbreak and blaming health care staff transmission on sexual relations. This led to the replacement of the Minister of Health and Sanitation and other top officials on August 29, 2014, and the creation of the new National Ebola Response Center (NERC) to coordinate efforts, under the leadership of the Minister of Defense with technical support from the UN and the UK.[21] Political influence had enabled the Minister of Health and Sanitation to ignore the existing national crisis architecture and create a new one that did not work. This led to an ineffective and slow response as well as financial losses, showing up the weakness of institutional and security sector reform that was only as deep as the paper on which it was printed.

A security sector network was also developed by NGOs in the post-war period, the West Africa Early Warning and Early Response

Network (WARN), by the West Africa Network for Peacebuilding (WANEP) in cooperation with a regional inter-governmental body, the Economic Community of West African States (ECOWAS). It also appears not to have been used effectively to help contain the epidemic or rather, not effectively re-purposed from a focus on political incidents with potential consequences for national stability, to epidemiological monitoring. In Nigeria, polio tracking technologies were used successfully to track and trace contacts of known EVD cases in real time, using GPS and mobile phone technology to break chains of transmission (WHO situation assessment October 20, 2014). However, my previous research indicates that there are reasons to be skeptical that security sector networks were ready for dual use in analogous ways: they are aimed at identification and containment of incidents that could become politicized and are a lot less fine grained and technologically advanced, lacking in tracing capacity.

After an initially slow response, the UK announced a large-scale intervention in September 2014. Although led by Public Health England, it depended on the construction by the UK Ministry of Defence (MOD) of the medical facilities for 700 additional beds in an operation codenamed "Gritrock." These beds would then be staffed by NGOs, so-called "implementing partners,"[22] whose apparent unreadiness led to much criticism in Sierra Leone. For instance, only 11 beds were operational by the end of November 2014 at Kerry Town Centre, the flagship facility run by Save the Children, and full capacity not reached until later in 2015. NGOs provided a large, and well-publicized, share of EVD care in Sierra Leone. Médecins Sans Frontières (MSF) alone managed around 40 percent of available beds at the end of 2014, compared with the less publicized 50 percent run by the Sierra Leonean Ministry of Health and Armed Forces, with some support from international agencies and governments like the UK, China, and Cuba (see MSF Briefing Paper December 2014). Many smaller NGOs also tried to help, which in turn caused coordination difficulties (see Ebola Partners Operational Plan, UNICEF, and Sierra Leone Ministry of Health and Sanitation 2014).

The providers of EVD care operated on an unequal playing field. Sierra Leonean health staff who provided the majority of care worked under poorer conditions, for longer hours, and with more basic safety equipment, and without being formally entitled to (and initially without receiving) the same standards of care as the foreign staff when they fell ill. Foreign staff were initially all evacuated to more advanced facilities abroad when they showed symptoms. However, by the end of 2014, the UK MOD had set up a special 12-bed facility at Kerry Town intended for UK and international health care workers and Sierra Leonean health care professionals working in UK-sponsored facilities, which they ran themselves, where in practice no Sierra Leonean health care professionals were turned away. Yet the willingness of Sierra Leonean health care staff to use this facility was severely compromised by negative perceptions of the UK MOD and by persistent rumors.

The US Center for Disease Control and Prevention (CDC) has been running a research program on another viral haemorrhagic disease, Lassa fever, in Sierra Leone since the mid-1970s. Kenema is an area with the highest incidence of Lassa fever in the world and it also became one of the earliest epicenters of the EVD in Sierra Leone. The fact that Kenema Hospital was close to this epicenter and also contained both a world-class research facility working on a haemorrhagic fever and an appalling public hospital wing, quickly gave rise to conspiracy theories that Ebola was a manufactured disease deliberately let loose on the population by local and international elites for medical testing purposes and to garner funds. (See Chapter 2 by Bah and Chapter 3 by Barry in this volume.) For decades the facility had demonstrated very visibly how the interests of the international public health community, in this case research, were prioritized rather than the wellbeing of local people. The government's decision to make this hospital its regional Ebola hospital also made it highly vulnerable, since it had extremely poor infection control routines, despite the haemorrhagic fever research and treatment experience. As Bausch (2015a), a key researcher working in Kenema with the World Health Organization during this period, points out: "24 (89%) of 27 health care workers working in the Ebola ward in Kenema have contracted Ebola virus, 19 of them fatally (case fatality rate = 80%), revealing the dismal state of infection prevention and control (IPC) at Kenema Government Hospital." In total 37 staff members died.

At the moment of writing, 11 Sierra Leonean doctors and 40 registered nurses had succumbed to the disease.[23] Before the outbreak, Sierra Leone, with a population of over six million people, was being served by approximately 100 doctors and fewer than 1,000 registered nurses and 100 midwives.[24] The vast majority of these health care workers were concentrated in the Western Area, in and around the capital, rather than the rural provinces (MoHS 2009). The issue of trust being undermined by not simply bad provision or a lack of development but by visible inequities in the allocation of resources in favor of external priorities such as medical research rather than local health care is central here. Disingenuous rhetoric, failed development, and even projects that are successful according to external priorities in the context of poverty and the widespread failures of projects that would have had more of an impact on ordinary people's lives threaten attempts to address public health weaknesses in fundamental ways.

There is already good evidence that more people have died as a result of excess morbidity from other diseases than from Ebola as a result of the epidemic: this is partly due to a loss of capacity and of scarce resources having been diverted from general health care, but even more dramatic has been the loss of trust. A careful situation analysis and population health needs assessment of Moyamba District shows a sharp increase in mortality affecting the prevention of death from curable diseases especially in maternity care and for young children:

> The data collected at individual health facilities for the period of the Ebola outbreak and the equivalent period the year before illustrate marked declines in overall attendance (by up to 73%), attendances for antenatal care (by 50%), deliveries (by 44%), paediatric admissions (by 75%), paediatric malaria admissions (by 80%), child health clinics, and general outpatient consultations (by over 50%), and also a reduction in vaccination coverage. Analysis of burial data indicates that *as many deaths were recorded in four months in Moyamba than in previous one year periods*. Forty percent of those dying at the current time are children under the age of five years. (Elston 2015, 1; emphasis in the original)

The breakdown of trust in Sierra Leonean health care provision is killing the country's children as people make the entirely rational but dangerous decision to stay away from facilities that were little more than death traps during the epidemic, due to nosocomial transmission (Kilmarx et al. 2014). The closure of schools for nine months has also affected teenage pregnancy rates, with an estimated increase of 25 percent, and led to an increase in STDs (Elston 2015, 3; Risso-Gill and Finnegan 2015). In a general sense, the devastating after-effects of the Ebola epidemic are the real-life manifestations of theoretical development studies debates. However, the context makes them unusually lethal; when most development projects go wrong they tend to "fail to complete," running out of funding. In the fast moving situation of the Ebola epidemic and its aftermath, which played out in the lean season before new crops were harvested when the rain also raised the disease burden of the ever-present malaria, policy and operational mistakes were counted in preventable deaths.

Securitization as another form of violence

Sierra Leone's health system has been portrayed as the failing link within a securitized global health response system; in the words of Anne Roemer-Mahler: "When it comes to the threat of lethal infectious diseases, the world is only as secure as its weakest link" (2015, 3). While this is doubtlessly true from a global containment perspective, when it comes to reducing the security threats and forms of violence experienced by those at the sharp end of the epidemic outbreak, everyday Sierra Leonean citizens, forms of securitizing discourses are not likely to be locally beneficial. I have sought to show how abstract academic analyses based on theories of structural violence can serve to obscure the issues at hand as much as clarify them, and how past forms of development intervention as security sector reform failed to protect Sierra Leone from the epidemic. There are also dangers associated with the way that the global response, when it finally came in the summer of 2014, was securitized and highly militarized, in a context of historical insecurity. In early September, US President Barack Obama described Ebola as a "global security threat with profound political, economic and security implications for all of us"; indeed a US "national security priority"[25] and the UN Security Council declared the Ebola outbreak in West Africa a threat to peace and security[26] soon thereafter. By the time the international community woke up to the crisis, EVD had reached the point of exponential growth, and the rapid deployment and logistical capabilities of the military seemed desirable.

Within the aid community, the humanitarian arm is historically particularly resistant to the threat of militarization – wary of association with military missions that would jeopardize their perceived neutrality and hence their ability to work in conflict zones and other complex emergencies. However, in recent years they have also been the types of organizations that have most needed military assistance in precisely these environments. The UK development community is also understandably wary of the militarization of aid for the entirely practical reason that the budget of the Department for International Development (DfID) has been ring-fenced whereas the Department of Defence's budget has not, since the Conservative government came to power in 2010, leading to the suspicion that military objectives and personnel may seek to dip into the development pot.

The EVD epidemic caused a number of changes in this relationship. From the start NGOs were amongst the most prominent actors, with MSF taking a leading role in calling attention to the outbreak, calls that their government and international partners ignored for a long time until the scale of the crisis became such that they begged for military intervention as the only partners they could conceive of with the logistical capacity to turn the tide.[27] Previous to the outbreak MSF were one of the humanitarian NGOs that would often be used as an example of an organization keen to keep its distance from the military; now they had to learn to cooperate closely with military partners. The UK mission announced in September 2014 was spearheaded by the MOD. As the MSF had pointed out, they had the logistical airlift capacity and biohazard response capabilities that civilian actors lacked, and they were also experts in crisis response. As one senior officer told me: "We found that doctors can't run a crisis response. We are still suffering from that early failure" (November 6, 2014).

The 104 Logistics Support Brigade arrived ahead of the DfID counterpart and established the Joint Inter-Agency Task Force Headquarters (JIATF HQ). The Army also sent the 22 and 34 Field Hospitals and the 5 Armoured Medical Regiment as well as the 170 Infrastructure Support Group. The Royal Air Force contributed a large transportation aircraft (the Boeing C-17A Globemaster III) that brought the first personnel and materials at the start of October. The Royal Navy contributed the RFA Argus, a large vessel to be used as a base, with hospital and aircraft carrying capacity and three Merlin helicopters. The latter enabled the Sierra Leonean President, Ernest Bai Koroma, who worked closely with the UK Joint Commander

Military Component, to visit the rural areas worst affected by the epidemic personally. (The Irish Defence Forces and the Canadian Armed Forces also provided Medical Units.)

The US response to Ebola in Liberia was even more militarized than the UK's efforts, with a larger contingent of troops who were more visibly at the forefront of delivery, although they also worked closely with NGOs and Liberian government partners. Obama had pledged 3,000 troops; in the end the deployment peaked at 2,800, of mostly reservists. This military contingent was complimented by the technical expertise of CDC and USAID staff, and they worked with the Liberian government, and with Liberian and international NGOs (White House 2015). The US Department of Defense (DoD) directly built ten of the 15 Ebola Treatment Units constructed as part of the response and in addition, like the UK MOD, a specialist unit for treatment of Ebola-infected health care workers, the Monrovia Medical Unit (MMU), which was staffed by the US Public Health Service Commissioned Corps (White House 2015).

The French response had to be less visibly dependent on its military component given the sensitivities of the difficult post-colonial relationship between Guinea and France. Despite the smaller number of army personnel deployed, the French Ministry of Defense played an important part. Its Military Health Service trained local health workers in cooperation with the Guinean Military Health Service at the Manéah site (in the suburbs of Conakry), while French health workers prepared for deployment to the Ebola Treatment Centers at the civil security unit in Nogent-le-Rotrou (150 km west of Paris). Like the UK MOD the French Ministry of Defense also set up a dedicated medical center for the treatment of health workers combating the epidemic in Guinea under their own management (staffed with over 110 soldiers, mainly from the Military Health Service).[28]

The EVD response not only depended on the military, it was also militarized in terms of the language used. Little heed seemed to be paid to the obvious downsides of this approach to "combating" the disease. Movement in and out of the affected countries became severely restricted, hindering the relief effort as well as general economic activity, and their nationals stigmatized, which was demeaning as well as impractical. As Benton and Dionne put it: "Western governments' designation of the Ebola crisis as a crisis of security for the West … seemed to put Africans who were ill or dying in the same category as politically motivated terrorists" (2015, 223). Although there was an important awareness-raising component to the response, which changed dangerous behaviors and may have turned the tide (for parallels with Liberia see also Nyenswah et al. 2016) the medical care on offer to those suspected of having the disease was forceful, and intimidating, and nosocomial transmission for a long time rendered hospital care a dangerous proposition. The broad coalition made up of Sierra Leone government agencies, international partners including the UK military, and NGOs needed to fight the disease nevertheless reinforced existing power inequalities and struggled to be perceived positively.

I have outlined how lack of trust in the health system killed more Sierra Leoneans than EVD (Elston 2015), the reluctance of even qualified Sierra Leonean health staff to undergo treatment at the UK MOD Kerry Town medical facilities, and how rumors portraying Ebola as a deliberately imported and propagated disease associated with external agents and elites gained credibility from the mismatch between their concerns and local priorities. The war has left a legacy of fear, suspicion, and unresolved tensions. An example of these tensions includes people's sensitivity to sudden loud noises, which led to hostility between local communities and the drivers of Ebola ambulances who would not turn off their sirens when traveling in the countryside on bad, and therefore slow, roads.[29]

There are also legal objections to the prominent role in humanitarian assistance missions played by the UK Armed Forces in recent years, including for example during Typhoon Haiyan in the Philippines (Operation Patwin), which make this trend a matter of internal as well as external controversy within the UK MOD. The Oslo Guidelines supplementing the Geneva Accords state that military resources should be used only in the last resort, if there are no other available civilian options.[30] Such doubts, taken together, add up to grave concerns in the academic community over the potentially counter-productive consequences of the militarization of relief assistance. Risks include more autocratic government, empowered by emergency legislation and funding, and a continued misplaced emphasis by donors on security sector reform and strengthening.

Given that perfectly rational suspiciousness brought about by heavy handed Ebola interventions by the state and its external partners, and dangerous compulsory hospital care, constitute a real and present form of harm there is an acute need to rebuild trust. While human security could be one way of introducing a more holistic perspective including health and other aspects of wellbeing that would fit within the current frames of analysis, academics should be aware that all forms of securitized discourses privilege "hammer versus nails" approaches by emphasizing compulsion and force. Even the structural violence approach suffers from this weakness. Although it starts out with the basic recognition of our indisputable equal human worth, and of the historical injustices that have produced a situation where the life chances of some are radically worse than others, this recognition does not in and of itself provide an answer as to how to change the status quo. As often observed, rights are only enforceable if there are matching obligations on a system to provide them. Currently there is no such global system and no indication that countries with the resources to underwrite such claims would do so. They do not accept the responsibility for one human being to help another as incontrovertible fact, nor that they have an historical obligation to do so because of past injustices and current righteous anger.

A strength of non-securitized development approaches, reflected in both Duffield's and Sen's writings, is their insistence on a welfare-oriented approach to human suffering, even when it reaches the level of an acute humanitarian emergency. By making welfare their focus, approaches such as those seeking the expansion of human capabilities provide ways of arguing for and acting in the interests of solidarity without universal agreement, without the scaremongering that dehumanizes victims of disease. Trust is a two-way relationship, which has to start with those seeking to govern Sierra Leoneans, nationally and internationally, investing more trust in them. This will lead to a situation where Sierra Leoneans can input their priorities and concern and help develop systems that are useful to them. Why not seek to build on the aspects of Sierra Leonean national identity that its citizens are consistently proud of, like a history of educational achievement, which includes their ownership of the first Western-style university in sub-Saharan Africa, and Pan African and South-to-South links and intellectual thought (Paracka, 2003), to inspire public debate about the best ways to strengthen emergency responses as well as provision of routine health and welfare?

Conclusion

The EVD epidemic of 2014–2015 was an unanticipated threat to Sierra Leone, where the disease was previously unknown. Yet it was the weaknesses of the response that turned the outbreak into an epidemic reflecting old, foreseeable problems. There were continuities with the everyday challenges of politics and development and some of these were legacies of the post-conflict choices by donors as well as politicians to prioritize national security over individual wellbeing. With the populations of Sierra Leone, Liberia, and Guinea in effect uninsured, these development strategies gambled on raising the countries to middle income status through economic development before any disaster struck. This gamble turned out to be misplaced as Ebola precipitated a humanitarian disaster. Once the health emergency became a threat to global security the large-scale interventions led by the UK, the US, and France in the affected countries were again military in nature, cementing the prioritization that had contributed to the problem in the first place.

The question now is whether that fundamental problem, of the lack of a basic safety net, will be addressed? Without the mining income, economic development will stall even if the affected countries overcome some of the setbacks caused by the EVD crisis. As Thornhill (2014) puts it in the context of Liberia: like the trodden-upon dust in Maya Angelou's poem, Liberians will always rise. But why should they have to? Why shouldn't their lives simply be tolerable?

Specific funds flooded in to deal with the emergency in the second half of 2014, but such flows have now dried up and most of the infrastructure created was temporary or impossible to repurpose. There are some additional funds and an extension of credit from the IMF (2015), but calls for economic reparations to address historical injustices of structural violence are unlikely to succeed, whatever their moral merits. If a focus on structural violence serves to maintain a development discourse of security and threats then the potentially counter-productive consequences could include more autocratic government, empowered by emergency legislation and funding. It could also foster a misplaced emphasis by donors on security sector reform and strengthening. Instead, the focus should be on rebuilding trust and improving existing welfare systems, which can both be achieved by prioritizing the input of the population who are its intended users. The priorities, perspectives, and wellbeing of the Sierra Leonean population must be given primacy in the aftermath of the EVD epidemic.

Notes

1 The Sierra Leonean governance system is mixed: the country is divided into three Provinces (Eastern, Northern, Southern) and the Western Area, which is the former Crown Colony of Freetown and its surrounds. The next administrative level is the 14 Districts with directly elected councils (who also, with the exception of the two districts of the Western Area, send their 12 elected paramount chiefs, to parliament) and then the 149 chiefdoms. Until 2004 when a World Bank sponsored program re-established elected Local Councils at this level, the chieftaincy was the main form of local governance in the rural areas and it remains strong (Reed and Robinson 2013). One hundred and twelve parallel electoral constituencies, based on resident numbers and sometimes made up of more than one chiefdom, each elect one MP to parliament.

2 All health care statistics presented here are from the WHO Global Health Observatory Data Repository, http://apps.who.int/gho/data/node.main.475?lang=en (last accessed September 26, 2016).

3 The WHO defines out-of-pocket expenditure as any direct outlay by households, including gratuities and in-kind payments, to health practitioners and suppliers of pharmaceuticals, therapeutic appliances, and other goods and services whose primary intent is to contribute to the restoration or enhancement of the health status of individuals or population groups. It is a part of private health expenditure.

4 Nussbaum (2000) outlines ten capabilities that all democracies should support for their citizens. The first and second of these, life (in the sense of being able to live to a normal life-span) and bodily health, obviously fell short.

5 China has increased its political standing through humanitarian support during the crisis. Like the UK, China has focused its efforts on building treatment facilities, but it has also sent medical teams, and its emergency aid has been worth a total of 700 million yuan (around 112.2 million US dollars), according to official Chinese sources, see http://www.xinhuanet.com/english/special/ebola/.

6 See WHO, http://www.who.int/features/2014/cuban-ebola-team/en/.

7 For more on Kenya's role in this AU-led mission see, for example, http://news.xinhuanet.com/english/africa/2014-12/17/c_133862211.htm.

8 See http://www.huffingtonpost.com/jeffrey-sachs/a-call-to-scale-up-commun_b_7584724.html.

9 Sierra Leone 2004 Population Census, http://www.sierra-leone.org/Census/ssl_final_results.pdf (last accessed September 26, 2016).

10 See World Bank data: http://data.worldbank.org/country/sierra-leone (last accessed September 26, 2016).

11 Prices went from $190 per ton in 2011 to around $60 per ton at the time of writing. See International Monetary Fund Country Report no. 15/76, March 2015, *Sierra Leone: Second Review under the Extended Credit Facility Arrangement and Financing Assurance Review, and Requests for Augmentation of Access under the Extended Credit Facility and Debt Relief under the Catastrophe Containment and Relief Trust – Staff Report, Press Release and Statement by*

the Executive Director for Sierra Leone, 4. Available at: http://www.imf.org/external/pubs/ft/scr/2015/cr1576.pdf.

12 See World Bank data: http://data.worldbank.org/country/sierra-leone (last accessed September 26, 2016).

13 See World Bank, "Update on the Economic Impact of the 2014 Ebola Epidemic on Liberia, Sierra Leone, and Guinea," December 2, 2014, http://www.worldbank.org/content/dam/Worldbank/document/Economic%20Impact%20Ebola%20Update%202%20Dec%202014.pdf.

14 IMF Country Report no. 15/323, November 2015, http://www.imf.org/external/pubs/ft/scr/2015/cr15323.pdf.

15 First one of the two iron ore mining companies, London Mining, a major employer in Marampa, was bankrupted by the twin pressures of Ebola-related closures and the low international price of steel, and then the other operator, African Minerals, who initially took over London Mining via a company owned by its chairman, shut its operations in Tonkolili in November 2014, finally going in to administration in March 2015 after failing to repay its partner, China's Shandong Iron and Steel Group (IMF 2015). Shandong then acquired the remaining 75 percent that it did not already own, pledging to invest and restart production. Production of iron ore restarted in 2016.

16 See "KPMG Pulls Out of Management of Ebola Fund," http://www.salonepost.com/sp/news/articles/article200.asp.

17 http://www.ibtimes.com/ebola-outbreak-2014-ebola-riot-turns-deadly-sierra-leone-town-1709771.

18 See Amnesty International statement released on the May 4, 2015, *Sierra Leone: Ebola Regulations and Other Laws Must Not Be Used to Curtail Freedom of Expression and Assembly*, https://www.amnesty.org/en/articles/news/2015/05/sierra-leone-ebola-regulations-and-other-laws-must-not-be-used-to-curtail-freedom-of-expression-and-assembly/.

19 This strategy was initiated already in 1996 when the international community helped the country to organize elections through the UN, with the UK as the major donor. These elections severely complicated and disrupted the first peace process, which broke down leading to the war's first amputation campaign and another six years of conflict (Amos 2011).

20 Cabinet Office briefing room A.

21 See Awareness Times, http://news.sl/drwebsite/publish/article_200525604.shtml.

22 UK Government Press Release, September 17, 2014, https://www.gov.uk/government/news/uk-to-increase-support-to-sierra-leone-to-combat-ebola--2.

23 The Sierra Leonean doctors who died from the disease were Dr. Modupeh J.H. Cole, Dr. Sahr Jimmy Rogers, Dr. Olivette Buck, Dr. Godfrey George, Dr. Martin Salia, Dr. Michael Kargbo, Dr. Aiah Solomon Konoyeima, Dr. Dauda Koroma, Dr. Thomas T. Rogers, Dr. Victor Willoughby, and Dr. Sheik Humarr Khan. Dr. Songo Mbriwa, an army captain and the ninth doctor to be infected, was the sole survivor. See Sierra Leone's State House Communications Unit: http://www.statehouse.gov.sl/index.php/office-of-the-chief-of-staff/1405-president-honours-ebola-warriors, and Sierra Leone Nursing Association: http://www.sierraleonenursesassociation.org/.

24 The latest available official Sierra Leonean statistics are from the 2009 *National Health Strategic Plan 2010–2015*, and tally well with the disaggregated number of registered nurses and midwives available through the WHO (922 and 95 respectively) for 2010, see the Global Health Observatory

Data Repository, from which all subsequent healthcare statistics are drawn: http://apps.who.int/gho/data/node.main.475?lang=en (last accessed September 26, 2016).

25 See http://edition.cnn.com/2014/09/07/politics/ebola-national-security-obama/.

26 See UN News Centre: http://www.un.org/apps/news/story.asp?NewsID=48746#.VYvXI1L_qCo.

27 See address by Dr. Joanne Liu international president of Médecins sans Frontières (MSF) to the UN, September 2, 2014, reproduced in full: http://www.msf.org/article/msf-international-president-united-nations-special-briefing-ebola.

28 See http://www.diplomatie.gouv.fr/en/french-foreign-policy/health-education-gender/fight-against-the-ebola-epidemic/events/article/fight-against-the-ebola-epidemic-19978.

29 Personal communication, Paul Richards, February 25, 2015.

30 See *Guidelines on the Use of Foreign Military and Civil Defence Assets in Disaster Relief*, "Oslo Guidelines," available at: http://www.refworld.org/pdfid/47da87822.pdf.

References

Amos (née Jönsson), Julia (2009a). "The Overwhelming Minority: Inter-Ethnic Conflict in Ghana's Northern Region," *Journal of International Development*, 21, 4: 507–519.

Amos (née Jönsson), Julia (2009b). *Voices of Reason: A Ghanaian Practice-Based Vision of Peacebuilding*. CRISE Working Paper no. 68.

Amos, Julia (2011). "Non-Profits of Peace: Two West African Case Studies of Mediation by Conflict-Resolution NGOs." Doctoral thesis, University of Oxford.

Amos, Julia (forthcoming). "Narratives of Peace and Conflict: A Ghanaian Example of NGO Peacebuilding," *World Development* (forthcoming).

Batty, Fodei (2014). "Reinventing 'Others' in a Time of Ebola," Fieldsights – Hot Spots, *Cultural Anthropology Online*, October. http://www.culanth.org/fieldsights/589-reinventing-others-in-a-time-of-ebola.

Bausch, Daniel G. (2015a). "The Year That Ebola Virus Took over West Africa: Missed Opportunities for Prevention," *The American Journal of Tropical Medicine and Hygiene*, 92, 2: 229–232.

Bausch, Daniel G. (2015b). "Sequelae after Ebola Virus Disease: Even When It's Over It's Not Over," *The Lancet Infectious Diseases*, April. http://dx.doi.org/10.1016/S1473-3099(15)70165-9.

Benton, A. and Dionne, K.Y. (2015). "International Political Economy and the 2014 West African Ebola Outbreak," *African Studies Review*, 58, 1: 223–236.

Bolten, Catherine E. (2014). "Articulating the Invisible: Ebola beyond Witchcraft in Sierra Leone," *Fieldsights – Hot Spots, Cultural Anthropology Online, October. https://culanth.org/fieldsights/596-articulating-the-invisible-ebola-beyond-witchcraft-in-sierra-leone.*

Drèze, Jean and Sen, Amartya (1991). *Hunger and Public Action*. Oxford: Clarendon Press.

Duffield, Mark R. (2007). *Development, Security and Unending War: Governing the World of Peoples*. Cambridge: Polity.

Duffield, Mark (2008). "Global Civil War: The Non-Insured, International

Containment and Post-Interventionary Society," *Journal of Refugee Studies*, 21, 2: 145–165.
Elston, James (2015). *Beyond Ebola: Rebuilding Health Services in Moyamba, Sierra Leone: A Situational Analysis and Population Health Needs Assessment*. Doctors of the World/Médicos Del Mundo.
Farmer, Paul (2004). "An Anthropology of Structural Violence," *Current Anthropology*, 45, 3: 305–332
Farmer, Paul (2014). "Diary," *London Review of Books*, 36, 20: 38–39.
Ferguson, James (2006). *Global Shadows: Africa in the Neoliberal World Order*. Durham NC and London: Duke University Press.
Ferme, Mariane (2001). C. *The Underneath of Things: Violence, History, and the Everyday in Sierra Leone*. Berkeley, CA and London: University of California Press.
Ferme, Mariane C. (2014) "Hospital Diaries: Experiences with Public Health in Sierra Leone," *Cultural Anthropology*, October 7. http://www.culanth.org/fieldsights/591-hospital-diaries-experiences-with-public-health-in-sierra-leone.
Gbla, Osman (2007). "Security Sector Reform in Sierra Leone," in Len le Roux and Yemane Kidane (eds) *Challenges to Security Sector Reform in the Horn of Africa*. Pretoria, South Africa: Institute for Security Studies, 13–36.
IMF (2015). Country Report no. 15/323, November. http://www.imf.org/external/pubs/ft/scr/2015/cr15323.pdf.
Keen, David (1994). *The Benefits of Famine: A Political Economy of Famine and Relief in South-western Sudan, 1983–1989*. Princeton, NJ: Princeton University Press.
Keen, David (2005). *Conflict and Collusion in Sierra Leone*. Oxford and New York: James Currey and Palgrave.
Kilmarx, Peter H. et al (2014). "Ebola Virus Disease in Health Care Workers: Sierra Leone," *Morbidity and Mortality Weekly Report*, 63, 49: 1168–1171.
McGovern, Mike (2014). "Bushmeat and the Politics of Disgust," Fieldsights – Hot Spots, *Cultural Anthropology Online*, October. http://www.culanth.org/fieldsights/588-bushmeat-and-the-politics-of-disgust.
Médecins Sans Frontières (2014). *Ebola Response: Where Are We Now?* MSF Briefing Paper, December. MSF.
Ministry of Health and Sanitation (MoHS) (2009). *Sierra Leone. National Health Strategic Plan 2010–2015*. Freetown, Sierra Leone: Ministry of Health and Sanitation.
Moran, Mary and Hoffman, Daniel (2014). "Introduction: Ebola in Perspective," Fieldsights – Hot Spots, *Cultural Anthropology Online*, October. http://www.culanth.org/fieldsights/586-introduction-ebola-in-perspective.
Nussbaum, M. (2000). *Women and Human Development: The Capabilities Approach*. Cambridge: Cambridge University Press.
Nyenswah, T.G. et al. (2016). "Ebola and Its Control in Liberia, 2014–2015," *Emerging Infectious Diseases*, 22, 2 (February): 169–177.
Opala, Joseph A. (1994). "'Ecstatic Renovation!': Street Art. Celebrating Sierra Leone's 1992 Revolution," *African Affairs*, 93: 195–218.
Paracka, D.J. (2003). *The Athens of West Africa: A History of International Education at Fourah Bay College, Freetown, Sierra Leone*. New York and London: Routledge.
Reed, Tristan and Robinson, James (2013). "The Chiefdoms of Sierra

Leone." Manuscript, Harvard University. http://people.fas.harvard.edu/treed/history.pdf.

Richards, Paul and Mokuwa, Alfred (2014). "Village Funerals and the Spread of Ebola Virus Disease," Fieldsights – Hot Spots, *Cultural Anthropology Online*, October. http://www.culanth.org/fieldsights/590-village-funerals-and-the-spread-of-ebola-virus-disease.

Richards, Paul et al. (2015). "Social Pathways for Ebola Virus Disease in Rural Sierra Leone, and Some Implications for Containment," *PLoS Neglected Tropical Diseases*, 9, 4: e0003567.

Risso-Gill and Finnegan (2015). *Children Ebola Recovery Assessment: Sierra Leone*. Freetown: Save the Children, World Vision, Plan International.

Roemer-Mahler, Anne (2015). Global Governance and the Limits of Health Security. IDS Practice Paper in Brief no. 17, February. Institute of Development Studies.

Sen, Amartya (1981). *Poverty and Famines: An Essay on Entitlement and Deprivation*. Oxford: Clarendon Press.

Shaw, Rosalind (2002). *Memories of the Slave Trade: Ritual and Historical Imagination in Sierra Leone*. Chicago, IL: University of Chicago Press.

Thornhill, Kerrie (2014). "Academic Questions about the Ebola Crisis," *Democracy in Africa*, October. http://democracyinafrica.org/academic-questions-ebola-crisis/.

UNICEF and Sierra Leone Ministry of Health and Sanitation (2014). "Sierra Leone Ebola Partners Operational Plan: Who Is Doing What and Where."

Venkatapuram, Sridhar (2011). *Health Justice: An Argument from the Capabilities Approach*. Cambridge: Polity Press.

White House (2015). "Fact Sheet: Progress in Our Ebola Response at Home and Abroad," February. https://www.whitehouse.gov/the-press-office/2015/02/11/fact-sheet-progress-our-ebola-response-home-and-abroad.

7 | "I AM A WOMAN. HOW CAN I NOT HELP?": GENDER PERFORMANCE AND THE SPREAD OF EBOLA IN SIERRA LEONE

Aisha Fofana Ibrahim[1]

Introduction

The Ebola Virus Disease (EVD) epidemic is quintessentially the story of women's vulnerability, survival, and resilience in Sierra Leone. That Ebola started with, and has disproportionately affected women should come as no surprise in a society such as Sierra Leone where gendered structural inequalities limit women's well-being and where the primary role of caregiving, which often leaves women vulnerable to many ills, has culturally been made the purview of women. Women's gendered experiences may differ by class, geography, economic status, and individual histories but it is safe to say that they all experience some form of state-supported gender discrimination and exclusion that is manifested socially, politically, and economically in the ways in which the state deals with issues around women's education, economic empowerment, rape, spousal battery/domestic violence, sexual harassment among many other issues that specifically affect women. As such, it can be argued that the vulnerability of women and girls during the epidemic is integrally linked to underlying gender inequalities in productive resources, societal norms, and their limited ability to negotiate safer sex practices.

Gender roles, underlined by notions of masculinities and femininities, became central to the response to Ebola. Often, violence against women emerges from a rigid construct of masculinity and as Risman contends, "the cultural significance attached to male bodies signifies the capacity to dominate, to control, and to elicit deference and such expectations are perhaps at the core of what it means for men to do gender" (Risman 2004, 448). It can be argued that men and women were exposed to different forms of danger and risk-taking behaviors mainly because of gender norms. Men were expected and encouraged to be tracers, members of burial teams and vigilante groups because of their perceived strength and fearlessness, while women were expected to care for the sick. Women were thus disproportionately affected by the economic and social impact of Ebola not only because they were 51 percent of the population that succumbed to the disease but also because they had to take care of sick relatives, and become bread winners and sole providers for children when husbands succumbed to the disease or were unable to provide for the sustenance of their families. In many ways the role of men in fatherhood and caregiving is relegated to financial support of the family and as such "most men are still not morally responsible for the quality of family life, and women have yet to discover how to avoid being held responsible" (Risman 2004, 442). The assumption of women's responsibility for children, their disadvantaged position in the workforce, and their physical vulnerability to male violence all contribute to giving them little bargaining room when their (or their children's) interests conflict with those of the men they live with, thereby in turn worsening their position relative to that of men (Okin 1994, 16–17).

This chapter examines the gendered experience of women during the EVD outbreak and shows how gender norms ensure the maintenance of social order, sanction deviance from those norms and produce inequitable dynamics that are often risky for women and girls as well as for men and boys (Keleher and Franklin 2008). It also shows that women were not only victims but also active agents in the fight against EVD as they mobilized variedly at the community level as well as nationally to bring an end to the spread of the deadly disease. The chapter is anchored on findings from an Ipas supported study conducted by the Women's Response to Ebola in Sierra Leone Campaign (WRESL) on the impact of EVD on women and girls in which I served as lead researcher. WRESL, a coalition of over 22 women's organizations, was constituted in June 2014 out of the realization that EVD was affecting women differently and that something needed to be done about it.

The coalition wanted the discourse to move from that of women as victims to that of women as agents in the fight against the disease. Noticing that a gendered response was neither part of the state's national Ebola response plan nor part of its implementation strategy, the coalition decided to focus on ensuring that the gendered nature of EVD was taken into account at all levels in the fight against the deadly virus. They were able to do so through advocacy and the provision of goods and amenities such as hand-washing stations to women affected by EVD. WRESL advocated for data to be disaggregated by gender and age on suspected and infected persons, fatalities, and survivors in all Ministry of Health and Sanitation (MoHS) Reports and Updates in order to identify and document the differences in gender roles, activities, needs, and opportunities for both men and women; for quarantined homes to be provided with not just food and water but also fuel for cooking, sanitary pads, and laundry and cleaning supplies, because women would have been under undue stress in the performance of their domestic duties; for the provision of alternative learning opportunities for students during the prolonged closure of schools because the probability of out-of-school girls falling pregnant was very high.

This study was conducted in eight of the hardest hit districts, with a focus on two of the most affected chiefdoms in each of these districts.[2] Informed by feminist epistemology and methodology, the study involved the use of interviews, focus group discussions, and a survey. A total of 1,317 people participated in the study: 661 took part in a survey, 512 in focus group discussions, 144 individuals were interviewed using a semi-structured interview approach. In each district, a total of 18 individual semi-structured interviews were conducted, comprising six women/girl survivors, six women community leaders (an organization leader, Sowei/Traditional Birth Attendant [TBA], and Mammy Queen), and six stakeholders (district task force Chief, councilor, teacher, health care worker, member of parliament, and religious leader). Eight focus group discussions were conducted in each district comprising eight people per group (traders, pregnant/lactating mothers, young women, farmers, security sector personnel, nurses, bike riders, media practitioners). Ten "her" stories were also recorded from women/girl EVD survivors in each district. Findings from this study indicate that women were disproportionately affected by EVD mainly because of structural inequalities they faced at all levels of society, and which is also closely tied to their role as caregivers.

The state, women, and gendered inequality in Sierra Leone

Even though Sierra Leone's rating on the UNDP Human Development Index (HDI) had moved by 1.28 percent between 1980 and 2014, it was still within the low human development category with a 0.143 index in 2014 and ranking 181 out of 188 countries. In terms of inequality, the HDI fell to 0.241 percent and in relation to the Gender Inequality Index (GII), which measures gender inequality in health, education, and command over resources, Sierra Leone scored 0.814 with 0.370 for females as opposed to 0.454 for males (UNDP 2016).

Women constitute nearly 51 percent of the population in Sierra Leone, but only receive 79.7 percent of what their male counterparts enjoy in education, health, and income.[3] The GII of 2014 ranked Sierra Leone 145 out of 188 countries in terms of attainment of the targets set out in the ranking system. The GII reflected gender-based inequalities in three areas, namely reproductive health, empowerment, and economic activity.[4] Successive governments have tried to support women's advancement but women still do not enjoy full gender equality in access to resources, representation, and power. The reasons for this include conflicting government policies, the deep-seated patriarchal attitude of male child preference, the continued practice of female genital mutilation (FGM), which many see as subordinating women and young girls in society, and the existence of discriminatory laws on inheritance and land tenure outside Freetown, the capital city. Also impeding gender equality are some legal statutes and portions of the 1991 Sierra Leone Constitution. For example, Section 8 of the Chieftaincy Act of 2009, provides legal backing to discriminatory customs and traditions; Section 7 of the Citizenship (Amendment) Act of 2006 allows for discrimination against women on issues of nationality; whilst Articles 27(d) and (e) of the 1991 Constitution of Sierra Leone makes provision for discriminatory legislation against women under certain circumstances.[5]

Official state policy and outmoded cultural practices have severely limited women's educational opportunities, resulting in high illiteracy levels, and a lack of qualifications and skills that can be used in the formal economy. As of 2015, the literacy rate for females aged 51 years and above in Sierra Leone was 38 percent, while the overall national literacy rate was 48 percent.[6] The number of women in leadership positions is small. Currently, there are only 14 women in a parliament of 124 and only five cabinet and seven deputy ministers out of 50 ministerial positions. Fewer women can also be found as heads of public and private institutions, or in senior management as members of boards or chairpersons of boards of directors. This can be attributed to a number of factors including: traditional cultural beliefs and practices bar women from taking part in decision-making and other forms of public participation; lack of political will; and resistance to the empowerment of women through education. Education for women and girls has often been hindered by early marriage, teenage pregnancy, and male child preference in many rural communities of the country. In essence, even though Sierra Leonean women make up over 60 percent of the labor force, as either farmers and/or petty traders, they have limited access to both material and financial resources and live below the poverty level.

Studies have shown that the level of education, choice, and agency of women can influence women's health outcomes as well as those of their children (World Bank 2011). The level of education of a woman can have a great impact on their mortality, as well as on those of their children (Kanu et al. 2014). With over 50 percent of women of childbearing age in Sierra Leone being illiterate, it is no wonder that the country has such high rates of infant and maternal mortality. The state's policy on free primary education for all, plus three years of junior secondary school education for girls, has made little or no difference in changing the educational status of girls and women in rural areas. Many see the free education as paradoxical because the cost of keeping a child in school – books, uniforms, lunch, and transportation – is much more than the free tuition being offered by the state. As such, where people have to make the hard decision of which children to send to school, girls are often not the preferred choice. Coupled with this male preference is the low quality of education in state-run schools especially in rural communities. Support from the state for these schools is meager and they are often ill equipped and staffed by unqualified teachers.

Even though many policy instruments geared towards the advancement and empowerment of women have been adopted over the years, the lives of women have not changed significantly partly because of lack of implementation, especially in the areas of monitoring and evaluation.[7] However, in spite of insurmountable challenges, women continue to advocate for gender equality and women's empowerment at all levels of society. As has been documented, women played an active role in the peace processes that ended the Sierra Leone civil war and have, since post-war, continued to push for the consolidation of peace and the creation of gender-sensitive laws and policies (Jusu-Sheriff 2000; Day 2008; Abdullah and Ibrahim 2010; Ibrahim 2015). Women's activism was apparent in the fight against EVD in which they mobilized not only to sensitize but also to provide material support for victims of the disease.

Women's health and the culture of care Over the years, Sierra Leone has earned the unenviable reputation of being one of the worst places to be a mother because of its high maternal mortality rate.[8] For the majority of women, deterrents for seeking help at health facilities include: obtaining permission from husbands to seek medical help, the cost of health care, the distance to medical facilities, transportation, and lack of trust in public health facilities that are usually understaffed and have a limited amount of drugs. The introduction in 2010 of the government's Free Health Care Initiative (FHCI) for pregnant and lactating mothers, as well as children under five years, saw increased access to maternal and reproductive health care and a reduction in maternal mortality on the eve of the EVD. The EVD outbreak, however, exposed the inadequacies of the health care system including women's access to sexual and reproductive health services. On the eve of the EVD outbreak the country could only boast of 136 medical doctors and 1,017 nurses and midwives (Wright and Hanna 2015).

Women are responsible for providing care not only for their children but also for the community at large. In communities with limited access to health care, women become the sole providers of health care services for their families. The fact that traditional African models of society have been shaped by rigid gender relations prevents many women from questioning their expected role of caregivers even when it makes them vulnerable and susceptible to ill health. As Judith Butler writes

> I think for a woman to identify as a woman *is* a culturally enforced effect. I don't think that it's a given that on the basis of a given anatomy, an identification will follow. I think that "coherent identification" has to be cultivated, policed, and enforced; and that the violation of that has to be punished, usually through shame. (Kotz 1992)

This is clearly manifested in the experiences of many women who had to take care of sick family members and relatives because they were expected to do so.

Feminists have differed on their stance on the theoretical debate around nature versus nurture. Some have argued that attributes such as nurturance constitute a feminine "essence," while others postulate that the only differences between men and women, that are not strictly biological, are mainly products of culture and history, and therefore socially constructed. In essence, the social construction of women's lives reflects their broader engagement with a gendered social system, which influences both individual-level risks and social and economic vulnerabilities to communicable and contagious diseases. It is therefore not surprising that the first person in Sierra Leone assumed to have contracted and spread the EVD was a female traditional healer who had crossed the border to neighboring Guinea to provide care for some sick relatives. As a healer, this woman provided not only consultation services for her sick relatives but also physically took care of her relatives for an illness with familiar symptoms and unpredictable consequences.

The traditional responsibility of women in performing rituals of birth and death and being primary care givers in the home, community, and health centers contributed adversely to their high infection rate during the EVD epidemic. Women were dominant in all aspects of the health system in both low-tier positions such as cleaners and birth attendants as well as the better paying positions of nurses and health practitioners. They were most vulnerable to infection in these positions given the lack of personal protective equipment (PPE) and their initial unfamiliarity with the disease and ways to halt EVD infection.

The closure of hospitals and community health clinics led to many health complications including Vesical Vaginal Fistula (VVF). The abandonment of pregnant women in some health centers led to prolonged labor, miscarriages, obstetric hemorrhage, and other complications. In many instances the "fear of transmission and stigma against potentially infected individuals at the community level made access to care for pregnant women even more difficult" (Menendez and Khatia 2015). Women were therefore left with the responsibility of providing antenatal and postnatal care in their communities. Thus a respondent poignantly recounted:

> A member of the community had returned home after spending a month with her grandmother in a hospital in one of the big towns. On her return, she complained about not feeling too good and was taken to a health center. While there, she had a miscarriage and was taken care of by her friend, the resident midwife in the clinic. After a lot of vomiting and running stomach, she passed away. No one suspected Ebola. When she died women in the community came together and performed expected funeral rites. A week or so later, the midwife and all those who took part in the burial ceremony started falling sick and dying. That was the start of Ebola in our community.

There is a pervasive sense of responsibility and obligation on women to take care of loved ones that are directly linked to gendered roles assigned by society. In addition, for the majority of women who live in rural areas, the rural–urban divide limits their access to information on health issues as well as knowledge on how to take control of their health. Like most people in the country, the women in this community had limited or no information on the symptoms of Ebola and how it is contracted. Interestingly, even when they had some information, their perceived role as women influenced their better judgment. According to an Ebola survivor:

> I suspected that my mother-in-law had Ebola but took care of her all the same. I am a woman, how can I see my loved ones suffering and not help? My husband and in-laws expected me to do my duty and I believe I had to do it. I would have been blacklisted in the community had I not done my duty.

As women put their lives at risk, they manifest what Butler describes as the repetitive performance of gender – the differentiating relations by which speaking subjects come into being. The women who put themselves at risk believe that caregiving is part of their being and therefore do not question the expectations of society. EVD is said to have a high case fatality rate (70 percent) and mostly affects people in the prime productive age, between 15 and 44 years of age. Nearly 57 percent of EVD cases were Sierra Leoneans within this age range.[9] Thus, young and healthy women who were obliged to provide care succumbed to the disease.

In a society where women's sexuality is constantly under surveillance and where they are expected to adhere to their partners' wishes, women's vulnerability to health complications related to sexual reproductive health was very much gendered. In Port Loko District, community respondents disclosed that contraception was seen as the woman's responsibility and men did not have to wear condoms. Not only does this have implications for women's own control over their reproductive cycle, but it also reflects a constrained ability to exercise their voice. Furthermore, it places women at greater risk of pregnancy and pregnancy-related complications and exposes them to the potential dangers of unsafe contraceptives.

With limited access to sexual reproductive health services, respondents indicated that many young women resorted to dangerous contraception and abortion practices. For example, women reverted to the use of TBAs who had been discouraged from attending to births under the Free Health Care initiative (FHCI), as they were seen as a potential source for the high mortality rate among pregnant women. The ban on TBAs failed to take cognizance of the significant gender role they play in society. On contraception, a respondent in Marampa chiefdom confessed:

> We used to have Marie Stopes in our community before Ebola. Though not every woman had access to the service, at least many did have access. Since Ebola we have not been able to go for our shots. I take my shots every six months and it is now due. I hear some of my colleagues have gone back to taking medicine from traditional birth attendants (TBAs). They either give a herb concoction or they give you a rope that you should tie around the waist. With the herbs, you are protected by the number of gulps you take. So if you take two gulps you will be protected from pregnancy for two months. With the rope, you are safe as long as you don't take it off. I also hear that some girls buy pills from "pepeh doctors" (drug peddlers).

According to another respondent in Masuba (Bombali):

> A lot of crazy things are going on. I know of someone in this village who tied bricks to her stomach and asked her friend to walk all over her stomach. She did abort but I think it's very

> dangerous. I hear a young woman in a village not far from here used ampiclox (antibiotics) to abort and another used some saline concoction to abort. There are also soweis who help young girls abort and they use a combination of herbs. There are also some nurses who are performing abortion in secrecy. They charge according to how far the pregnancy has gone. So if you are one month pregnant they ask you to pay Le100,000, if two months, it's 200,000, and so on.

Gender norms also create a dominant male masculinity that sustains male risk-taking behaviors, such as unsafe sexual practices, that impact on women as well as on men's vulnerability to morbidity and mortality. As such, structural factors such as masculine sexual privilege, expectations of female sexual passivity, and domestic violence exacerbate women's infection vulnerabilities. Thus, even though there is evidence of sexual transmission of Ebola after recovery from the disease, many women had no choice but to engage in sex with their partners. In many cases, refusing a spouse or boyfriend sex can result in physical, emotional, and/or economic abuse. Women are raised to not deny sex and in many cases are solely dependent on the man for their survival.

The traditional practice of polygamy does not help either. As women compete for the attention and support of a single man, they do all in their powers to outdo their co-wives. Thus, when one wife denies her spouse sex, he can always go to the other wife or wives. A number of female survivors interviewed indicated that they contracted the disease from their husbands who had refused to adhere to the prescribed 90 days of sexual abstinence after recovering from Ebola. A 22-year-old woman in Masuba recounted her experience:

> My husband left Mauban not feeling too well and came back after two months claiming that he had been working in Makeni and had been taken care of by my co-wife. He never contacted the kids and me since he left and I had the suspicion that he might have been in an Ebola treatment center. I had no proof and when I asked him he got so furious and threatened to go back to Makeni to my co-wife where he is appreciated. He forced me to have sex with him and a week later I became ill with Ebola.

The above respondent is in a relationship in which the man seems to have neither an obligation to explain to his wife his whereabouts nor the moral obligation to inform her that he is an EVD survivor. Instead, he uses his society-approved power to blackmail his wife and in the process demand sex. The power imbalance works at different levels in this scenario. The woman is young and married to an older man, already has a baby, and is not educated and not financially independent. To make matters worse, she lives in a community in which staying married and "respect" for the spouse is paramount. This respondent is in every way trying to comply with what she is expected to do not only as a woman but also as a much younger person in an unequal relationship. In most cases age and gender confer power on some over others. Her husband can go and come as he wishes, she can be left alone for long periods of time to raise their children; her husband is allowed to marry other women and to demand sex from his spouses but the respondent is expected to only perform the expected gender role of a dutiful wife. She performs gender even in the face of oppression. As Butler reiterates, "performativity has to do with repetition, very often the repetition of oppressive and painful gender norms ... This is not freedom, but a question of how to work the trap that one is inevitably in" (Lotz 1992).

Four women's voices: femininity as vulnerability and agency

The four testimonies presented below capture the real experiences of four female survivors: two from the original epicenters of Kailahun and Kenema in the eastern region of Sierra Leone, and two from the subsequent epicenters of Port Loko and Bombali in the northern region of the country. And all four testimonies demonstrate caregiving as integral to the pervasive performance of femininity in Sierra Leone: a disease engulfed a community and women were suddenly thrust into the frontline because of their culturally constructed roles as caregivers. Teneh in Bombali was summoned by her husband to provide care for her mother-in-law; Finda in Kailahun had to fulfill her familial "duty" to her mother who was sick with Ebola without her knowledge; Fatmata from Kenema contracted the virus from a sick visitor from the village who was under the care of her grandmother; and Yeabu from Port Loko took ill after being infected by a visiting brother who had contracted the disease. All were infected and recovered within three months after EVD officially became known in Sierra Leone.

These four testimonies in key areas of the country are arguably insufficient to warrant any hard and fast generalizations about how and why EVD engulfed the country within four months of its official discovery. Yet, they present us with a suitable point of departure to begin to think about the disease and the geography of death that it carved as well as its impact on the collective conscious of communities. Teneh had to be moved from one part of the country to another because there were no treatment centers in the north when she got infected. Her refusal to go to the nearest health center also raises fundamental questions about why the hospital, a site of treatment and potential healing, came to represent death in a time of crisis. Not only were some of the women afraid of seeking medical assistance when it was available, they were also unsure of its availability. Yeabu in Port Loko had to wait for an ambulance for eight days; Fatmata in Kenema and Teneh in Bombali were reluctant to seek medical assistance: one had to run away and hide while the other had to be convinced she would survive if she went to a treatment center. From reluctance to visit medical centers to dying while waiting for an ambulance to coming to terms with the prevalent belief that EVD was witchcraft, we begin to see multiple layers within which to make sense of the Ebola holocaust.

As these testimonies reveal, EVD was not just about catching a virus, being sick, and going to the hospital. EVD was also about trying to fathom the causes of your ailment, accessing the nearest health center, and finding the necessary support and resources to do so. It was about thinking of how the disease had affected a survivor's sense of self, their perceptions of how they are viewed by others, and how well they are able to reinsert themselves into their communities.

Tenneh Conteh, Bombali District My name is Teneh Conteh and I live at 14 Samuel Street, Teko, Makeni, Bombali District. I have a four-month old baby. One night my husband received a call from her sister informing him that his mother was sick. The next day, my husband told me to prepare light soup and take it to her (my mother-in-law), so I did. On the second day of her illness, I went to check on her and to assist her if needed. At this time, she was getting worse so I had to spend the rest of that day in her house. A nurse was called upon to examine her. I never knew that it was Ebola. The nurse gave her an IV fluid also not knowing that she had Ebola. Three days later, my mother-in law passed away. Immediately after this tragedy, I also started experiencing fever, diarrhea, and vomiting.

During the three-day shut down, the search and sensitization team came to our place but I was afraid to report myself; so I hid. Unfortunately, after the three-day exercise, my sickness became worse, so I finally reported myself to my uncle, a health worker, who called the ambulance and I was taken to the paramedical holding center. My blood sample was collected and the result came back positive. The next day in the early morning hours, I was told that I would be taken to Kailahun for intensive treatment. Upon hearing this, I started crying, thinking that I would never see my children again. But my uncle gave me words of encouragement and hope. He told me to have faith and that all is going to be well and nothing wrong is going to happen to me. I believed and trusted in God. We were seven in the ambulance and the journey was terrible for us. Sadly, one of us (a woman) died on the way to the Kailahun treatment center.

Upon our arrival at the Kailahun treatment center, we were received well, treated well until we were finally cured of the Ebola virus. In my family, we were seven in number who contracted the virus, painfully only two of us, a small boy, survived and myself. When I was discharged I was given a certificate and I was told by the medical practitioners that I must abstain from sexual activities for 90 days because they said the virus is very active in the vaginal fluid and semen and can be transferred to a sexual partner. So I did as I was told.

The same day, we returned home. Some of the community people received us well including the chief. A woman who is one of my neighbors, who used to plait my hair before I got sick, refused to do so after I came back from the treatment center. I have been having problems with my left eye and have visited the hospital for medicines to relieve the pain. I was given some eye drops. In addition to that, I am also experiencing pain in my knees and toes but I have no money to pay the hospital because all my property was burnt down and now I can't do any business. I used to sell food but people will not buy from me now and my husband has lost his job because he was taking care of the children when I was in the hospital. Please I'm asking anyone who has empathy to help us with medication and scholarship for our children and for me to engage in business to keep my family going.

Finda Hermore, Kailahun District I am Finda Hermore and from Buedu, Kissy Teng Chiefdom, Kailahun district. I am 14 years old and a JSS 3 student awaiting BECE[10] results. I don't remember when I was admitted to the treatment center as I was unconscious but I was discharged on July 11, 2014. I was infected by my sick mother for whom I was the caregiver. My duty as a daughter compelled me to do things for my mother because there was no one else to care for her. I did not know that my mother was Ebola positive. Other family members did not contract the disease.

Although everything was done at the treatment center to help me survive, I still remained discouraged. Later on I summed up courage and made up my mind to live again. This change in attitude greatly helped me to respond to treatment. However, I have been experiencing aches and pains since my discharge from the center.

The 90 days' abstinence rule for survivors is a valuable measure for preventing further infection but I think that the stigmatization of survivors needs to be discouraged.

I am now committed to advising people to continue to obey the rules for preventing Ebola. They should wash their hands frequently. As far as I am concerned, all the preventive measures should be sustained well beyond the Ebola outbreak.

Fatmata Koroma, Kenema District I am Fatmata Koroma and I am 16 years old. I live in Kenema. I am a seamstress and I attended school up to JSS 2. I was in hospital between June and August 2014. I contracted the disease through one of my aunt's relatives who came to our home from the village complaining of sickness. Little did we know that she was carrying the Ebola virus. My grandmother was directly responsible for treating her but we all lived in the same house. We did not report that our aunt was sick but the neighbors did so. By the time the ambulance arrived she had died. All of us ran away from our house out of fear of being taken away. While in hiding, many of us became ill. My parents died and four of my aunt's children also died. At this point I reported at the hospital and convinced my aunt to do the same. My aunt and I survived.

Before my admission, I experienced frequent bowel movements, weakness, body pain, loss of appetite, and vomiting. By the time I got to hospital I had rash all over my body and was bleeding from my nose. They began to give me a drip and I was advised to drink plenty of water. I did not eat well while in hospital but later regained my appetite after my discharge.

I was discharged from hospital on the day H.E. President Koroma visited Kenema hospital. I was given 60,000 Leones ($10). I decided to go to our village instead of staying in Kenema town. The villagers rejected us out of fear of being infected. I returned to Kenema and stayed with my aunt. I need assistance to buy a sewing machine so I will be in a better position to help my younger sisters who are attending school.

Yeabu Kanu, Port Loko District My name is Yeabu Kanu and I live at Petifu Bana, Buya Romenda Chiefdom, Port Loko District. I am 55 years old and I engage in petty trading and farming and never attended school. I was admitted on August 3, 2014 and discharged on September 5, 2014. The first I heard about the Ebola virus was that we were told that if this disease should come to our village we should not wash dead bodies, we should not visit or touch sick people and we should avoid body contact. I contracted the disease through my brother who was sick when I visited him in another village.

Initially we did not believe it was the Ebola virus because a lot of people in Komrabai village had confessed that a plane, associated with witchcraft, had crashed and that a lot of people would consequently die. As a result, when my elder brother became ill I thought he was among those who were on the plane. I became infected before he died. My children and mother were also infected through me.

My mother treated me with herbs in our village before I was taken to the holding center. I spent eight days in my village waiting for an ambulance to pick me up. A lot of people died within this period. I also spent another five days at the holding center where I was treated with few tablets and porridge with no proper care. The nurses were afraid of us and simply threw food at us. If you were not strong enough to walk and collect your own food you would starve. Things were different at the treatment center where I was given enough care, food, and medication.

When I returned home upon my discharge from the treatment center, my family received me well – they were very happy for me. The community and my friends treated me a little bit better but many people were afraid of me. I faced a lot of stigmatization. I am amongst the first people who contracted the Ebola virus disease in my community. We became part of the social mobilization team and we sensitized other communities and villages about the disease. Today I am happy because I survived but sad as well because I have lost my loved ones. I also have problems with my eyesight, since my discharge. I am afraid that if I remain ill, I will not be able to work or feed myself.

I would like to see greater support for survivors, improved access to health services, and I want everyone to adhere to the public health messages on infection prevention control. I would like to get a job so I can feed myself.

Stigmatization, exclusion, and exploitation: the struggle for dignity and livelihood after EVD

As women and girls dealt with relationship issues, they also had to, as EVD survivors or as members of households of EVD-affected persons, deal with stigmatization at both the inter-communal and intra-communal levels. Some households were helped by community members to fetch water, wood, and perform other chores that quarantine prevented them from doing while others did not get such support from members of their community. This kind of stigmatization and exclusion is a rarity in close-knit communities where social relations form the base of solidarities and function as the chief source of safety nets in the absence of a welfare state. This became a source of anguish for many women, as expressed by a respondent:

> I thank God for surviving Ebola but I will never forget how we were treated when we were in quarantine. I am really hurt and do not understand why the people in the house two doors from our house were helped and we were not. We lived in peace with all in this community but when our household was in quarantine we were discriminated against … no one came to help us fetch water, wood, or buy goods for us in the market. Twenty-two people died in our household and people go around saying we brought Ebola to this community. It is not fair.

Survivors were also stigmatized and accused of spreading the disease through sex and this has led to many single women being shunned by potential partners. The stigmatization of women in relation to spreading the disease is a continuum in the metaphor of women's bodies and sexuality as diseased. Medically, the Ebola virus is said to be active in the semen of men for 90 or more days after surviving Ebola but interestingly, female survivors are mostly being accused of spreading the disease through sex, a position that leaves them vulnerable to exploitation and abuse by men and women alike. Indeed, sexualization in patriarchal societies involves a loss of female power, autonomy, and efficiency, and an imposition of norms and restrictions that are internalized by both men and women (Lee and Sasser-Coen 1996).

Stigmatization also led to loss of income for many women. At the inter-communal level, people in quarantined communities faced stigmatization and exclusion from neighboring communities. This has had particularly adverse consequences on women due to their dependence on agriculture and trade for income generation. Women from EVD-affected communities were denied entry into EVD-free communities and prevented from selling their wares and farm produce in these communities, leaving many families desperate. Those who practiced trades such as hairdressing also lost their clientele and source of income.

Women's unequal access to and control over productive resources and their greater presence in economically risky activities such as petty trading contributed to their vulnerability during the EVD outbreak. As farmers, petty traders, and artisanal miners, the ban on trading and travel restrictions resulted in economic hardship in many surveyed communities. This is also true for women in service sector jobs such as catering, hairdressing, petty food distribution, and sex work, especially at the height of the EVD epidemic when physical contact was strongly discouraged and people were literally afraid to touch one another.

As primary providers of food for the family, the abandonment of farms meant that women could neither grow nor harvest their crops and therefore were unable to feed their families. In some cases, they could not take their farm and other goods to weekly markets because of the ban and in extreme cases because of stigmatization. There was a time when people refused to buy farm produce and cooked food from women from affected communities in the markets. The collapse of village savings and loan schemes due to the death of participants and the inability to repay microfinance loans worsened women's economic conditions. For many families, economic difficulties led to a reliance on children for economic assistance. Residents of nearly all communities in this study mentioned that poverty rates as well as school closures had affected "parent–child" relationships, leaving parents unwilling or unable to monitor their children. Some parents turned a blind eye to their children's commercial and sexual activities due to issues of poverty. This relaxation of discipline included allowing their school-going sons to become commercial bike riders and their daughters to co-habit or stay overnight with men who could afford to take care of them.

Economic hardship also left women and girls susceptible to sexual abuse or resorting to transactional sex, given the limited available options to secure their livelihood and that of their families. Respondents reported that the high incidence of poverty among girls made them particularly vulnerable to sexual violence and exploitation, and contributed to an increase in the already high pregnancy rate for teens. A witness revealed:

> We have over ten girls in this village who have become pregnant. This is the case in all the neighboring villages, some lost all adult family members and became the head of their households and have to fend for their younger siblings. They engage in sex for money or goods and end up pregnant … I think the closure of schools and lack of access to contraceptives also contributed to the high rate of teenage pregnancy.

The economic situation in the country has created a system in which many are chronically impoverished, while a few have sufficient financial resources. This creates a power dynamic in which the most vulnerable group, often women, become susceptible to exploitation and oppressive relationships. An increase in teenage pregnancy was reported across all communities, with the prevalent assumption that this was directly related to the twin issues of poverty and school closure. Transactional sex, often connected with poverty, has been an issue of concern in Sierra Leone and many other African countries. Many of the young women in our study who became pregnant before or during the EVD epidemic can attribute their pregnancies to transactional sex.

There is a plethora of studies that have examined why young girls and boys exchange sex for money and other gifts (Ankomah 1998; Longfield et al. 2002; Temin et al. 1999; Bledsoe 1990; Calves et al. 1996; Hulton et al. 2000; Nyanzi et al. 2001; Gregson et al. 2002; Meekers and Calves 1997). Reasons range from getting funds to cover education-related expenses, making connections for social networking and advancement, to peer pressure to acquire luxury items, such as expensive clothing, jewelry, cell-phones, fashionable hairstyles, accessories, and makeup. Interestingly, findings from these studies suggest parental pressure to engage in transactional sex is often implicit rather than explicit, and parents seek to obtain funds to finance their child's education-related expenses, luxury items, and necessities for the household (Chatterji et al. 2004). That some parents encouraged or turned a blind eye to the activities of their daughters even in the midst of a deadly epidemic such as EVD shows the value placed on women in Sierra Leone – how devalorization occurs through cultural scripts associated with femaleness and how women themselves have internalized this discourse. As Lee and Sasser-Coen assert, "the disciplinary practices of femininity, and the language, words, gestures used to describe women's bodies create the discourses of the body politic and structure our thinking, communicating, and acting" (Lee and Sasser-Coen 1996).

Conclusion

This chapter has tried to show how gender ideologies are inscribed into male and female subjectivities, traditional constructions of gender roles reinforce unequal power relations, and men's power within the family is often legitimized by highly patriarchal cultural norms.

Moreover, the myopic view that the spread of EVD was mainly because of backwardness, superstition, and ignorance clearly ignores the intricacies of the political economy of the spread and control of the disease. It fails to acknowledge other factors such as the lack of trust of citizens in the state and health care system, the element of fatalism, and the gender dynamics of the disease and its contagious effects (Batty 2014; Ferme 2014). The state's response to the epidemic was clearly manifested by the then Minister of Health, Miatta Kargbo, who while testifying to parliament on the uncontrollable spread of EVD on June 7, 2014, blamed it on ignorance of the people and their refusal to seek medical help. She further went on to blame two nurses who she claimed had contracted and spread the virus while engaged in promiscuous sex. Ms. Kargbo's testimony in parliament brought out two major issues. One was her inability to address the structural inequalities that contributed to the spread of the disease, especially the state's failure over time to invest in the health care system of the country, which culminated in an understaffed and underequipped and completely broken health care system. Thus for the majority of Sierra Leoneans, who are poor, and for the vast majority of women who are even poorer, the decision to seek help from broken public health facilities remains a problematic proposition.

The second issue was that of scapegoating – "the opportunity to reinvent others and blame them for the calamity" (Batty 2014). In this case, the minister blamed the female nurses, but not their male partners, for promiscuity and spread of the disease. This is very much in line with women's additional burden of blame for society's evils that goes back thousands of years. In most religious texts, the female is associated with sex and sin much more so than men. This cultural blame is so ingrained in the psyche of both men and women that it is not surprising to see the minister blame the nurses rather than their sex partners. Minister Kargbo reproduced the very discourse that subordinates women as second-class citizens in a context that doubly presents their oppression and exploitation as cultural – a product of a tradition invented by another to subject the other.

The EVD epidemic has affected Sierra Leoneans variedly. It is clear that structural factors such as poverty and cultural expectations, which place the burden of responsibility on women and girls for caring for the family, contributed to making them more vulnerable to the disease and therefore disproportionately affected.[11] Women will continue to suffer, post-EVD, if the structural and institutional barriers that impede their empowerment and full participation are not addressed. As it is, EVD survivors interviewed for this study experience weakness, dizziness, and giddiness, joint pains in the knees and limbs, back and side pains, and loss of/and reduced vision.

Emotional trauma was also widely reported, and survivors say they continue to experience different kinds of anxieties. They are plagued by sadness at the death of loved ones as well as their own experience of the harrowing disease. They also reported depression from the stigmatization faced on their return, financial ruin, and the lack of economic compensation from the government.

In a society where the literacy rate of women is below 40 percent and where the dropout rate of teenage girls is twice as high as those of boys, the banning of pregnant girls from returning to school and/or taking public exams that determine their entrance into high school or tertiary institutions is counterproductive. It will have a devastating impact on the development and empowerment of women and girls, ranging from high rates of maternal and infant mortality and morbidity, increased sexual and gender-based violence, low literacy levels, and low economic advancement. Disadvantaged culturally, socially, and economically, EVD has heightened women's vulnerability in a country whose post-Ebola economic prospects are still uncertain.

Notes

1 I would like to thank my fellow researchers on this project – Ms. Rosalyn McCarthy, Ms. Eileen Hanciles, Dr. Fredline MCormack-Hale and Ms. Finda Koroma – for their invaluable contributions to the project.

2 The study was conducted in Western Urban (Mount Aureol–Allen Town and Kroo Bay–Aberdeen), Western Rural (Waterloo and environs and Grafton to Funkia), Bo (Bompeh and Kakua chiefdoms), Moyamba (Lower Banta and Fakunya chiefdoms), Kenema (Lower Bambara and Nongowa chiefdoms), Kailahun (Kissi Teng and Jawei chiefdoms), Port Loko (Marampa and Buya Romende chiefdoms), Bombali (Bombali Sheborah and Makari Gbanti chiefdoms).

3 The provisional data from the 2014 Census shows that Sierra Leone's population grew 4,976,871 in 2004 to 7,075,641 in 2015, at an average annual growth rate of 3.2 percent. Females were 50.9 percent of the population, while males were 49.1 percent. https://www.statistics.sl/wp-content/uploads/2016/06/2015-Census-Provisional-Result.pdf (accessed October 16, 2016).

4 UNDP Human Development Reports, http://hdr.undp.org/en/composite/GII (accessed October 16, 2016).

5 See The Constitution of Sierra Leone, 1991: http://www.sierra-leone.org/Laws/constitution1991.pdf (accessed October 16, 2016).

6 See data at World Bank on literacy rates: http://data.worldbank.org/indicator/SE.ADT.LITR.FE.ZS?locations=SL (accessed October 16, 2016).

7 The National Policy on the Advancement of Women (2000), The National Gender Strategic Plan (2010–2013), and The Sierra Leone

Action Plan on Gender Based Violence (2012–2016). See also Sierra Leone National Action Plan for the full implementation of United Nations Security Council Resolutions 1325 (2000) and 1820 (2008). www.peacewomen.org/assets/file/NationalActionPlans/sierra_leone_nap.pdf (accessed October 16, 2016); The Government of Sierra Leone (n.d.); Ministry of Social Welfare, Gender and Children's Affairs (2014).

8 Save the Children (2014). A more recent Africa Confidential publication puts the number of medical personnel at 275 doctors and 9,008 nurses when the outbreak began. *Africa Confidential* 57, 4 (February 19, 2016), www.africa-confidential.com.

9 See WHO Ebola Data and Statistics, http://apps.who.int/gho/data/view.ebola-sitrep.ebola-summary-age-sex-20160511?lang=en (accessed October 16, 2016).

10 JSS is Junior Secondary School and BECE is Basic Education Certificate Examination.

11 See the study conducted by African Development Bank (2016).

References

Abdullah, Husainatu, and Ibrahim, Aisha Fofana (2010). "The Meaning and Practice of Women's Empowerment in Post-conflict Sierra Leone," *Development* 53, 2: 259–266.

African Development Bank (2016). *Women's Resilience: Integrating Women in the Response to Ebola.* Abidjan: ADB. http://www.afdb.org/fileadmin/uploads/afdb/Documents/Generic-Documents/AfDB_Women_s_Resilience_-_Integrating_Gender_in_the_Response_to_Ebola.pdf (accessed October 16, 2016).

Ankomah, Augustine (1998). "Condom Use in Sexual Exchange Relationships among Young Single Adults in Ghana," *AIDS Education and Prevention* 10, 4: 303–316.

Batty, Fodei (2014). "Reinventing 'Others' in a Time of Ebola," Hot Spots, *Cultural Anthropology Online*, October 7, 2014. http://www.culanth.org/fieldsights/589-reinventing-others-in-a-time-of-ebola.

Bledsoe, Carolyn (1990). "School Fees and the Marriage Process for Mende Girls in Sierra Leone," in Peggy Reeves Sanday and Ruth Gallagher Goodenough (eds) *Beyond the Second Sex: New Directions in the Anthropology of Gender.* Philadelphia, PA: University of Pennsylvania Press, 283–309.

Calves, Anne Emmanuele, Cornwell, Gretchen T., and Enyegue, Parfait Eloundou (1996). *Adolescent Sexual Activity in Sub-Saharan Africa: Do Men Have the Same Strategies and Motivations as Women?* University Park, PA: Population Research Institute.

Chatterji, Minki, Murray, Nancy, London, David, and Anglewicz, Philip (2004). *The Factors Influencing Transactional Sex among Young Men and Women in 12 Sub-Saharan African Countries.* USAID Policy Report.

Day, Linda R. (2008). "'Bottom Power': Theorizing Feminism and the Women's Movement in Sierra Leone," *African and Asian Studies* 7: 491–513.

Ferme, Mariane (2014). "Hospital Diaries: Experiences with Public Health in Sierra Leone," Hot Spots, *Cultural Anthropology Online*, October 7, 2014. http://www.

culanth.org/fieldsights/591-hospital-diaries-experiences-with-public-health-in-sierra-leone.

Gregson, Simon, Nyamukapa, Constance A., Garnett, Geoffrey P., Mason, Peter R., Zhuwau, Ton, Carael, Michel, Chandiwana, Stephen K., and Anderson, Roy M. (2002). "Sexual Mixing Patterns and Sex-Differentials in Teenage Exposure to HIV Infection in Rural Zimbabwe," *The Lancet* 359: 1896–1903.

Hulton, Louise A., Cullen, Rachel, and Khalokho, Symons Wamala (2000). "Perceptions of the Risks of Sexual Activity and Their Consequences among Ugandan Adolescents," *Studies in Family Planning* 31, 1: 35–46.

Ibrahim, Aisha Fofana (2015). "Whose Seat Will Become Reserved? The 30% Quota Campaign in Sierra Leone," *African and Asian Studies* 14: 61–84.

Jusu-Sheriff, Yasmin (2000). "Sierra Leonean Women and the Peace Process," *Accord* 9: 46–49.

Kanu, Joseph Sam, Tang, Yuan, and Liu, Yawen (2014). "Assessment on the Knowledge and Reported Practices of Women on Maternal and Child Health in Rural Sierra Leone: A Cross-Sectional Survey," *PLoS ONE* 9, 8 (August): 1–14. http://journals.plos.org/plosone/article/asset?id=10.1371/journal.pone.0105936.PDF (accessed September 26, 2016).

Keleher, H. and Franklin, L. (2008). "Changing Gendered Norms about Women and Girls at the Level of Household and Community: A Review of the Evidence," *Global Public Health* 3, S1: 42–57.

Kotz, Liz (1992). "The Body You Want: Liz Kotz Interviews Judith Butler," *Artforum* 31, 3 (November): 82–89.

Lee, Janet and Sasser-Coen, Jennifer (1996). *Blood Stories: Menarche and the Politics of the Female Body in Contemporary U.S. Society*. New York and London: Routledge.

Longfield, Kim, Glick, Anne, Waithaka, Margaret, and Berman, John (2002). *Cross-Generational Relationships in Kenya: Couples' Motivations, Risk Perception for STIs/HIV and Condom Use*. Working Paper no. 52. Washington, DC: PSI Research Division.

Meekers, Dominique and Calves, Anne-Emmanuele (1997). "'Main' Girlfriends, Girlfriends, Marriage, and Money: The Social Context of HIV Risk Behaviour in Sub-Saharan Africa," *Health Transition Review* 7 (Supplement): 316–375.

Menendez, Clara and Munguambe, Khatia (2015). "Ebola Crisis: The Unequal Impact on Women and Children's Health," *The Lancelet Global Health*, January 22. http://dx.doi.org/10.1016/S2214-109X(15)70009-4.

Ministry of Social Welfare, Gender and Children's Affairs (2014). *Country Report by Sierra Leone on Implementation of the Beijing Platform for Action (1995) and the Outcome of the Twenty-Third Special Session of the General Assembly (2000)*, June. http://www.unwomen.org/~/media/Headquarters/Attachments/Sections/CSW/59/National_reviews/Sierra_Leone_review_Beijing20.pdf (accessed October 16, 2016).

Nyanzi, S., Pool, R., and Kinsman, J. (2001). "The Negotiation of Sexual Relationships among School Pupils in South-western Uganda," *AIDS Care* 13, 1: 83–98.

Okin, Susan Moller (1994). "Gender Inequality and Cultural Difference," *Political Theory* 22, 1: 5–24.

Provisional data from the 2014 Census. https://www.statistics.sl/

wp-content/uploads/2016/06/2015-Census-Provisional-Result.pdf (accessed October 16, 2016).

Risman, Barbara J. (2004). "Gender as a Social Structure: Theory Wrestling with Activism," *Gender and Society* 18, 4: 439–450.

Save the Children (2014). *State of the World's Mothers*. http://www.savethechildren.org/atf/cf/%7B9def2ebe-10ae-432c-9bd0-df91d2eba74a%7D/SOWM_2014%20_EXEC_SUMMARY.PDF (accessed August 27, 2015).

Temin, Miriam J., Okonofua, Friday E., Omorodion, Francesca O., Renne, Elisha P., Coplan, Paul, Heggengougen, H. Kris, and Kaufman, Joan (1999). "Perceptions of Sexual Behavior and Knowledge about Sexually Transmitted Diseases among Adolescents in Benin City, Nigeria," *International Family Planning Perspectives* 25, 4: 186–190, 195.

The Constitution of Sierra Leone (1991). http://www.sierra-leone.org/Laws/constitution1991.pdf (accessed October 16, 2016).

The Government of Sierra Leone (n.d.). *The Agenda for Prosperity: The Road to Middle Income Status: Sierra Leone's Third Poverty Reduction Strategy Paper (2013–2018)*. http://www.undp.org/content/dam/sierraleone/docs/projectdocuments/povreduction/undp_sle_The%20Agenda%20for%20Prosperity%20.pdf (accessed October 16, 2016).

UNDP (2016). *Human Development Report 2015: Work for Human Development: Briefing Note for Countries on the 2015 Human Development Report: Sierra Leone*. http://hdr.undp.org/sites/all/themes/hdr_theme/country-notes/SLE.pdf (accessed February 19, 2016).

World Bank (2011). "Education and Health: Where Do Gender Differences Really Matter?" in *World Development Report 2012: Gender Equality and Development*. Washington, DC: The International Bank for Reconstruction and Development\World Bank, 104–148.

Wright, Simon and Hanna, Luisa (2015). *A Wake Up Call: Lessons from Ebola for World Health Systems*. London: Save the Children. https://www.savethechildren.net/sites/default/files/libraries/WAKE%20UP%20CALL%20REPORT%20PDF.pdf (accessed October 16, 2016).

8 | "GOD BLESS WHATSAPP": NEOLIBERAL EBOLA AND THE STRUGGLE FOR AUTONOMOUS SPACE IN SIERRA LEONE

Ibrahim Abdullah

> Not even the most repressive regime can stop human beings from finding ways of communicating and obtaining access to information.
>
> Nelson Rolihlahla Mandela

Introduction

The increasingly contentious debate to grant Ernest Bai Koroma the unconstitutional bid for a third term in office, that started barely a year after his re-election as president of Sierra Leone, was momentarily drowned in 2014 by the war against the lethal Ebola Virus Disease (EVD), a neoliberal scourge that had engulfed the nation. EVD wrecked the nation's already skeletal and broken health care system, exposing its inability to cope with the mounting infections. Confronted with an unwinnable war, as the regime characterized the EVD scourge, the government imposed a state of emergency, which deterred popular, open forms of civic protests, and made it possible to detain individuals without charging them to court. A popular radio journalist was detained for allegedly violating the state of emergency regulations, generating widespread public cries for his release. Denied the right to free expression in the name of a state of emergency, individuals and civic groups sought autonomy in cyber space to freely express their views on the state of the nation, the EVD scourge, and the defense of democratic rights and civil liberties. What does this switch from overt to covert claim-making tell us about how individuals and groups organized to articulate their interests around combating EVD and holding the ruling class of Sierra Leone accountable? To what extent did the new liberation technology, the Internet and other communication apps, especially WhatsApp, create new spaces for sustaining/expanding claim-making movements or networked activism in a context of a constricting public sphere?

This chapter argues that the switch from overt to covert claim-making, characterized by the proliferation and popularity of WhatsApp groups, though partly occasioned by the declaration of a state of emergency, might just turn out to be the way of the future for claim-making organizations in contemporary Sierra Leone. The safety in numbers in the virtual realm; the anonymity of participants across space and time; the linkages between individuals and groups across party, location, gender, and ethnicity; the connections between home and diaspora; created a bonding that made it possible for them to express themselves without fear of being arrested or arraigned. Covert claim-making, I argue, is consistent with the fundamental tenets of democracy in a modern state. In the context of the Ebola epidemic it provided a safe and secure space within which to organize and challenge the official narrative about the disease and official actions to contain the scourge. The popularity of WhatsApp went far beyond the imagination of activists and officialdom. The availability of cheap smart phones armed with cameras and Internet friendly led to the proliferation of WhatsApp groups when the medium became the most cost-effective avenue to communicate and get things done. In post-Ebola Sierra Leone it has seemingly attained the height of a sacred space wherein issues are discussed and decisions taken on important matters of national concern.

The chapter is divided into four sections. The first section lays out the context within which cyber activism evolved to become the most popular and acceptable norm for networked activism as the mode of covert claim-making. The second section deals with the broken health infrastructure that provided the objective basis for these WhatsApp groups to emerge and to challenge the actions of state officials in the declared war from above against the deadly Ebola virus. The third section examines the operation of WhatsApp groups in the context of Ebola and the kinds of conversations that animated cyber/digital activism. The final section discusses the popularity of WhatsApp groups in post-Ebola Sierra Leone – their hegemonic position as the medium of choice – and the attempts from above by officials of state to control the newfound weapon of cyber activists in the name of the general good.

Context: the truth behind the fastest growing economy and the third-term bid

The strident call by the party faithful and fellow travelers for an extension of the presidential tenure started gaining ground after the All Peoples Congress (APC), the ruling party, won the general elections in November 2012. The move, organized by the ruling APC, was anchored on party sentiments that had swayed the gullible electorate regarding the extraordinary performance of the president in providing the proverbial public good. A party apparatchik who was later appointed as minister after been sacked for allegedly engaging in sharp practices subsequently repackaged this party position, which the opposition Sierra Leone People's Party (SLPP) challenged. The president, the minister informed the nation, belonged to a special species of leaders that are "transformational" in the sense that they rarely ever happened in history. Because of their alleged rarity in politics, he told the nation, such individuals should be kept in power to allow them to fulfill their "transformational" agenda.[1] This transformational tag, clearly the sole basis for demanding an extension of the presidential tenure, rests on a shaky neoliberal construct which the government had been using to market itself as a "progressive" regime committed to fulfill its electoral mandate to satisfy the public good.

Sierra Leone, the president and officials of state kept reminding its citizens, has had the fastest growing economy in the world. According to this narrative, the country has moved forward steadily, from civil war to post-conflict reconstruction, and is now on its third poverty reduction strategy paper – The Agenda For Prosperity. From 2007 to 2011 it registered impressive growth rates: an average of 5.3 percent. The economy's alleged growth rate of 15.2 percent in 2012 was higher than that of any other country in Africa (*Africa Focus Bulletin* 2015). This, however, dropped to about 10 percent in 2013, but was estimated to hover around 11.3 percent in the first quarter of 2014 (*Africa Focus Bulletin* 2015; Government Budget, November, 2014). Yet these impressive growth rates, the ideal neoliberal marker that enables officials to access bilateral and multilateral funding, only tell half of the story – a story that hardly includes the grinding abject poverty that characterizes the majority of Sierra Leoneans. What then is the problem with impressive growth rates amidst mass poverty, broken health facilities, and high unemployment, as justification for a third-term bid? Budget Advocacy Network (BAN), a Freetown-based research outfit put out a counter-narrative that explained, and ultimately raised questions about, the much touted success story of Sierra Leone as the world's fastest growing economy (*Africa Focus Bulletin* 2015). BAN and the National Advocacy Coalition on Extractives (NACE) – two claim-making networks – conducted a survey of mining companies operating in Sierra Leone and discovered that though revenues from mining have increased four times since 2011, they still constitute a "small part of the economy" (*Africa Focus Bulletin* 2015). The reason why this was so has to do with the terms under which mining capital, especially in iron ore, was allowed to operate in an enclave economy desperate to attract foreign capital. The tax break and other incentives designed to attract capital are literally bleeding the nation. In 2012 alone tax breaks for six firms were equivalent to 59 percent of the total state budget, and more than eight times greater than the expenditure on health (*Africa Focus Bulletin* 2015). These incentives range from exemptions on customs duties, payments of the Goods and Services Tax (GST), mandatory in all transactions, together with reductions in the rate of income tax payable by the mining companies. It is not surprising that because of these illegal arrangements (they were not sanctioned by parliament as required by law), Sierra Leone was only able to raise 10.9 percent of its GDP from taxes – almost 50 percent short of the UN estimate of 20 percent of GDP from taxes to meet the then Millennium Development Goals (MDGs) by 2015. Growth rates might be impressive in projecting a positive image to foreign investors and an undiscerning public, but the reality on the ground suggests that the operations of mining capital, the alleged source of the double digits growth, does not benefit the country. On the contrary, mining capital undermines economic sovereignty and impoverishes the majority of Sierra Leoneans. The extreme dependence on receipts from primary exports is a shameful continuation of the colonial political economy of an import–export model. Having no control over external demand, the economy remained extremely vulnerable to any changes at the international level.

The missed opportunities occasioned by a blind faith in the neo-liberal agenda to deliver the public good in a laissez faire manner has enormous implications for governance and democracy in Sierra Leone. The illegal arrangements with mining companies commenced in 2009 when ministers and key officials issued concessions to companies without any strictures from either the executive or legislators; thus flouting the constitutional provision that enjoins them to seek parliamentary approval. Neither the National Revenue Authority (NRA), the sole institution mandated to monitor such transaction, nor the Ministry of Finance, another oversight agency, were privy to the numerous tax exemptions granted to companies since 2009. And the losses, from all indications, continue to mount because other interests have emerged in allowing the new situation to continue. While the NRA is mourning the loss of needed revenue, mining capital continues to make huge profits in the context of an iron ore boom. It is estimated that the state will lose $131 million from 2014 to 2016 from corporate income tax incentives granted to five mining companies (*Africa Focus Bulletin* 2015). And this does not include the loss from GST and customs duties. This colossal revenue loss could easily be invested in social services – particularly health and education – and agriculture, where the bulk of the working population make their living. Lack of transparency and discretionary tax incentives subvert democracy and accountability.

BAN's strident advocacy in the area of "promoting popular participation, transparency and accountability in both the national and local budget processes" is beginning to raise awareness on revenue availability and its abuse by the Sierra Leone political class (Abdullah 2013, 97). But such research and advocacy should be linked to the neoliberal paradigm, which constitutes the very foundation for such laissez faire policy as tax incentives in the name of attracting capital. By linking such ad hoc and discretionary actions to the prevailing mantra of free market it becomes possible to engage the public on the wider implications of a proposed government plan to institute tuition fees for university education at a time when the majority of college graduates go for two to three years without a job. Put differently, there is a direct connection between tax incentives, youth unemployment, privatization of higher education, and broken health and social services. The strident advocacy by BAN which prompted officials to slash the budgetary allocation to health – from 11 percent in 2011 to 7.4 percent in 2012; and up again to 10.5 percent as a result of advocacy and agitation – was in the best tradition of a social movement committed to change. The neglect of social services, particularly health and education, was to hit hard when Ebola struck in the second quarter of 2014.

Neoliberal Ebola and broken health infrastructure

Waxing confident in his budget speech at the end of 2014, the then Minister of Finance and Economic Development, Mr. Kaifala Mara, informed the nation that the "unprecedented outbreak of the Ebola Virus Disease has created a devastating social and humanitarian crisis with severe negative economic impact, thus, reversing the impressive economic growth we have achieved in recent years" (Government Budget, November 2014, 1). The "combined effect" on all sectors of the economy, he continued, "has significantly lowered the growth prospects of the economy." Thus, economic growth, he forecasted, "will slow down to 4.0 per cent compared to the original projection of 11.3 per cent" (Government Budget, November 2014). The World Bank, the principal watch dog over the economy, fingered Sierra Leone as having "suffered the greatest economic losses" from the Ebola scourge (*Africa Focus Bulletin* 2015, 1). According to the Bank, the economic growth rate "estimated at a 11.3 per cent in the first half of 2014, contracted at a 2.8 per cent annual rate in the second half of the year, and was projected to drop another 2 per cent in 2015" (*Africa Focus Bulletin* 2015, 1). The devastating impact on all sectors of the economy also witnessed the depreciation of the national currency – 9.2 percent in the formal sector and 13.2 percent in the parallel market – due to the inordinate demand for hard currency. The almost partial shutdown of the economy raises fundamental questions about the nature of the much-touted economic growth as well as the political economy of development underpinning such anti-people policies.

Narratives about Ebola have been as varied as the impact of the disease on the societies and polities of the three Mano River Union states (MRU). Yet one recurring, but externally derived, factor that has been constant in all the narratives has been the historic involvement of the three countries with IMF conditionalities. These conditionalities, which amount to a rolling back of the state and massive cuts in key areas like health and education, were compounded by long civil wars in Sierra Leone and Liberia, and the chronic instability and economic crisis in Guinea. How this deadly cocktail of IMF prescription, war, and economic crisis created a context for Ebola to flourish has been the staple of most commentaries on the Ebola scourge in the name of political economy. Privileging the above in explaining Ebola might help in understanding the Ebola scourge; even so, it must be acknowledged that it only tells half the story. The other half, which has to be part of the conversation, has to do with the anti-modernist nature of a top-down politics and its exclusionary practices, which condemns the majority to live on the fringes of history without the benefits of modernity. Ebola, it could be argued, might have been quickly contained in its original epicenter if the bulk of the population were involved as active participants in matters affecting their quotidian existence.

Ebola allegedly surfaced in Guinea in December 2013 with confirmed cases recorded in March 2014 (see Bah, Chapter 2 of this volume and Barry, Chapter 3 of this volume). By May, when Sierra Leone allegedly recorded its first Ebola infection, absolutely nothing had been done to prepare to respond to the disease. In the interim, things seemingly went back to business as usual as if nothing was happening in distant Kenema, the original epicenter of the disease, some 304 km away from Freetown. When in July 2014 the only virologist in the country, Dr. Umar Khan, the frontline general in the battle to contain the scourge, got infected and passed away, EVD was catapulted to a household word that evoked fear, terror, and death amongst the citizenry. In this grim situation, the presidency went into overdrive. Mirroring government actions in neighboring Liberia, a state of health emergency was declared in a televised address to the nation, and strident efforts were made locally and internationally to attract attention and support. The palpable lack of capacity to contain the disease in its original epicenter in the southeast – inadequate medical personnel; lack of laboratory facilities; treatment/holding centers; hospital beds; ambulances; protective clothing; and even gloves and stretchers – and the total lack of leadership or direction from the Sierra Leone Ministry of Health ensured that the disease would engulf the whole nation within four months, bringing everyday life to a complete halt, with schools and college on a prolonged vacation (see Abdullah and Kamara in Chapter 5 of this volume). Six months after the first recorded case, Ebola, historically a mainly rural disease, would be ensconced in the ghettos and high-density areas of Freetown, the center of power.

Freetown became the epicenter and the main battleground in the now declared war against Ebola, and increased support – in the form of more medical personnel, mobile laboratories, and personnel equipment, construction of more holding and treatment centers – was mobilized from outside. By November 2014 the donor community and other do-gooders had pledged almost $790 million, even though less than 40 percent of this amount had reached Sierra Leone by January 2015 (Government Budget, November 2014). As at November 2014, the government claimed to have disbursed Le 80 billion – Le 9.9 billion directly to the Ministry of Health and Sanitation, Le 40 billion to Ebola response, and Le 30 billion for hazard pay incentives into the dedicated Ebola account at the Sierra Leone Commercial Bank (Government Budget, November 2014, 3). The internal donations and pledges to the president from individuals and institutions became an eyesore on national television as they continued to mount *parri passu* with the daily infection in the country. By the end of November Sierra Leone recorded the highest infection rate in a single month in the history of Ebola epidemic – 2,150 – more than the then total official death toll in neighboring Guinea.

Like the civil war of the 1990s that preceded it, the war against Ebola provided an ideal moment for the nation, sans fratricidal bloodshed, to fight as one, in the name of the mythical patria. Indeed committed patriots rallied to the call only to be edged out by the extreme partisanship, which the evolving war came to assume (see Barry, Chapter 3 of this volume). And, like all wars, the war on Ebola opened up avenues for people to make money, for corruption to thrive, and for unscrupulous contractors to get fat. The resounding refrain from the general public that state officials and so-called civil society activists were using Ebola as a cover to access funding that would be converted to personal use went unheeded. The apparent availability of funds to "sensitize" the public about the EVD, especially on the dos and don'ts of the disease, made headline news. "Sensitization," the official buzzword for public campaigns about the disease, later turned out to be a code word, for accessing and converting Ebola-related funds into personal use.

The public awareness campaign that went on in the name of "sensitization" was taking place at a time when the generals in the war had no army to deploy. The Ministry of Health and Sanitation did not demonstrate the desired leadership, with respect to command and control, in the war from above, nor did the Ebola Response Committee (ERC) subsequently set up after the minister, Miatta Kargbo, was disgracefully dropped and her deputy installed. Even the National Ebola Response Center (NERC) later constituted with the substantive Minister of Defense, Pallo Conteh, as CEO initially operated without a clear-cut strategy about how to win a war that appeared unwinnable.[2] The lack of equipment and the necessary resources to conduct the war – there were only five ambulances in a nation of seven million when the disease broke out – ensured that the generals remained safely ensconced in their bunkered headquarters in the capital city passing commands to those in the frontline who had no clue about what they should do without necessary equipment and logistics. The incessant commands from above therefore came to naught: they did not produce the desired results; consequently numbers kept rising. This failure to contain the disease sans equipment and personnel opened the doors to civil society activists and their "sensitization" campaign.

The "sensitization" campaign centered on basic hygiene – wash your hands with chlorine; do not touch corpses; call 117 to attend to the dead; and report all sick persons in your household – turned out to be a market place to make money. Members of parliament and traditional rulers were provided with funding to conduct so-called "sensitization" in their areas even though some of them hardly spend time in their respective constituencies. The disbursement of funding for "sensitization"; the awarding of contracts to import ambulances and to construct holding and treatment centers, witnessed the transformation of war to a veritable money-making business. The auditor general's report covering the period May–October 2014 clearly reveals the high level of corruption involved in the war against Ebola. Civil society activists, contractors, and ministry officials gulped the Le 84 billion disbursed by the state. Not only were supporting documents (receipts, invoices, delivery notes) not tendered to justify how tax payers' money was being spent but procurement rules and procedures were routinely flouted in the name of emergency to deliberately defraud the state (Audit Service Sierra Leone 2015). The coordinator of Health for All Coalition (HFAC), the leading civil society organization in the health sector, had checks issued in his name and also contracted a loan from the Ebola funds without any agreement on when the said loan would be repaid. A parliamentarian who had received approximately Le 63 million for constituency sensitization got another Le 110 million three days later "in respect of daily subsistence allowance (DSA) and fuel to facilitate the same community sensitization" for which he had collected money earlier (Audit Service Sierra Leone 2015, 9). Members of the security services, deployed to hospitals, collected money from their areas of deployment as well as from their respective units. Fictitious names appeared in payment vouchers for hazard allowances for health workers. To crown it all no taxes were deducted from any of the transactions in the period under review.

The auditor general's report galvanized activists and patriots across party lines at home and in the diaspora demanding justice. But long before the report was even published, a popular radio journalist, David Tam Baryoh, had been asking troubling questions about how the war was conducted and why things were done in particular ways. He queried the management of Ebola funds and who was getting contracts and under what conditions. His *Monologue* program, which many citizens avidly looked forward to every Saturday night, dealt with governance and other topical issues affecting the nation. He was picked up early November 2014 and incarcerated for ten days at the maximum-security prison in Freetown. The official explanation from the office of the attorney general and minister of justice alleged that he had "made disparaging and inflammatory statements that in no way would aid the collective efforts we are making as a nation in the fight against the Ebola virus disease." The Minister of Justice and Attorney General, Frank Kargbo, charged that the journalist was undermining the war against Ebola by suggesting that government was "using the ongoing constitutional review process to perpetuate itself in governance rather than fighting the Ebola virus disease" (Government of Sierra Leone, Chambers of the Attorney-General 2014). The arrest and incarceration of the journalist under the Public Health Emergency decree was widely condemned by civil society activists and the media. It took a sustained campaign by civil right activists to secure his release under stiff conditions that were allegedly against the law. His detention revealed the extent to which officialdom would go in securing consensus in the war against Ebola. Asking troubling questions had become a problematic pastime that irked officials. In the context of the then state of emergency, officials were in effect saying that all civil rights were suspended. It was in this context of constricting political space that cyber activists reclaimed the Internet and its limitless possibilities for communication and networked activism.

Multiple transgressions as communication: the making of an autonomous public sphere

Arguably, one of the most enduring outcomes to emerge from the war against Ebola is the struggle for an autonomous discursive space owned and operated by digital activists – at home and in the diaspora – yearning for meaningful and qualitative change. The proliferation of WhatsApp chat groups in the first half of 2014 was given a major boost with the outbreak of Ebola and the subsequent demand for credible information. A veritable cyber-community of Sierra Leoneans had emerged during the civil war around discussion forums where issues dealing with the war were avidly debated and solutions proffered. But these were the privileged few who had access to the Internet when it was not popular or readily available. Globalization created an organic linkage between home and diaspora that was unprecedented; this communication network was given a revolutionary fillip with the mass circulation of the mobile phone, particularly the smart phone, which heralded the dawn of communication as a symbolic trope. The numerous Sierra Leonean chat groups that dotted the cyber world went into overdrive to mobilize resources and pose poignant questions about the state of the state when the Ebola epidemic broke out in May. By the time David Tam Baryoh was arrested, cyber activists were already making claims and questioning the legitimacy of the regime – these conversations shifted from the overt Facebook to the covert WhatsApp platform and networked activism. Indeed the covert movement bordering on transgressive political claims that emerged as a result of the Ebola epidemic was WhatsApp based. Some of these groups pre-dated the Ebola epidemic but they got to establish their political mark and modus operandi within the framework of Ebola and a repressive and intolerant state apparatus.

The WhatsApp groups or forums come in different shades and are organized in specific ways that allow for close monitoring of members and their postings. Some of these WhatsApp groups are occupation-specific such as the Sierra Leone Association of Journalists (SLAJ), Another Forum, or the Fourah Bay College, Academic Forum, consisting of faculty members, at the university. Others are exclusively constructed around activism, like the Native Think Tank (NTT), a consortium of civil society activists, or the Malen Jailed Activists forum – set up to mobilize support for activists incarcerated for defending the rights of peasants farmers dispossessed by

SOCFIN – Human Rights Briefs, and Civil Society Caucus. Most of these groups are trans-gender, trans-national – involving Sierra Leoneans at home and in the diaspora – trans-political party affiliation, and doggedly pro-change – change in the loose sense of an alternative to the status quo. There are also student groups scattered all over the country that include the unemployed – recent graduates still out there without any source of making a living. The gradual ballooning of groups and their ubiquitous presence seemed to have followed the trajectory of the Ebola virus. The more the virus spread among the population the more WhatsApp groups proliferated, popping up everywhere, as if to counter and engage the deadly virus in a mortal combat.

A WhatsApp group quickly emerges when folks with similar interest decide to share information of mutual importance: this could be political, social, or personal. Once constituted with an administrator, groups expand to include members across/around the country and in the diaspora. The key link in WhatsApp group participation is information sharing and activism. And what better information was there to share outside Ebola and how it was ravaging the land that they love? Only the group administrator(s) can enlist membership and therefore knows every member in the group. Group members occasionally use their real names but others prefer to use a title or *nom de guerre* – for example "digital politician," "goggle technician," "leggo me," "AK 47," "visionary," "hakuna matata." These are some of the types of designation in the covert world of cyber activism. A claim-making organization, apparently based in the UK – United Sierra Leone – recruits members by urging them to "take action, report, join WhatsApp Groups" (United Sierra Leone WhatsApp chat forum 2014). Before long WhatsApp chat groups, relatively marginal to mainstream society as a chat house and source of information, became central as a source of accessing and disseminating information critical of state and society. By the last quarter of 2014 all government press statements and those of international organizations appeared on WhatsApp. Even the daily Ebola updates appeared on WhatsApp, with key institutions setting up WhatsApp accounts to receive and access information. This move from the periphery to the center was no doubt a reflection of the incendiary nature of cyber activism, as the place to inform and be informed, in the wake of Ebola.

All WhatsApp cyber activist groups are about change in the broadest sense of the term. From political satire to parody, public officials, particularly the president and his ministers, are the butt of hilarious jokes. Lampooning public officials is also a strategy employed by cyber activists to drive home their political message. These animated political conversations are enlivened with short video clips or audio messages, mostly from Sierra Leoneans in the diaspora, which occasionally go viral in the world of cyber activism. Most of these images deal with corruption, Ebola funds, and the ineptitude of the regime in fighting/winning the war against Ebola. The heightened interest and involvement of diasporan Sierra Leoneans in cyber activism is unprecedented in the history of the country and is reflective of the enormous capacity of cyber technology as it dissolves space and unites entities within the stream of information flow. WhatsApp is not simply a medium of opposition to counter the official narrative from above; it is also an advocacy medium to mobilize independently of the state and to get officials to act on issues activists consider to be in the best interest of the general public. The constant reference to democratic norms and practices as the framework of all state actions is a pointer to their unambiguous commitment to democratic change.

As one commentator revealed in relation to the popularity of WhatsApp as the medium of communication in Ebola Sierra Leone, social media "is quickly overtaking the radio as the de facto source for news" (Mccordic 2014). Yet another chimed in: "social media has sidestepped the mistrust, political bias and vested interests of much traditional media, to become the people's political megaphone of choice" (Forna 2015). It is hardly coincidental that when Dr. Modupeh Cole, one of the leading physicians in the war against Ebola got infected with the virus, the campaign to get the experimental drug, ZMapp which was administered to two Americans who later survived, was launched on a WhatsApp forum. A message on the Health Workers on WhatsApp forum read:

> Friends, it is with saddened hearts that we announce that a senior Physician Specialist attached to the Connaught Hospital has tested positive for Ebola. *We hereby appeal to the US research laboratory to please make the drug, ZMAPP available for Dr. Cole's use.* We do not want to loose yet another colleague. We want all

> those concerned to see this message. Please share or repost if u want him to survive.

Later, another message was posted:

> Confirmed Report.
>
> Dr. Cole of Connaught Hospital had been taking to d isolation unit in Kailahun 4 treatment. He has been confirmed Ebola positive.
>
> He is a Sierra Leonean USA trained physician. He treated a patient at d Annex ward at Connaught Hospital who also had been confirm positive but die later. The Annex Ward is closed to public now. (Mccordic 2014)

Dr. Komba Songu-Mbriwa, the only senior medical personnel who got infected and survived, revealed in an interview how he got to learn that he was Ebola positive from a WhatsApp forum. His serum was collected with his middle name to conceal his identity but someone in the know decide to make it public even before he was officially informed. Feeling unwell, he opted to stay at the Hastings Treatment Centre – the only center operated by Sierra Leone medical personnel under the military – only to learn from his wife that he was Ebola positive. Such "disturbing" circulation of classified information breaching patient confidentiality was common during the war against EVD.[3] And its lingering existence in different forms in post-Ebola Sierra Lone underlines the "other" side of WhatsApp and social media.

These kinds of messages were posted and cross-posted all over WhatsApp groups to spread the word about everyday happenings in a situation where death lingered in the minds of all, and people came to rely on networked communication to share information. The sharing of information on WhatsApp forums in the name of the collective good took a bizarre turn when the nation woke up to an early morning message on August 10, 2014, enjoining compatriots to bathe with lukewarm salt water. Many heeded the call – bathe in lukewarm salt water – without verifying the authenticity of the source. But the prescription allegedly came from a so-called prophet in Nigeria, T.B. Joshua, where there was no Ebola epidemic (Kamara 2014; Lipton 2014). WhatsApp had indeed become the medium for national Ebola awareness.

A Freetown blogger, who correctly identified Facebook and WhatsApp as the most influential media – "topping the list" – during the war against Ebola, missed the overarching importance of this new medium by claiming that its use is restricted to "about 15% of the population," "the minority literate population who live in Freetown and other cities" (Kamara 2014). His Luddite invocation to go to "the basics of information sharing" – "the use of town criers and chiefs" – is as laughable as it is pathetic in this age of networked communities (Kamara 2014). The new "liberation technology," to borrow Larry Diamond's formulation, has changed politics in authoritarian contexts in complex and contradictory ways (2010). The restriction of movement occasioned by the state of emergency and the prohibition of public gathering, catapulted the phone, particularly the smartphone, and with it the WhatsApp platform, into public memory and everyday life. As one observer remarked, "WhatsApp is as much of a forum for spreading jokes, stories, and satire, as it is a genuine vehicle for informing and mobilizing, to the extent that the distinctions become blurred and permeable" (Lipton 2014).

The WhatsApp platform mobilizing potential and its covert and exclusive format are consistent with the collective need of activists to pursue their clandestine objective of networked activism. It is precisely this clandestinity and its concomitant license to transgress that has continued to worry officialdom. The restriction on public gathering and movement might have occasioned the popularity of WhatsApp as the medium of popular anger, mobilization, and protest against the state in a crisis situation. A press statement issued by Amnesty International called on the government to "stop using emergency regulations brought in to combat Ebola as a pretext to restrict freedom of expression and peaceful assembly" (Ogundeji 2015). The organization also alleged that "a man was charged with insulting the president after having forwarded a WhatsApp message he did not author." The everyday transgression by cyber activists drew adverse publicity in the wake of the war against Ebola and put officials on the spot to defend their draconian actions. The protest marches mounted by Sierra Leoneans in the diaspora against the "sacking" of the vice-president; protests against the president in Washington and New York; and the arrest of ten protesters in front of the US embassy in Freetown have been singled out as evidence of networked activism – mobilization via social media (Conversation with a senior police officer, March 2016).

Cyber activists/activism challenged state officials by presenting a counter-script, an alternative communication network/universe that subverts and undermines the status quo. From challenging the number of daily infections put out by the Ministry of Health and Sanitation, activists questioned the strategy and tactics of the war against Ebola, the awarding of contracts to political cronies, and the general ineptitude of the state to stem the tide of the infection, especially after the epicenter swung from the south-east to the north-west. The discrepancy between the total number of infections claimed by the ministry and the WHO – a difference of 2,000 – appeared as a deliberate attempt by state officials to cover up the magnitude of the scourge. The autonomy of cyber activists and the anonymity of membership were of concern to officialdom. The neat network within and between groups makes it easy to cross-post or forward information with images and occasionally audio clips to multiple networks. These occasionally go viral depending on the issue and information being conveyed. By the end of 2014 state officials publicly expressed their disappointment in containing the other virus in cyber space: cyber activists and their transgressional claims. What officials least realized was that they were fighting on two fronts: the war from above against Ebola and the unwinnable war against cyber activists.

When the auditor general's report was bought to the nation's attention by BAN, cyber activists went to war. The attempt by the majority leader in parliament, backed by the speaker, to prohibit public discussion on the issue by advancing a spurious procedural argument was thrown out of court. Cyber activists countered these arguments by emphasizing the supremacy of the constitution and the right to freedom of speech and freedom of the press. Other groups, including the official opposition party, took up the gauntlet by affirming the supremacy of the constitution, the right to freedom of expression, and the limits of parliamentary control. Even the normally quiescent Sierra Leone Bar Association came out strongly against the majority leaders' interpretation of the constitution (Press Release: WhatsApp). In the wake of the controversy the Anti-Corruption Commission (ACC) that had earlier asserted its mandate to investigate the allegations in the auditor general's report, without parliamentary interference, had to back down by conceding to collaborate with parliament to investigate the matter. While home-based cyber activists challenged the right of parliament to prohibit public conversation on the auditor's report, diaspora groups threatened to secure permission to mount pickets in Sierra Leone missions abroad. Others even went further to demand the resignation of the president and his entire cabinet for their alleged role in mismanaging Ebola funds. The mountain of open letters to the president calling for immediate investigation and justice is unparalleled in the history of Sierra Leone.

As Ebola continued to ebb in the first two months of 2015 amidst a major controversy over citizens' right to discuss allegations of massive fraud and corruption in the auditor's report, officials of state were expressing deep concern over cyber activism and its potential to subvert activities of state. A senior government spokesperson was quoted as saying that "government will develop a cyber-security law to protect the image and integrity of not only individuals and institutions but more so to protect the country against any form of terrorism or cross border crimes" (Karim 2015). The Criminal Investigation Department (CID) will collaborate with the international police, Interpol, "to get the job done; monitor, track down, and arrest and prosecute offenders": "if you commit an offence on WhatsApp or Facebook, the law will not protect you" (Karim 2015). The war against "terrorism" (cyber activism?) might turn out to be the next frontline in what would appear to be a new Sierra Leone in a perpetual state of war. How that war will be fought and won depends on how cyber activism repositions itself in post-Ebola Sierra Leone.

"God bless WhatsApp":[4] cyber activism and the continued struggle for an autonomous space in post-Ebola Sierra Leone

The popularity of WhatsApp as the communication medium of choice, and of covert activism, is captured in everyday life in the city of Freetown and other urban centers. "Sapping" has become the mode of communication for activists as well as non-activists. The ubiquitous market women/petty traders, a key group in testing the popularity of any regime in power, are aware of the importance of WhatsApp as the medium of covert and not so covert communication.

An inscription emblazoned on the back of one of Freetown's most popular forms of public transportation, the *poda-poda* mini-bus – "God Bless WhatsApp" – underlines the widespread popularity of WhatsApp as the medium of communication. The "blessing" heaped on WhatsApp by the *poda-poda* driver/owner could be read as a tacit affirmation of its importance in social networking in a moment of crisis.[5] There is a WhatsApp restaurant on the highway, at Waterloo in rural Freetown, not too far from the cemetery where Ebola bodies were interned in their thousands. Another WhatsApp restaurant, located close to the original Kingtom cemetery, where Ebola bodies were initially interned, seems to recall the dreadful moment of the Ebola holocaust. Both WhatsApp and Ebola have entered the popular imagination as key markers of a moment of crisis that has a special place in the individual and collective memories of several communities.

That memory is arguably central to understanding why WhatsApp groups have continued to operate as they did under the state of emergency that came into force after Sierra Leone lost its only hemorrhagic fever specialist Dr. Khan. The state of emergency still in force as Ebola ebbed together with the relaxation on free movements as communities ravaged by Ebola began the eventual countdown to zero, did not translate to a total lifting of the emergency regulations. Even when schools and colleges were scheduled to resume, officials still balked at rescinding the emergency regulation. This refusal to lift the emergency regulation impinging on freedom of expression was interpreted as a deliberate attempt to stifle freedom of speech. Some have even argued that the preferential application of the emergency regulations targeted the opposition broadly defined, that is to say, all those who appeared, and are seen, based on an interpretation of their actions and utterances, as anti-government. Keeping the Ebola emergency regulations in force appears as a measure to stifle the public sphere – in particular cyber activism. Official response to the mounting attacks on social media, which became strident under Ebola, now assumed a different face: social media must be "regulated."

Even so, the debate that started around the regulation of social media under Ebola has to be understood within a particular context – the context of changed circumstances, warranting a changed modus operandi for WhatsApp groups. And the dogged insistence by cyber activists that officials were out to stifle freedom of expression has some merit. But post-Ebola Sierra Leone, still under a health state of emergency, presented a different situation. The liberty to publish as they deem fit, to circulate information in closed WhatsApp groups, to cross-post important news items and analysis on current political issues, to discuss advocacy options, and mobilize resources for press conferences, came to dominate most activist groups in post-Ebola Sierra Leone. A popular radio journalist at Culture Radio, an FM station with a phone in program – *Burning Issues* – created a group linked to his program with the same name – "Burning issues!" Members are mostly avid listeners who send SMS messages and phone in to participate in his lively evening conversation on topical issues. His WhatsApp group quietly sucked in members nationally linking the forum with the radio conversation. Similarly, NTT, a research consortium focusing on topical issues of concern to the general citizenry, inducted more participants and expanded its activities to include the monitoring of every activity that impinges on everyday life: from the unauthorized hike in electricity tariffs to excessive charges and poor service from cellphone companies; from concern with IMF/WB prescription to fuel subsidy; and from police brutality to gang violence among marginal youth. Other WhatsApp groups administered by journalists and other civil society activists usually circulate information questioning official actions and putting forward alternative ideas. There are several overlapping WhatsApp groups dedicated to political debates on important national happenings. Others are simply monitoring outlets, disseminating information of interest to the public. The view expressed by some practicing "professionals," that WhatsApp groups are taking over the dissemination of information in contemporary Sierra Leone, is closer to the truth than most would acknowledge.

And that popularity has gone beyond discussion to active participation in shaping the outcome of events through cyber mobilization and the pooling of resources from group participants globally. Images and audio clips of a recent police shooting of people demonstrating in Kabala, Koinadugu District, against the re-location of a youth center to another district went viral after activists linked up with participants to tell their own story. NTT was in the forefront of the Kabala killing of two students: it continuously covered the incident with video and audio clips which were subsequently cross-posted to other groups; it mobilized resources and dispatch field workers to conduct on-the-spot investigation into what really happened. It also sent representation to the subsequent consultative meeting involving the police and community and wrote a report chronicling police brutality and impunity since 2007. And these are precisely the kind of publicity, video, and audio clips that officials would rather not have in the public domain: it not only questions the professionalism of the police but also raises questions about justice and the rule of law. As it turned out the two students gunned down had nothing to do with the demonstration. Others are replicating the activities of WhatsApp groups like NTT in civil society as they employ the new technology of liberation to make their presence felt.

Yet the ideals, which animate such activists' agendas – freedom of expression and democratic rights broadly defined – and the covert mode of operation are not exclusive to organized groups like NTT. Concerned citizens armed with smart phones are also active in exposing police brutality and other sharp practices involving state officials – from messengers and drivers to senior civil servants and minsters of state. There are many video clips of traffic violations, police brutality, and lawlessness, citizens' anti-social activities, and the conversion of public goods to private use, that normally make the rounds on the numerous WhatsApp forums that are trans-national – involving Sierra Leoneans at home and abroad. These activities and happenings generate lively discussions centered on active citizenship and the meaning of democracy. Some observers have fingered the never-ending parody and lampooning of public officials as the most worrisome aspect of WhatsApp postings and discussion groups. And these faux pas have degenerated into what one blogger recently referred to as "revenge porn" – the posting of nude photographs of public officials (Forna 2015). To be sure this "kind of paparazzi culture," which has allegedly "gripped the country," no doubt calls for a "regulatory mechanism" to check the "worst excesses of such behavior" (Massaquoi 2014). Exposing the bodies of Ebola victims might offend our collective sensibility just as the posting of nude photographs violates the privacy of individual citizens. Yet these actions by allegedly aggrieved and outraged citizens are not peculiar to Sierra Leone, nor are they sufficient grounds on which to justify cyber censorship. The effective use of smart phones to expose societal ills is now part of everyday life in contemporary West Africa

– from Dakar to Lagos to Conakry and Douala – and it continues to yield positive dividends with regard to the law, order, and justice (Searcey and Barry 2016). Brima Kamara, a spokesperson for the Sierra Leone Police, is a member of a WhatsApp group – "Talk With the Police" – made of up citizens, politicians, and police officers. He is of the view that "videos help improve the police force in a nation still recovering from a brutal civil war" (Searcey and Barry 2016).

When on August 8, 2016 the newly appointed minister of information and communication appeared on a popular radio program – *Good Morning Sierra Leone* – unveiling what appeared to be an outline of a proposed government policy on social media, his emphasis was not on censorship and control but on regulation in the interest of the general public. A Sierra Leonean "digital activist" resident in the US, who described himself as a "blogger, political, social activist, a satirist and co-founder of *Makoni Times*," an-online newspaper in the US, was not impressed with what the minister had to say. For him, the proposed policy "would ban anonymity online, punish people who commit libel against public officials, and create a way for the government to monitor social networks for offenses and establish a database of the Sierra Leone diasporans who are active on social media" (Foryoh 2016). The minister, he alleged, is so determined to "create a government task force or cyber police" that no "human right or left group will tell him what to do" (Foryoh 2016). Seemingly determined to subvert the alleged draconian measures, the blogger supplied a list of possible alternatives – use of proxy servers/VPN/ultraSurf/ ultraReach and others – to "get around social media blockades" if and when such a policy becomes operational.

The debate around social media, which started under Ebola, pitting cyber activists and civil society activists against the state, has seemingly peaked in post-Ebola Sierra Leone with all parties committed to regulation in the interests of the public good. Yet how that regulatory mechanism should operate, and in whose interest, remains unresolved as cyber activists and professional journalists continue to bemoan the shrinking space in the public sphere. The President of the Sierra Leone Association of Journalists, Kelvin Lewis, expressed his concern at the association's general meeting late last year. "The space we have to work is shrinking," he emphasized, urging his colleagues to "employ professionalism and deprive anti-press freedom agents the excuse for their actions" (Cham 2015). The Deputy Minister of Information and Communication, Theo Nicol, who was present at the meeting defended the need for control and censorship to stop activists from "posting all sorts of unacceptable materials" (Cham 2015). From control to regulation, the debate has now shifted to responsibility and acceptability. But who determines what is acceptable still remains problematic as cyber activists battle over unrestricted freedom in the name of democracy.

When the National Telecommunications Commission (NATCOM) unveiled its proposed pathway to tackling what has become an official obsession with social media activism, the issue of security and privacy loomed large in their expressed concern with regulation. If the politicians had been circumspect with their real intentions, the technocrats at NATCOM were not so sanguine. At a consultative meeting held in September the NATCOM Director of Consumer and Corporate Affairs was unequivocal: "We are talking about invasion of privacy. We are talking about incitement. We are talking about immorality and all of it" (Cham 2016). He made it clear that the two most popular social media platforms – WhatsApp and Facebook – have been contacted about their intention to "police" cyberspace. They will go ahead, he informed a journalist, with plans to set up an Internet Exchange Point (IXP) – a monitoring infrastructure that would enable NATCOM to track users using specific language. This will make it possible for officials to take action against such individuals. The NATCOM boss was more guarded in his pronouncement; they are not out to block or ban social media, he informed the gathering. "It is time for users to take responsibility for their actions and posts on social media," he declared (Cham 2016).

The apparent seesaw, from one public official to another, reads like an opinion poll on how they individually interpret the transgressive communication strategy of cyber activists in post-Ebola Sierra Leone. On the extreme right is the deputy minister of information and communication who has publicly endorsed what he dubbed the "Chinese way": a restrictive space owned and controlled by state power. "While it is not our wish to stifle free expression," the minister cautioned, "we are also mindful of our responsibility as a government to ensure that the fundamental rights, especially the part that deals with privacy of individuals, are respected." Occupying the middle ground are the technocrats at NATCOM and the security buffs at the Office of National Security (ONS), flagging control and monitoring technology as a bulwark against cyber activism. As state officials continue their forward march to "gag" cyber activism, civil society activists concerned with the shrinking public sphere have stepped up their campaign to resist any imposition from above. All are concerned that a fundamental aspect of liberal democracy – freedom of expression – is under threat on the eve of a general election. A leading human rights lawyer and respected civil society activist, Emmanuel Saffa Abdulai, expressed his concern on the proposed policy: "When you come out with a law blazing to control social media you basically send a chilling effect out to the public that you cannot now go on Facebook and WhatsApp and criticize government" (Cham 2016). In the immortal words of Nelson Mandela: "Not even the most repressive regime can stop human beings from finding ways of communicating and obtaining access to information."

Conclusion

The evolution of an imagined community of networked activists, at home and in the diaspora, dedicated to change in the broadest sense of the term, is arguably consistent with democratic principles in the liberal tradition. From questioning the right of the ruling party to use its majority in parliament to extend the presidential tenure, claim-making organizations have moved ahead to even question parliament's interpretation of the constitution with respect to freedom of expression to discuss the auditor general's findings on the use and disbursement of Ebola funds. Such transgressive politics are in the best tradition of liberal democratic practice; they enhance democracy and are an intrinsic part of the democratic culture. In the context of the Ebola scourge and a state struggling to limit freedom of expression, by claiming it is a public good that has to be monitored in the interests of the general public, such transgressions are seen as an infringement on the power of the executive to secure the public good in the interest of all. Who has the right to do or say what and how is the major question (quandary) that cyber activists are posing as they struggle clandestinely but not so clandestinely in the safety of their numerous WhatsApp groups, to expand the constricting public sphere within which they are allowed to operate under a state of emergency.

The stridency and popularity of WhatsApp as the current mode of choice guaranteeing freedom of expression – God Bless WhatsApp – runs counter to the state project of what constitutes the limit to such rights. The conversation about limiting freedom of expression in the interests of the public good amidst claims and counter-claims about what is desirable and acceptable has repositioned social media at the center of the discourse on democratic change. How this struggle – to deepen democracy or curtail civil liberties and constitutional rights? – will pan out in post-Ebola Sierra Leone amidst dwindling economic fortunes and an austerity regime depends on the balance of forces on both sides of the divide, and what each will be willing to concede in the interests of the collective good. "In the twenty-first century, social movements are an integral part of functioning democracies because democratic regimes often do not function very well" (Johnston 2014, 159). Whether state officials will concede to such persuasive reframing of the problematic remains to be seen. With elections slated for early 2018, the struggle in cyberspace by digital activists and their interlocutors will continue to rock state and society until an acceptable modus is agreed upon.

Notes

1 The current Minister of Information, Mohamed Bangura, recently told the nation in a popular radio program that the APC will be in power for the next 50 years (Radio Democracy: July 2016).

2 Conversation with United Nations Mission for Ebola Emergency Response (UNMEER official): Amadu Kamara, November 2014.

3 Interview: Sierra Leone's only Ebola surviving Doctor, *Politico*, November 2, 2015.

4 "God Bless WhatsApp": an inscription on the back of a city commuter bus in Freetown, Sierra Leone. Such inscriptions, very common in contemporary Africa, advertise the popular in everyday life; they can be found in every city in Africa. See Lawuyi (1997).

5 Conversations with commuter drivers about the inscriptions on their vehicles and their multiple meanings.

References

Abdullah, I. (2013). "Towards an Understanding of Social Movements in Contemporary Sierra Leone," in Sylla, Ndongo (ed.) *Liberalism and Its Discontents: Social Movements in West Africa*. Dakar: Rosa Luxembourg Foundation, 74–105.

Africa Focus Bulletin (2015). "Sierra Leone: Losing Out," January 6.

Audit Service Sierra Leone (2015). *Report on the Audit of the Management of the Ebola Funds, May to October 2014*. Freetown: ASSL.

Cham, K. (2015). "Space for Free Expression Shrinking: SLAJ President Laments," *Politicosl.com*, June 9.

Cham, K. (2016). "Sierra Leone Moves Ahead with Controversial Plan to 'Control' Social Media," *Politicosl.com*, October 7.

Diamond, Larry (2010). "Liberation Technology," *Journal of Democracy* 21, 3 (July): 69–83.

Forna, Memuna (2015). "Sierra Leone's Social Media Must Live Up," *Politicosl.com*, August 14.

Foryoh, Patric (2016). "Help Stop Mohamed Bangura from Banning Social Media in Sierra Leone," *Makoni Times*, August 10.

Government Budget and Statement of Economic and Financial Policies, November 2014.

Government of Sierra Leone, Chambers of the Attorney-General (2014). Press Release on the Arrest and Detention of Dr. David Tam Baryoh, November.

Johnston, Hank (2014). *What Is a Social Movement*. Cambridge: Polity Press.

Kamara, Alpha (2014). "Sierra Leone: How Influential Are Facebook and WhatsApp?" *IDGConnect.com*, May 22.

Karim, R. (2015). "The Call for a Cyber Law Is Timely," WhatsApp, February.

Lawuyi, Olatunde Bayo (1997). "The World of the Yoruba Taxi Driver: An Interpretative Approach to Vehicle Slogans," in Barber, Karin (ed.) *Readings in African Popular Culture*. Bloomington, IN: Indiana University Press, 146–150.

Lipton, Jonah (2014). "Mixed Messages: Social Media, Rumours and Responses to the #Ebola Outbreak in #SierraLeone's Capital, Freetown," *Africa at LSE*, August 19.

Massaquoi, I. (2014). "Ebola and the Ethics of Social Media in Sierra Leone," *Politicosl.com*, September 18.

Mccordic, Chad (2014). "Ebola Frontline: Social Media Is Raising Ebola Awareness in Sierra Leone," *Newsweek*, August 13.

Ogundeji, Olusegun Abolaji (2015). "Social Media Plays Central Role in Sierra Leone Political Crackdown," *PCWorld* / IDG News Service, May 7.

Searcey, D and Barry, J.Y. (2016). "Inspired by the US, West Africans Wield Smartphones to Fight Police Abuse," *The New York Times*, September 16.

Various statements from different groups in several WhatsApp forums, 2014/2015.

PART FOUR

TRANSNATIONAL ACTORS AND THE POLITICS OF CRISIS RESPONSE

9 | AFRICAN UNION, ECOWAS, AND THE INTERNATIONAL POLITICAL ECONOMY OF THE EMERGENCY RESPONSE TO EBOLA

Semiha Abdulmelik[1]

Introduction

The outbreak of the Ebola Virus Disease (EVD) in Guinea, Liberia, and Sierra Leone, including the detection and containment of a small number of cases in Nigeria, Mali, and Senegal, since December 2013 became a litmus test of the ability of African continental and regional organizations to respond effectively to a major health and security crisis. The international response to the crisis was tardy; it took nearly nine months from the first set of cases in Guinea in 2013 for the World Health Organization (WHO) to declare the outbreak a public health emergency of international concern (PHEIC). However, the Economic Community of West African States (ECOWAS) had declared the outbreak "a serious threat to regional security" in March 2014, and had started mobilizing resources and international support. The African Union (AU) followed on the heels of ECOWAS with the mobilization of African health ministers, and the subsequent creation of the African Union Support to Ebola Outbreak in West Africa (ASEOWA) – an unprecedented civilian-military mission to help in the containment of the epidemic.

This chapter analyzes the effectiveness of ECOWAS and the AU in dealing with the complex health, humanitarian, and security challenges posed by the EVD epidemic in West Africa. It examines the extent to which these responses are embedded within, or deviating from, the already existing international response architecture. It pays particular attention to the degree to which the consolidation of emerging thinking, institutional experimentation, and innovative practice that are the hallmarks of the ECOWAS and AU responses to this unprecedented crisis presents an opportunity to operationalize African solidarity. In this regard, it analyzes three critical issues at the heart of the crisis: the ability to raise financial and other resources internally to support its responses without resorting to or depending primarily on external donors; capacity to anticipate, plan, and respond in a timely manner to any major crisis of this magnitude; and division of responsibilities and relationships between the two organizations as well as other governmental and non-governmental organizations in responding to major health and security crises on the continent.

It argues that despite the rhetoric about regional and continental unity, the AU and ECOWAS responses to the pressing challenges faced by the continent continue to be embedded in, and mediated by, the international political economy and the Western-designed architecture of humanitarian responses to "crisis" in Africa. The Ebola response then constitutes a mid-way attempt at "accommodating" a semblance of African ownership, leadership, and solidarity, within the existing model of (largely) external funding of these institutions' crisis response initiatives. It will demonstrate that despite the separate responses to the Ebola crisis by the AU and ECOWAS, they both demonstrate that African solidarity initiatives are still a reflection of the existing global crisis response architecture. Even so, both institutions show a break with the crisis-oriented architecture by also addressing and focusing attention on structural issues. Lastly, it argues that both institutions have made attempts at consolidating this emerging capacity and experience to build institutional early warning and rapid response capacity for emergencies. Until issues of financing and subsidiarity are taken seriously, there is a risk of replicating the tensions of the global system regionally, and maintaining the current status quo, which ties African institutions and their *raison d'être* to the vagaries of the international response architecture.

The context of the pan-African responses

Though there have been outbreaks of the EVD in the Democratic Republic of Congo, Gabon, and Uganda since the 1970s, these had been localized and contained relatively quickly. The outbreak in Guinea, Liberia, and Sierra Leone had a number of features, which shaped the continental and regional responses to it. First, it was unprecedented in scale and virulence. Second, the governments and health systems in the affected countries were inadequate to meet the scale of the medical challenge (see WHO and the Governments of Guinea, Liberia and Sierra Leone 2014). Third, it displaced thousands of people and severely affected the movement of populations and goods within and outside the affected countries. Finally, having crossed national borders, EVD threatened to become a major regional, and even global, crisis beyond the three affected countries.

The magnitude and virulence of the Mano River Union (MRU) Ebola outbreak caught the international community and African states completely by surprise. By August 2014, when WHO declared its PHEIC, it was clear that the current Ebola outbreak was "unprecedented in scale and geographical reach," with a higher caseload than all previous outbreaks combined and with significant and broader impact on security, livelihoods, and economies of not just the affected countries, but of the West African region (UNOCHA 2014, 3). By the end of August 2015, there were 3,685 cases of EVD in West Africa, and 1,841 deaths – an overall fatality rate of 53 percent. During this time, the three affected countries were also experiencing a dramatic increase in cases, with "widespread and intense transmission, both inland and in the capitals" (WHO 2014a, 2). Indeed, in September 2014, the Centre for Disease Control's (CDC) Ebola modeling tool projected that "extrapolating trends to January 20, 2015, *without additional interventions or changes in community behavior* [emphasis mine] (for example, notable reductions in unsafe burial practices), the model also estimates that Liberia and Sierra Leone will have approximately 550,000 Ebola cases (1.4 million when corrected for underreporting)" (Meltzer et al. 2014).

These apocalyptic projections of the CDC were made in light of the sub-regional crisis in the health sector of Sierra Leone, Liberia, and Guinea that pre-dated the epidemic.[2] The "under-resourced, under-staffed, and poorly equipped" (Save the Children 2015, vii) health systems of these countries had one to two doctors available per 100,000 people, and with a heavy urban bias (WHO 2014b). Hospitals and clinics were poorly maintained and lacked basic medical supplies. The rapidly unfolding EVD outbreak had a devastating impact on local health care workers. By August 2014, over half of the more than 240 health care workers who had contracted the disease in Guinea, Liberia, Nigeria, and Sierra Leone, had died (WHO 2014b). A lack of protective equipment, proper training, and poor working conditions contributed to the heavy toll, while also generating greater anxiety among the population. The death toll amongst health workers deprived the affected countries of one of the most vital components required for responding to the outbreak – a trained and capable work force. The lack of health workers, or reluctance by the besieged health workers to come to work, led to the closure of medical facilities in some areas, impacting both Ebola and non-Ebola medical services. Ultimately, local responses were seriously hampered, and the crisis could not be "quickly contained, reversed, or mitigated" due to weak national health systems (Save the Children 2015, vii).

The inability of the governments of Liberia, Sierra Leone, and Guinea, through their health systems, to contain the Ebola epidemic in a rapid and timely fashion led to the displacement and imposition of major restrictions on free movement of people, infected and non-infected, within and across their borders. The Internal Displacement Monitoring Centre (IDMC) tracked displacement patterns due to the disease and identified five categories: populations fleeing to avoid exposure; those fleeing quarantine measures; those seeking health care from better served areas (not just from rural to urban areas, but also between the affected countries); those forcibly evicted or fleeing stigma due to their previous Ebola status; and those fleeing violence and rights violations (IDMC 2014). These displacement patterns largely reflect measures to restrict or prevent movement internally to avoid exportation of the disease from one community/area to another by the national authorities of the affected countries. These measures – often enforced by military personnel, as well as frustration and lack of trust in the governments – exacerbated fear and social tension and led to a deterioration of security in many communities within the affected countries (ACAPS 2014).

The restriction on the movement of people was not only limited to the borders of the affected countries. The threat and fear of importation of EVD led to a wide range of travel bans, restrictions, and land border closures, as well as suspension of direct air links with Sierra Leone, Guinea, and Liberia by some of their neighbors as well as others within and outside Africa, despite recommendations by the WHO to the contrary (Galatsidas and Anderson 2014). These measures not only affected trade, livelihoods, and the movement of people, leading to shortages of fuel, food, and basic supplies, but also humanitarian operations. Indeed, when Chad closed its border with Nigeria, it noted that despite the economic costs to the region, the decision was necessary on public health grounds (MacDougall 2014).

The context in which the African continental and regional responses were exhibited and visible was then one of increasing frustration over the lack of a "robust, prompt, and efficient response by the international community" and "governments' poor management of the epidemic" (ACAPS 2014).

The continental and regional approaches to the epidemic

ECOWAS: framing EVD as a regional security threat ECOWAS undertook the first set of African regional efforts to respond to the Ebola epidemic in Sierra Leone, Liberia, and Guinea. Between March and August 2014, the leadership of the regional body framed the Ebola epidemic as a transnational security threat, advocated for and mobilized resources, strengthened their coordination efforts, and pushed for the continuance of travel and trade with the affected countries. In March 2014, months before the WHO declared the Ebola outbreak in West Africa an PHEIC, ECOWAS, through its Mediation and Security Council, declared Ebola to be a "serious threat to regional security," and thus called for a "regional response to the crisis" (ECOWAS 2014a). The AU and UN subsequently echoed this securitization of the outbreak. While the AU and UN would subsequently create and deploy special missions to the affected areas, the Council urged the ECOWAS Commission to "take appropriate action in collaboration with the relevant health institutions in the region to mobilize stakeholders and resources to stem the spread of the epidemic" (ECOWAS 2014a). The initial ECOWAS response then was primarily routed via its existing specialized health agency, the West African Health Organization (WAHO), and focused on two principal issues: the immediate mobilization and disbursement of funds for epidemiological and surveillance support in the affected countries and the provision of information and guidelines to ECOWAS Member States on mitigation actions and the evolving status of the outbreak in the region.

As the crisis intensified, ECOWAS also stepped up its advocacy and resource mobilization efforts. It established a Solidarity Fund, which quickly generated 8 million USD from ECOWAS Member States (ECOWAS n.d. a). The funds were then disbursed as direct support to the affected countries, as well as for broader efforts and initiatives by WAHO. In May 2014, ECOWAS signed a tripartite agreement between WAHO, WHO, and the African Development Bank (ADB) for "exceptional and urgent assistance for the fight against the Ebola outbreak in the affected and neighboring countries" to the value of over 3 million USD. The ADB provided an additional 5.9 million USD in October 2014 to support the deployment of health personnel. As EVD engulfed the sub-region, and the need for a more comprehensive response plan, both national and regional, became evident, ECOWAS assisted Member States to formulate national action plans as well as a regional multi-sectoral plan/roadmap. This plan was shared with major partners and it formed the basis for mobilization of greater resources and advocacy regionally and internationally. Faure Gnassingbé, the President of Togo, who had been appointed as the regional coordinator for the ECOWAS response, John Dramani Mahama, the President of Ghana and then Chairman of ECOWAS, and Kadré Ouedrago, the President of the ECOWAS Commission engaged in high-level advocacy internationally at the UN General Assembly (Mahama 2014). They also partnered and coordinated the regional response with UN offices such as the UN Office for West Africa.

A strong component of the ECOWAS response was its efforts to strengthen coordination, as well as national and regional leadership with regards to the Ebola response. A meeting of ECOWAS Health Ministers convened in Monrovia on April 11–12, 2014 emphasized vigilance not only in the affected countries but also in the sub-region as a whole in combating the disease. This meeting was followed by an extraordinary emergency session of the ECOWAS Health Ministers on August 28, 2014 in Accra to further enhance coordination. The ministers decided, among other things, to put in place two regional monitoring and coordination mechanisms: the Ministerial Coordination Group and the Multi-Sectoral Technical Group (ECOWAS n.d. b). At the national level, it provided technical and financial support for the establishment of national coordination entities. President Mahama of Ghana, then chair of the ECOWAS-led efforts against Ebola, worked to ensure that there would be strategic level coordination and coherence between ECOWAS and the UN Mission for Ebola Emergency Response (UNMEER), created in September 2014. More broadly, ECOWAS hosted a high-level coordination meeting dubbed ECOWAS Partners Forum in

January 2015, bringing together the major regional and international responders and donors to discuss the ongoing response as well as post-Ebola recovery efforts (ECOWAS 2014b).

Apart from the initial response, and the subsequent monitoring and technical support to the affected countries, ECOWAS continued to push for the gradual but full resumption of trade and travel between the affected countries and the wider region as well as a normalization of air transport routes. This push was in recognition of the socio-economic impact that the crisis had wrought on the affected countries and the broader West African region. Looking beyond the Ebola crisis, and the need to strengthen future crisis response, the regional body wanted to move ahead to institute mechanisms to facilitate rapid deployment and preventative capacity as well as formulating plans for a regional surveillance and disease prevention center. More broadly, there was a strong consensus on the need to strengthen the region's health systems, make them more robust and resilient, and ensure they were adequately financed by Member States.

African Union: formation and deployment of ASEOWA In response to the actions undertaken by the ECOWAS leadership to coordinate regional efforts and mobilize international support, the AU revved up its own efforts to assist in the containment of the epidemic. It issued a call for assistance from its Member States and authorized the creation of an unprecedented civilian-military humanitarian mission. The organization also called for the speedy operationalization of the proposed African Centre for Disease Control and Prevention, and pushed for debt cancellation for the affected countries. The first concrete action undertaken by the AU was to convene, with the assistance of WHO, a meeting of all African Ministers of Health in Luanda, Angola on April 14–17, 2014. The meeting followed closely on the heels of a similar gathering of MRU ministers, which was noted earlier in the chapter. The final communiqué from the Angola meeting called for the mobilization of funds and assistance from states with experience in handling Ebola.

On August 19, 2014, back-to-back with the AU's commemoration of World Humanitarian Day, the Peace and Security Council (PSC) of the AU met and authorized the immediate deployment of an AU-led military and civilian humanitarian mission, the African Union Support to Ebola Outbreak in West Africa (ASEOWA) (AU 2014c).

Another layer of response then complemented this action, with the United Nations Security Council approval for the UN Mission for Ebola Emergency Response (UNMEER) in mid-September 2014. The concept of operations for the AU mission envisaged the deployment of 1,000 health workers (from public health officers to epidemiologists), as well as mission support staff, in the three affected countries for a period of six months (December 2014–May 2015), to be reviewed only when the countries were declared Ebola-free. Dr. Oketta, who as a Major General led the Regional Reserve Forces Command when the Uganda People's Defense Forces assisted in combating the Ebola epidemic in Northern Uganda and was serving most recently as the Director of the National Emergency Coordination and Operations Center in the Office of the Prime Minister of Uganda, was appointed to head the mission.

The focus on deployment of health workers was an explicit recognition that sufficient and well-resourced health personnel were critical to abating the crisis. The first group of volunteers for ASEOWA consisted of 86 health workers from diverse African countries including Burundi, Congo, Democratic Republic of Congo, Ethiopia, Kenya, Rwanda, Tanzania, Rwanda, Uganda, and Zimbabwe. Various African governments subsequently contributed contingents of health workers to the ASEOWA effort. By the end of January 2015, ASEOWA had screened, trained, and deployed 835 health workers to the three countries: 345 to Sierra Leone, 331 to Liberia, and 151 to Guinea (AU 2015g). In Sierra Leone, Liberia, and Guinea, the ASEOWA teams were involved in managing Emergency Treatment Units (ETUs), providing epidemiological support and equipment, supporting the reopening of hospitals, training local health workers, and leading national awareness campaigns.

In terms of strategic orientation then, the AU – through ASEOWA – served as a hub for advocacy (for lifting of travel and border measures and restrictions by Member States against the affected countries and cautioning against stigmatization and isolation),[3] mobilization (of primarily health care personnel, financial resources, and broader technical assistance), and coordination (of pledged assistance) in support of the response by affected Member States.

The PSC's decision to authorize ASEOWA is notable for a number of reasons. For one, it is the first time that the AU organ has invoked the provisions of the Protocol Establishing the PSC (Article

6 h), which outlines its mandate regarding humanitarian action and disaster management and the African Standby Force (ASF) in emergency situations, to authorize humanitarian action. Second, the PSC, like its counterparts at ECOWAS and the United Nations, acknowledged that the Ebola crisis was not just a humanitarian and public health emergency, but also a crisis with serious security implications. Cognizant that the three initially affected countries are in a post-conflict situation, the PSC was concerned that the epidemic would roll back the social, economic, and political progress that the three countries had made. Indeed, two of the three countries – namely Liberia and Sierra Leone – are part of the AU's pilot post-conflict reconstruction and development support (AU 2013c). This concern was not only limited to these two countries, but extended to the wider region, which has faced a number of multi-faceted security and development challenges. Ultimately, it is not just the "securitization" of a public health emergency by ECOWAS, AU, and subsequently UN that is noteworthy, but the corresponding authorization, a first for both institutions, of missions for a public health emergency. The Ebola crisis clearly pushed the AU and its security architecture in terms of its practice and thinking of responses to emerging challenges, which do not necessarily fit the conventional understanding of security.

In addition to the PSC's authorization of ASEOWA, during the 24th AU Summit held at the end of January 2015, AU Heads of State made a number of broader decisions prompted by the Ebola crisis (AU 2015e). First, AU Member States pushed for debt cancellation for the affected countries by international financial institutions. Second, Member States called for speedy operationalization of the proposed African Center for Disease Control and Prevention to strengthen continental resilience to similar crises. The Center, slated to be up and running by mid-2015, would have a coordination hub at the AU Commission and eight regional technical hubs to support Member States, with early warning as a first priority. It is envisaged that the Center will build on existing Center for Disease Control (CDC)/Public Health Center (PHC) capacities, nationally and regionally. NEPAD, an organ of the AU, through its African Medicines Regulatory Harmonization (AMRH) program, is also undertaking work to build regional and national capacity for regulatory oversight and ethical standards for clinical trials of vaccines.[4] The Summit also launched an Ebola Fund for financing the immediate response and long-term reconstruction needs of the affected countries. A stakeholders' meeting was convened on the margins of the Summit to survey and coordinate recovery efforts – with affected countries in the driving seat – all in a bid to strengthen the short-term response plan for long-term rebuilding. In the same vein, the Summit requested Member States with experience in dealing with Ebola to assist affected countries, and recommended the convening of a Global Conference on Ebola later in the year.

The 25th AU Summit held in June 2015 reviewed the situation in the three countries, and the Ebola response. It agreed, first, that given the declaration of Liberia as Ebola-free, ASEOWA would have to wind up by August 2015, but with continued support to strengthening the health systems of the affected countries. Second, it called on Member States to participate at the highest levels in the International Conference on Africa's Fight against Ebola being organized under the theme: "Africa Helping Africans in the Ebola Recovery and Reconstruction" on July 20–21, 2015. This conference, which was held in Malabo, Equatorial Guinea, resulted in the adoption of the Statute of Africa CDC by AU Ministers of Health, and called for direct budget support to affected countries, and the cancellation of their debts.[5] Last, the Summit requested the AU Commission, in collaboration with Member States and partners, to establish an African Volunteer Health Corps to be deployed during health emergencies.[6]

Operationalizing African solidarity: an analysis of key issues

The responses by AU and ECOWAS to the Ebola crisis elaborated in the preceding sections reveal the inherent complexities in operationalizing African solidarity in practical terms. The following section discusses three critical issues arising from this regional and continental response: the ability to raise financial and other resources internally to support its multiple projects without resorting to or depending primarily on external donors; the capacity to anticipate, plan, and respond in a timely manner to major crises; and the consequent division of responsibilities and relationships between the two organizations as well as other governmental and non-governmental organizations in responding to major health and security crises on the continent.

The ability to raise financial and other resources internally to support crisis response In part because of their chronic inability to raise funds – a reflection of the dependent nature of Africa's political economy – the bulk of the emergency efforts undertaken by the AU and ECOWAS have been funded by external international donors. For instance, from 2008 to 2011, AU Member States, through voluntary and statutory means, only contributed 2 percent to the AU's Africa Peace Facility, which funds the organization's peace and security efforts. The remaining 98 percent was funded by international bilateral and multilateral donors (Gilpin and Swearingen 2013). The 25th AU Summit held in June 2015 has authorized that this amount be gradually increased to 25 percent within the next five years, commencing 2016 (AU 2015d). The broader AU program budget also continues to be heavily dependent on external support, with Member States contributing only 7 percent of the program budget in 2011 and 2012 (AU 2012), and even less in 2013–2014 (AU 2014e). The financial situation in ECOWAS is considerably different. Its unique financing mechanism makes provision for the levying of taxes on goods imported from outside the region, meaning that the regular ECOWAS budget and activities are funded almost 98 percent by ECOWAS Member States (AU 2013d). In spite of this seemingly self-sufficient financial mechanism, the regional organization still relies to a large extent on partners to address and fund emergency, extraordinary, efforts and initiatives, as highlighted by the Ebola crisis.

Dependence on external sources of finance gives partners influence over these regional/continental bodies, which can hamper the autonomy, ideas, agenda and actions of these organizations, especially if they are "too fully brought into the same international bureaucracy, with its established norms, processes, and priorities, as most other actors in the sector" (Zyck 2013, 28). Donor influence may pressure or incentivize organizations to take up issues for which they are not adequately prepared or which do not reflect the interests of their secretariats or Member States. This is not to say that regional organizations are merely implementing agencies for the UN or Western donors (Baert, Felicio, and De Lombaerde cited in Zyck 2013). Some have taken concrete or symbolic actions that are contrary to donor priorities and agendas (Baert, Felicio, and De Lombaerde cited in Zyck 2013).

Conscious of the limitations imposed by the constraints of external funding, some scholars argue that African countries have espoused the idea of a Pan-African international political economy. The Solemn Declaration made by AU Heads of State during the OAU's 50th Anniversary (2013) pledged to "foster self-reliance and self-sufficiency," particularly through "tak[ing] ownership of African issues and provid[ing] African solutions to African problems; mobiliz[ing] our domestic resources, on a predictable and sustainable basis to strengthen institutions and advance our continental agenda" (AU 2013a). The Solemn Declaration contains three principles underpinning these professed ideals: "collective self-reliance and self-sustaining development, and economic growth; and prospects of 'delinking and autocentricity' vis-à-vis African global economic engagement" (Edozie 2013). Even so the billion-dollar question remains unanswered: can the global economy help Africa? Put differently, what does Africa want from the global economy (Edozie 2013)?

There has been some disquiet about the strong presence of development partners and externals in the financing and operationalization of ASEOWA. The official ASEOWA dashboard as of January 27, 2015 (AU 2015a)[7] lists the donors to ASEOWA as the European Union, United States, China,[8] Norway, and the AU; with the World Health Organization, Center for Disease Control, USAID, International Federation of the Red Cross, UN Office for the Coordination of Humanitarian Affairs, and African Humanitarian Action (the only African institution) as technical assistance partners. Of the 13.1 million USD available to ASEOWA at that material time, the AU had only contributed 1.2 million USD. This AU funding was drawn from a number of existing sources, including 1 million USD from the Union's Special Emergency Assistance Fund for Drought and Famine in Africa and 100,000 USD from the IDPs and Refugees Special Fund. This small sum underscores not just the paucity of resources at the disposal of the organization, but also questions the various funds' fitness for the purposes for which they were designed. The September 2014 Extraordinary Meeting of the Executive Council not only asked for these exhausted funds to be replenished, but also demanded that the mandate of the fund be expanded to include public health emergencies and other emergencies.

Others have argued that the strongest impetus for the AU to act on the Ebola crisis, in the manner it did, came from partners. This exemplifies a skewed global architecture and relationship among international actors, which are disproportionally interested in immediate crises rather than long-term root causes and structural problems. Crises, in this architecture and for these actors, allows for (arguably) easier mobilization of resources (Centre for Global Health Policy 2014). While undoubtedly, bilateral and multilateral partners largely financed (particularly the first phase) and provided the technical backstopping for the Ebola response, it would be difficult to argue that this agenda is not the AU's or that it did not demonstrate ownership and leadership in response to the Ebola crisis. One of the AU's most powerful and authoritative organs, the PSC, and the highest levels of the AU Commission, the Chairperson's Office, rallied around the efforts to tackle the epidemic. The Ebola response then constitutes a mid-way attempt at "accommodating" a semblance of African ownership, leadership, and solidarity, within the existing model of (largely) external resourcing of the institution.

The AU financing problems are long-standing, and they reflect the shortcomings of the organization's current funding and expenditure streams, which include multiple and cumbersome bureaucracies resourced by voluntary or low Member State contributions. The organizational structures simply do not reflect the emerging challenges and realities of crisis the AU is increasingly tasked with addressing. This has provided greater impetus for putting in place innovative financing mechanisms and solutions at a continental level. The full scope of the AU's funding crisis was articulated in the seminal report by the High Level Panel[9] on Alternative Sources of Financing the African Union, chaired by Former President Obasanjo (AU 2012). Though the report acknowledges the organization's donor-dependent program budget is problematic, it points out "successful interventions – be they medical, humanitarian, military or police – are expensive. Africa simply can't afford to address major crises on its own" (Allison 2014). At the Extraordinary Meeting of the Executive Council on the Ebola Virus Disease (EVD) Outbreak in September 2014 (AU 2014d), ministers expressed their "concern over the current financial situation in the AU," and stressed the "critical importance of the timely payment of assessed contributions to the AU Budget for the implementation of all AU programmes, including confronting all humanitarian challenges such as the Ebola Crisis" and urged "Member States to pay up their due contributions to the AU Budget in a timely manner to enable the Commission to carry out effectively its mandate."

The 21st AU Summit approved the report in principle, and the Assembly of Heads of States and Government retained two of the financing options that were proposed, a $2 dollar levy per stay in a hotel and $10 on flight tickets to and from African destinations (AU 2013d). It requested that the AU Commission submit a report for consideration to the AU Extraordinary Conference of Ministers of Finance and Economic Planning for proposals on modalities of the two options (AU 2013b). The Extraordinary Conference of Ministers took place in March 2014 (AU 2014f), and its report tabled at the 24th AU Summit, the following year. The Summit did not advance the conversation, and, at worst its decision can be read as reversing the momentum gained on this issue. The Summit took note of the report, as opposed to adopting it, and focused on establishing a "binding" minimum agenda by "urging all Member States, that have not yet done so, to honor as soon as possible their contributions and arrears to the Union." It provided a loophole for Member States on the implementation of the broader alternative financial sources agenda: "Member States are giving the flexibility of its implementation" and requesting that a specialized committee "propose non-exhaustive and non-binding basket of options … on the understanding that Member States preserve their sovereign rights of adding new options/measures deemed convenient to them" (AU 2015f).

Ultimately, this decision may be a reflection of what is currently feasible and politically acceptable to Member States of the AU, despite the ascendancy of the discourse of alternative financing at the continental level. As with other key deliberations and policy discussions at the AU, rhetorical political consensus at the continental level often dissipates or even faces opposition when it comes down to implementation at the national level. One of the arguments adduced for this disjunction between continental aspiration and national action is that many African states have yet to be fully convinced about the benefits of membership in the AU (particularly vis-à-vis sub-regional organizations) and therefore the increased cost of membership (Fabricius 2015). Moreover, in this particular case there has been disquiet in certain Member States about the implications of the proposals being put forward due to the belief that they will be disproportionally affected given the structures of their economies (especially, those which are dependent on tourism). As long as this financial state of affairs remains unresolved, the AU will be hampered in its ability to act autonomously and decisively especially on critical humanitarian and security issues in the continent. The AU will continue to be subject to the vagaries of the international political economy of intervention in African developments in general, and in prominent emergencies and crises (especially those deemed of sufficient concern to the international community).

Renewed momentum for the domestic resource mobilization agenda came from another track, late in 2015, with the initiative of the AUC Chairperson to appoint an AU High Representative for the Peace Fund, whose mandate would be to mobilize additional resources for AU peace and security related efforts. This initiative was endorsed at the 547th meeting of the PSC at the level of Heads of State, held on September 26, 2015 (AU 2015c). On January 21, 2016, the Chairperson appointed Dr. Donald Kaberuka, the outgoing president of the ADB as the High Representative of the Peace Fund. The choice of representative, with strong international standing and track record, commitment to the continent, and extensive experience in development financing, sent a strong message on the AU's commitment to re-engaging and working towards finding sustained, predictable, and flexible funding mechanisms. The High Representative spent an extensive amount of time on outreach with Member States and other key stakeholders, and close to six months after his appointment, presented his Report on Financing the African Union and the African Union Peace Fund at the 27th AU Summit. The Summit encouragingly take note of the report without reservation and, more importantly, decided "to institute and implement a 0.2 percent Levy on all eligible imported goods into the Continent to finance the African Union Operational, Program and Peace Support Operations Budgets starting from the year 2017" (AU 2016). This decision represents a significant step in the AU's stated aim of achieving economic independence. The challenge ahead, once the modalities and systems are put in place, will be to operationalize and program these funds effectively and efficiently and ensure accountability.

Beyond AU Member States, broader domestic resource mobilization and private sector engagement are outlined as cornerstones of the AU Commission's 2014–2017 Strategic Plan and Agenda 2063 – Africa's forward looking development agenda. There have been a number of previous attempts, arguably with limited success, to mobilize private sector resources and encourage participation in the AU's various initiatives and responses. The African Solidarity Initiative Conference is a case in point. The private sector outreach for ASEOWA was successful in raising around $31 million from corporate entities in the telecommunications, banking, energy, manufacturing industries as well as the African Development Bank (AU 2014b). Though very much reactive and ad hoc, the initiative was indicative of the growing and enhanced relationship between AU and the African private sector. It also highlights the largely unnoticed but significant growth of African philanthropy (as opposed to philanthropy in Africa) through foundations, high net worth individuals, and other forms of private sector giving across the continent in its various manifestations, including an estimated upwards figure of 7 billion USD annually in donations from high net worth individuals on the continent (African Grantmakers Network 2013). In addition to private sector giving, the AU has also focused on citizen giving as part of its fundraising efforts, launching a continent-wide mobile (SMS) giving platform modeled after the 2012 Kenyans 4 Kenya campaign.[10]

The campaign illustrated not just the potential of innovative/mobile giving but that citizen giving, despite its small discrete amounts, can in aggregate amount to a substantial sum. The importance of such citizen engagement in fostering a sense of African citizenship and participation in the AU, as well as giving expression to African Solidarity, or *Ubuntu*, cannot be overstated. Nevertheless, these forms of private sector and citizen giving are significantly sensitive to demonstrated accountability, transparency, and programmatic capacity and efficiency, which the AU needs to pay particular attention to. Translating these reactive, issue-based initiatives into a more sustainable revenue stream for the AU's programs may go a long way in disentangling the AU from its deep reliance on international partners to finance its efforts and priorities. In this regard, and arguably from the impetus of the Ebola experience, the AU in January 2015 launched the AU Foundation, which was decided upon by AU Heads of State in May 2013 to "enable voluntary contributions towards the financing of priority areas of the African Union. The Foundation will strive to engage Africa's private sector, African citizens, communities, and leading African philanthropists to generate resources and provide valuable insight on ways in which their success can accelerate Africa's development" (AU 2015b).

The capacity to anticipate, plan, and respond to crises Much attention has been placed on African regional institutions' funding dilemma; although related and dependent, much less emphasis has been put on these institutions' capacity to prevent, anticipate, prepare for, and respond to public health and humanitarian crises. To some extent this is linked to the fact that the founding *raison d'être* of these organizations is (conventional) security or economic, which has influenced their policy and institutional evolution. While the policy scope of these organizations has broadened in the past decade, institutional mechanisms have not necessarily been in step to reflect the changed situation. Both responses demonstrate enormous reliance on ad hoc political measures rather than formal institutional mechanisms, exemplifying lack of readiness and robustness to deal with crises of such magnitude. The ECOWAS response arguably exhibited and made use of a greater degree of its political leadership. Thus ECOWAS Heads of State appointed the Togolese President Gnassingbé to head the region's Ebola response, while the Ghanaian President and ECOWAS Chairperson Mahama[11] and the ECOWAS Commission President Ouédraogo undertook solidarity visits to the affected countries and spearheaded high-level coordination meetings and outreach efforts to engage partners. On the other hand, the AU's Ebola response was championed primarily through the Commission, with Chairperson Zuma providing the high-level visibility for the Union's response. Interestingly the EVD crisis came on the heels of a number of decisions and recommendations pending implementation made at both the continental and regional levels to build surveillance/ early warning and response capacity, such as the establishment of an African Center for Disease Control and Prevention.

The PSC decision authorizing ASEOWA in mid-August 2014 did not result in deployment of health care workers to the affected countries until December 2014, although the ASEOWA Secretariat was in the process of being set up as early as October 2014.

Arguably the AU was quick to react, and less so to act. This has been acknowledged by the Chair of the PSC for the month of August 2014, Burundi's Permanent Representative to the AU, who presided over the PSC's Ebola deliberations and mission authorization (ISS 2014). This can be explained by two factors. The first is the limited presence of the AU in Member States, making on-ground efforts difficult and slow. The second, critically, is that the AU is not "operational" per se; that is, it currently has no standing emergency response capacity despite the reference to the ASF in the ASEOWA authorization. This is an important indication of where practice is ahead of policy; the ASF had not been declared fully operational and guidelines for humanitarian assistance and natural disaster support (HANDS) had yet to be adopted. Moreover, while the constitution of Emergency Response Teams (ERTs) is enumerated in the AU Commission's 2014–17 Strategic Plan, it is yet to be implemented. ASEOWA then relied solely on the impromptu mobilization of Member State public health capacity (for which there was no precedent), including the development of procedures, protocols, and coordination for the same, which understandably required some time. Moreover, given the very unique nature of ASEOWA, a degree of institutional experimentation and interdepartmental cooperation has been required by the AU. This mission drew on the planning and deployment experience of the Peace and Security Department, the public health expertise of the Department of Social Affairs, and the high-level mobilization and advocacy capacity within the leadership of the AU Commission (Chairperson's Office).

That the AU was able to mobilize sizable Member State contributions in the form of technical assistance and deployment of health care/response personnel, which formed the backbone of the response, is notable. The response by Member States is revealing – local response capacity does exist on the continent and this should be the focus of short-to-medium-term efforts: to have standing and readily deployable response capacity. This experience by the AU has the potential to provide lessons and impetus for speeding up the operationalization of mechanisms such as the ASF and standing ERTs, as well as requisite guidelines and policies. The AU response highlights the limitations of existing structures and mechanisms for early warning, preparedness, and response to public health and humanitarian emergencies at the continental level. This, along with other factors, arguably explains its lack of a timely response. Within its existing capacity and with a degree of institutional experimentation, it exhibited strong ad hoc mobilization capacity, which allowed for an appropriate immediate response – the deployment of health personnel to the affected countries.

ECOWAS presents a rather different picture. ECOWAS took cognizance of this health emergency early, having the advantage of a specialized public health institution through which it could undertake surveillance/early warning and drive its response. Thus ECOWAS's early warning capacity allowed the organization to act early, both in terms of declaring the epidemic to be a security threat as well as responding through advocacy and mobilization activities. The experience, programs, and expertise of WAHO also meant that ECOWAS provided a degree of technical leadership to the affected countries and had "internal" capacity to guide policy and decision makers. While the initial response focused on getting funds released for the affected countries and undertaking epidemiological and surveillance activities, the scale of the unfolding crisis and the incapacity of the affected countries' health systems to deal with the crisis – finances notwithstanding – led ECOWAS to adapt its strategy to a more comprehensive approach, which was outlined in the regional roadmap. ECOWAS nonetheless seemed to have better coordination capacity and mechanisms, both political and technical. Arguably, both ECOWAS and the AU sought a coordinating and advocacy role for international support; and partners either aligned themselves with one or the other in a kind of "forum shopping," or engaging and positioning themselves with both, such as the African Development Bank.

Global capacity to deal with major emergencies and crisis is skewed towards rapid response rather than the development of long-term capabilities. Given this prevailing global emergency architecture, there is a tension as to whether this capacity should be built locally or globally (Centre for Global Health Policy 2014) – or as the AU and ECOWAS responses highlight, continentally or regionally. The WHO has admitted that the conditions in the affected countries "made it difficult for WHO to secure support from sufficient numbers of foreign medical staff" and it presented the AU initiative to recruit health care workers from among its Member States as noteworthy in closing this personnel gap (Centre for Global Health Policy 2014).

Regardless of this improvised success, both the AU and ECOWAS do not currently have standby institutional rapid response capacity, and are pursuing an agenda to enhance response capacity at the respective levels, as well as surveillance and prevention capacity.

Beyond crisis

The roots of the EVD crisis clearly transverse failings in multiple policy areas. Both Sierra Leone and Liberia are long-standing and significant parts of the international community's post conflict reconstruction and development (PCRD) project and "investment." Both countries are, as noted earlier, also part of the AU's pilot PCRD purview. Despite this, the crisis has uncovered the absence of institutions and infrastructure to handle such crisis. It is not surprising then, that the initial criticism about the inadequate national response to this crisis has focused on the failure of PCRD in the affected countries, notably Sierra Leone and Liberia. This also informed the calls for debt relief for the affected countries. Subsequently, there has also been greater focus on issues of inadequate health spending. In 2001, AU Member States, in the Abuja Declaration committed to 15 percent budgetary allocation for health. At Abuja + 12, only six countries had met this target – and the affected countries were not among those six. As such, the two institutions have called for a renewed commitment to the Declaration, but also pointed out the need for greater and united leadership for a healthy Africa; generating innovative financing streams; strengthened health personnel; and not just greater but also smarter health investments (UNAIDS and AU 2013).

The responsibilities and relationships between the two organizations, as well as with other global organizations in crisis prevention, preparedness, and response The foregoing demonstrates that we can locate different capacities within the AU and ECOWAS; they are uneven and not corresponding capacities. Despite the rhetoric of Regional Economic Communities (RECs) such as ECOWAS, as "building blocks of the AU," there is no equivalence of early warning or crisis response structures at the different levels. This raises the critical question of the division of responsibilities and relationship between the two organizations. The "collaborative" relationship between the UN and the AU and the AU and sub-regional organizations is in theory governed by the principle of subsidiarity, that is, allocation of power from global levels downwards. The AU notes "three elements in the application of subsidiarity: decision making mechanisms, burden sharing and division of labour" (De Sousa 2013, 62). This is outlined in the Memorandum of Understanding on the Cooperation in the Area of Peace and Security between the African Union and the Regional Economic Communities (2009) (AU 2008), and was further reiterated and fleshed out at the September 2015 Abuja Retreat involving the AU PSC and the RECs, that

> taking into consideration *the overall responsibility of the PSC* as stipulated in its Protocol, the PSC and the RECs/RMs *shall apply the principles of subsidiarity, complementarity and comparative advantage on a case by case basis*, taking into account the peculiarities of each conflict/crisis situation. *In cases where the REC/RM concerned does not have a common approach on how to address a specific conflict/crisis situation, the peace-making responsibility shall revert to the PSC.* (AU 2015h, 2; emphasis added)

More salient, is how the principle of subsidiarity plays out in practice, in this instance between the AU and ECOWAS. According to Boadu, some African regional institutions and organizations may have perceived the EVD Crisis emergency as "an opportunity to jockey for prominence and leadership in the response to the crisis (and in the African (health) governance architecture)" (Boadu 2014). Leadership in global governance occurs in the context of both formal and informal processes of organization and decision making; and as multiple actors (both state and non-state) involved in solving the problem at hand, leadership is continuously being produced and reproduced (Dingwerth and Pattberg 2006). This was evident in the case of the different responses to the EVD outbreak. Nevertheless, it is difficult to know precisely the division of labor between the two organizations, and whether it merely emerged organically, through conscious orchestration, or mediation by international partners. At times, ECOWAS and the AU jointly organized the training and deployment of health workers to the affected countries, but at others, the AU appeared as just another partner at coordination meetings convened by ECOWAS. The concurrent and parallel deployments of health personnel and logistics by ECOWAS and AU response clearly demonstrated an understanding that the Ebola crisis was extensive, and had implications well beyond West Africa. Even though the relation between the two organizations seemed unclear in the heat of the crisis, the response model that emerged was arguably largely effective and significant, and AU efforts complemented those of ECOWAS. The issue of subsidiarity in practice (typically in the management of conventional security threats) has always strained AU–REC relations, and crises such as the EVD outbreak are bound to complicate understandings and operationalization of this relationship if they are not clarified and systematized based on lessons learned. The principles and "practice" of subsidiarity, though constantly invoked by the AU and RECS, remains under-theorized and poorly fleshed out.

More broadly then, EVD has put a spotlight on the issue of global disease prevention and health governance, and the responsibility of global, continental and regional organizations in preventing, responding to, and containing epidemic diseases. The involvement of several organizations, governmental and non-governmental, including the UN, AU, ECOWAS, WHO, CDC, and Médecins Sans Frontières (MSF) among others, also raises the issue of subsidiarity – de facto and de jure. More attention needs to be paid to clarifying and distributing roles and responsibilities to the complex groups of actors that are now involved in dealing with international emergencies.[12] The question of who is best placed to respond, and how, to the emerging challenges in Africa – which have both regional and global repercussions – and the need for coherence of response, coordination, and strategic division of responsibilities is pressing. There are then a number of critical questions raised by the Ebola outbreak for global health governance, and its fitness for purpose given the nature of contemporary challenges and the rise of regional institutions. In the case of global health governance, the WHO International Health Regulations (IHR) presents a framework for Member States to work together for global health security. The IHR focuses on states as the implementers and does not clearly spell out a role for regional organizations. This is problematic for a number of reasons. First, because as demonstrated by the affected countries, some states have poor public health capacity; second, some regional organizations such as ECOWAS, have public health architecture that sits parallel to the WHO regional health infrastructure and may be a source of duplication; and third, because it ignores the importance of collective and mutual interests – such as that found in regional groupings – to assist in mobilizing action and support by other states.

Conclusion: the way forward

The ECOWAS and AU responses to the Ebola crisis represent concrete attempts at operationalizing African solidarity and leadership in response to a serious transnational health and security crisis faced by a small group of its Member States. The responses, while anchored on existing mechanisms of collective consultation within these organizations, also contained indications of new approaches to dealing with the crisis, and the larger security threat that it posed to other Member States. Even with institutional constraints, ECOWAS and AU tried new ways of mobilizing financial as well as human resources to support the continental and regional response. The experience should provide lessons as well as impetus for speeding up the operationalization of mechanisms such as the ASF and standing ERTs. It also offers opportunities for broadening ECOWAS and AU thinking about regional and continental security as well as the institutional norms, arrangements, and practices within the two organizations. The response to the crisis necessitates that the AU should continue to deepen its cooperation with sub-regional organizations like ECOWAS, not just in traditional security matters but also public health and humanitarian emergencies.

If the crisis provided new ways of strengthening the AU and the sub-regional organizations, it also exposed the chronic problem that they have with adequately funding their operations and programs. Resource availability and preparedness autonomy became critical markers through which we can understand different limitations in the regional response to the Ebola crisis. The crisis showed that AU and ECOWAS are still trapped between dependence on the financial largesse of our contemporary international political economy and Pan-African aspirations of continental self-sufficiency; between unequal emergency response capacities and the autonomy to shape its own options. Systematic, targeted, and sustainable financing and (technical) resourcing of the AU's support to Member States, through domestic sources, are priority agenda issues as the AU seeks to consolidate its position as the premier African institution. The subsequent decision of the 27th AU Summit, on the 0.2 percent levy holds significant promise for the AU in this area.

On an optimistic note, the outreach to, and engagement with the African private sector and citizens to support regional and continental efforts to deal with the Ebola crisis is promising. However, strong capacity and resilience cannot be around high-profile appeals and donations during crisis, they need to be anchored on solid financial ground. The AU as custodian, and ECOWAS as sub-regional champion, continued to call on its Member States to adhere to the Abuja Declaration for budgetary allocations, pay their dues and contributions regularly, and strengthen national health systems. The AU in particular, using the collective voice and political clout of at the time 54 Member States, has used the crisis to highlight broader structural issues around the continent, such as debt burden and the ineffectiveness of current post-conflict reconstruction and peace-building approaches.

Lastly, notwithstanding an examination of the actual response, much has been made of the exceptional nature of the PSC decision to deploy ASEOWA. While this was enabled by a combination of the unique and extraordinary challenge presented by the EVD crisis, partner advocacy, and evident gaps in international response, parallel but related developments around the operationalization of multidimensional standby capacities under the ASF, finalization of HANDS policy, progress on securing sustainable and adequate funding under the Peace Fund for AU operations, and increasing consideration of the PSC of non-traditional security threats facing the continent – and non-security (or not purely security) tools to address them – may see the conditions under which the PSC deploys a similar – if better structured – response in future.

Notes

1 Semiha Abdulmelik is an alumnus of the African Leadership Centre. This chapter is an adaptation of a presentation given by the author at a public seminar in London, UK, organized by the African Leadership Centre, King's College London, in February 2015.

2 See chapters on the three affected countries in this volume.

3 During the Extraordinary Executive Council Meeting in September 2014, a decision called on "Member States to urgently lift all travel bans and restrictions to respect the principle of free movement and urge that any

travel related measures be in line with WHO and ICAO recommendations, in particular proper screening" (AU 2014d).

4 The African Centers for Disease Control held its inaugural meeting on May 9, 2016 in Addis Ababa. It endorsed Kenya, Nigeria, Gabon, Egypt, and Zambia as the Regional Collaborating Centers (RCCs) for the Africa CDC. Africa CDC (2016).

5 See International Conference on Africa's Fight to End Ebola, "Africans Helping Africans," http://www.au.int/en/newsevents/27027/international-conference-africa%E2%80%99s-fight-against-ebola-%E2%80%9Cafrica-helping-africans (accessed September 22, 2016).

6 http://summits.au.int/en/25thsummit/events/25th-assembly-african-union-commits-mainstreaming-women.

7 The Dashboard also lists the pledgees from the private sector roundtable.

8 Figures available list the US as pledging $10 million, the EU $5 million, and China, $2million. Louw-Vaudran (2014).

9 The Panel was established by a decision of the AU Assembly (Heads of State) at the 17th AU Summit the previous year.

10 http://www.africaagainstebola.org/SMS-Campaigns.php.

11 Until May 2015.

12 The WHO attempted to provide a clarification of roles and responses in their *Ebola Response Map*, August 28, 2014, but this was produced in the middle of the crisis.

References

ACAPS (2014). *Ebola in West Africa: Protection and Security*. Briefing Notes, October 14, 2014. https://www.acaps.org/country/guinea/special-reports#container-650 (accessed October 16, 2015).

Africa CDC (2016). "1st Governing Board Meeting of the Africa Center for Disease Control and Prevention Endorses Five Regional Collaborating Centers," Press Release, May 13, 2016. http://au.int/en/pressreleases/30318/1st-governing-board-meeting-africa-center-disease-control-and-prevention (accessed September 22, 2016).

African Grantmakers Network (2013). *Sizing the Field: Frameworks for a New Narrative of African Philanthropy*, April 1. http://wings.issuelab.org/resource/sizing_the_field_1 (accessed October 11, 2015).

Allison, S. (2014). "Think Again: In Defense of the African Union," Institute for Security Studies, September 9. http://www.issafrica.org/iss-today/think-again-in-defence-of-the-african-union (accessed October 16, 2015).

AU (2008). "Memorandum of Understanding on Cooperation in the Area of Peace and Security between the African Union, Regional Economic Communities, and the Coordinating Mechanisms of the Regional Standby Brigades of Eastern Africa and Northern Africa." http://www.peaceau.org/uploads/mou-au-rec-eng.pdf (accessed October 12, 2015).

AU (2012). "Progress Report of the High Level Panel on Alternative Sources of Financing the African Union Chaired by H.E. Olusegun Obasanjo, Former President of Nigeria Consultations with Member States." http://ccpau.org/wp-content/uploads/2014/03/Obasanjo-Panel-Progress-Report-Assembly-AU-18-XIX-2012-_E.pdf (accessed October 11, 2015).

AU (2013a). "50th Anniversary Solemn Declaration." http://agenda2063.au.int/en/sites/default/files/50th%20Anniversary%20Solemn%20DECLARATION%20En.pdf (accessed October 2015).

AU (2013b). "Decisions, Declarations, Resolutions," Assembly of the Union Twenty-First Ordinary Session, May 26–27. http://au.int/en/sites/default/files/decisions/9654-assembly_au_dec_474-489_xxi_e.pdf (accessed October 12, 2015).

AU (2013c). "First Progress Report of the Chairperson of the Commission on AU's Efforts on Post-conflict Reconstruction and Development in Africa," January 16. http://www.peaceau.org/uploads/psc-352-report-pcrd-16-01-2013.pdf (accessed October 12, 2015).

AU (2013d). "Modalities of Implementation of the Two Options Retained by the Assembly of Heads of State and Government of the African Union on Alternative Sources of Financing the African Union," Department of Economic Affairs. http://ea.au.int/en/sites/default/files/Alternative%20Sources%20_E.pdf (accessed October 13, 2015).

AU (2014b). "African Union Rallies Private Sector to Fight Ebola on 8 November in Addis Ababa," Press Release no. 305/2014, November 6. http://pages.au.int/ebola/events/african-union-rallies-private-sector-fight-ebola-8-november-addis-ababa (accessed October 12, 2015).

AU (2014c). "Communique," Peace and Security Council 450th Meeting, August 19. http://www.peaceau.org/uploads/psc-com-450-ebola-outbreak-19-8-2014.pdf (accessed October 16, 2015).

AU (2014d). "Decision on the Ebola Virus Disease (EVD) Outbreak," Executive Council Sixteenth Extraordinary Session, September 8. http://pages.au.int/sites/default/files/Final%20Decision%20Ext%20EX%20CL_E.pdf (accessed October 16, 2015).

AU (2014e). "Decisions and Recommendations," Executive Council Twenty-Fourth Ordinary Session, January 27–28. http://au.int/en/sites/default/files/decisions/9660-ex_cl_dec_783-812_xxiv_e.pdf (accessed October 16, 2015).

AU (2014f). "Extra-Ordinary Conference of African Ministers of Economy and Finance (CAMEF) to be held from 21 to 24 March 2014 in Abuja, Nigeria." http://ea.au.int/en/content/extra-ordinary-conference-african-ministers-economy-and-finance-camef-be-held-21-24-march-20 (accessed October 12, 2015).

AU (2015a). "ASEOWA Dashboard as of 27th January." http://pages.au.int/ebola/news/aseowa-dashboard-jan-27th-2015 (accessed October 13, 2015).

AU (2015b). "AU to Launch Foundation, and Introduce Ebola Solidarity Fund," Press Release no. 11/24th AU SUMMIT, January 27. http://pages.au.int/ebola/events/au-launch-foundation-and-introduce-ebola-solidarity-fund (accessed October 12, 2015).

AU (2015c). "Communique," Peace and Security Council 547th Meeting, September 26. http://www.peaceau.org/en/article/the-peace-and-security-council-of-the-african-union-au-at-its-547th-meeting-adopted-decision-on-the-funding-of-au-led-peace-support-operations-undertaken-with-the-consent-of-the-un-security-council (accessed October 11, 2015).

AU (2015d). "Decisions, Declarations, Resolutions," Assembly of the Union

Twenty-Fifth Ordinary Session, June 14–15. http://www.au.int/en/sites/default/files/decisions/9664-assembly_au_dec_569_-_587_xxiv_e.pdf (accessed October 14, 2015).

AU (2015e). "Decisions, Declarations, Resolutions," Assembly of the Union Twenty-Fourth Ordinary Session, January 30–31. http://summits.au.int/en/sites/default/files/Assembly%20AU%20Dec%20546%20-%20568%20(XXIV)%20_E.pdf (accessed October 14, 2015).

AU (2015f). "Decisions," Executive Council Twenty-Sixth Ordinary Session, January 26–27. http://summits.au.int/en/sites/default/files/EX%20CL%20Dec%20851%20-%20872%20(XXVI)%20_E.pdf (accessed October 12, 2015).

AU (2015g). "Fact Sheet: African Union Response to the Ebola Epidemic in West Africa." http://pages.au.int/sites/default/files/FACT%20SHEET_1.pdf (accessed October 12, 2015).

AU (2015h). "Retreat of the Peace and Security Council on Enhancement of Cooperation between the African Union Peace and Security Council and the Regional Economic Communities and Regional Mechanisms for Conflict Prevention, Management and Resolution in the Promotion of Peace, Security and Stability in Africa," PSC/Retreat/8, September 14–16, Abuja. http://www.peaceau.org/en/article/conclusions-of-the-retreat-of-the-peace-and-security-council-on-enhancement-of-cooperation-between-the-aupsc-and-the-recs-rms-in-the-promotion-of-peace-security-and-stability-in-africa (accessed October 12, 2015).

AU (2016). "Decisions and Declarations," Assembly of the Union, Twenty-Seventh Ordinary Session, July 17–18. http://au.int/en/sites/default/files/decisions/31274-assembly_au_dec_605-620_xxvii_e.pdf (accessed October 12, 2015).

Boadu, N.Y. (2014). "A Preliminary Assessment of the African Ebola Response," *International Health Policies*, December 17. http://www.internationalhealthpolicies.org/a-preliminary-assessment-of-the-african-ebola-response (accessed October 16, 2015).

Centre for Global Health Policy (2014). *The Ebola Crisis: An International Relations Response?* Workshop Summary, November 28, Sussex University. https://www.sussex.ac.uk/webteam/gateway/file.php?name=ebolacrisisir--worskhop-summary.pdf&site=346 (accessed October 16, 2015).

De Sousa, R.R. (2013). *African Peace and Security Architecture (APSA) Subsidiarity and the Horn of Africa: The Intergovernmental Authority on Development (IGAD)*. Lisbon: Center of African Studies, University of Lisbon.

Dingwerth, K. and Pattberg, P. (2006). "Global Governance as a Perspective on World Politics," *Global Governance*, 12: 185–203.

ECOWAS (n.d. a). "Status of the Regional Solidarity Fund," in *The Fight against Epidemic of the Ebola Virus Disease within ECOWAS*. http://www.ecowas.int/ebola/ (accessed October 16, 2015).

ECOWAS (n.d. b). "Strengthening Coordination and National and Regional Leadership," in *The Fight against Epidemic of the Ebola Virus Disease within ECOWAS*. http://www.ecowas.int/ebola/ (accessed October 16, 2015).

ECOWAS (2014a). "ECOWAS Ministers Call for Regional Response to Deadly Ebola Outbreak," no. 055/2014. http://reliefweb.int/

report/guinea/ecowas-ministers-call-regional-response-deadly-ebola-outbreak (accessed October 16, 2015).

ECOWAS (2014b). "Final Communique: High Level Coordination Meeting of ECOWAS Partners," no. 009/2015, January 16. http://news.ecowas.int/presseshow.php?nb=009&lang=en&annee=2015 (accessed October 16, 2015).

Edozie, R.K (2013). *New International Political Economy of Africa: A Pan-African Perspective*. http://ssrn.com/abstract=2336739 (accessed October 16, 2015).

Fabricius, P. (2015). "The AU Starts to Put Its Money (Closer to) Where Its Mouth Is," Institute for Security Studies, February 12. http://www.issafrica.org/iss-today/the-au-starts-to-put-its-money-closer-to-where-its-mouth-is (accessed October 16, 2015).

Galatsidas, A. and Anderson, M. (2014). "West Africa in Quarantine: Ebola, Closed Borders and Travel Bans," *The Guardian*, August 22. http://www.theguardian.com/global-development/ng-interactive/2014/aug/22/ebola-west-africa-closed-borders-travel-bans (accessed October 16, 2015).

Gilpin, R. and Swearingen, M. (2013). "Financing and Refocusing the African Union's Peace Fund," USIP International Networks for Economics and Conflict, June 24. http://inec.usip.org/blog/2013/jun/24/financing-and-refocusing-african-unions-peace-fund (accessed October 16, 2015).

IDMC (2014). *Displaced by Disease: 5 Displacement Patterns Emerging from the Ebola epidemic*, November 20. http://www.internal-displacement.org/blog/2014/displaced-by-disease-5-displacement-patterns-emerging-from-ebola-epidemic/ (accessed October 16, 2015).

ISS (2014). "Interview with H.E. Alain Aimé Nyamitwe," *Addis Insights*, October 21. http://www.issafrica.org/pscreport/addis-insights/interview-with-h-e-alain-aime-nyamitwe (accessed October 16, 2015).

Louw-Vaudran, L. (2014). "The AU's Ebola Mission: It's Not All about the Money," Institute for Security Studies, September 22. http://www.issafrica.org/iss-today/the-aus-ebola-mission-its-not-all-about-the-money (accessed October 16, 2015).

MacDougall, C. (2014). "Africa Tightens Ebola Travel Curbs as Affected Countries Face Food Shortages," *Reuters*, August 21. http://www.reuters.com/article/2014/08/21/us-health-ebola-travel-idUSKBN0GL23V20140821 (accessed October 16, 2015).

Mahama, J.D. (2014). "Statement of the President of the Republic of Ghana on the Occasion of the 69th Session of the United Nations General Assembly," September 25. http://www.un.org/en/ga/69/meetings/gadebate/pdf/GH_en.pdf (accessed October 16, 2015).

Meltzer, M.I., Atkins, C.Y., Santibanez, S., Knust, B., Petersen, B., Ervin, D., Nichol, S.T., Damon, I.K., Washington, M.L. (2014). "Estimating the Future Number of Cases in the Ebola Epidemic: Liberia and Sierra Leone, 2014–2015," *MMWR Supplements*, 63, 3: 1–14. http://www.cdc.gov/mmwr/preview/mmwrhtml/su6303a1.htm (accessed October 16, 2015).

Save the Children (2015). *Wake-up Call: Lessons from Ebola for the World's Health Systems*. https://www.savethechildren.net/sites/default/

files/libraries/WAKE%20UP%20CALL%20REPORT%20PDF.pdf (accessed October 16, 2015).

UNAIDS and AU (2013). "Abuja + 12: Shaping the Future of Health in Africa." http://www.unaids.org/sites/default/files/media_asset/JC2524_Abuja_report_en_0.pdf (accessed October 16, 2015).

UNOCHA (2014). *Ebola Virus Disease Outbreak: Overview of Needs and Requirements*. http://docs.unocha.org/sites/dms/CAP/Ebola_outbreak_Sep_2014.pdf (accessed October 16, 2015).

WHO (2014a). *Ebola Response Roadmap Situation Report 2*, September 5. http://apps.who.int/iris/bitstream/10665/132687/1/roadmapsitrep2_eng.pdf?ua=1 (accessed October 16, 2015).

WHO (2014b). *Situation Assessment*, August 25. http://www.who.int/mediacentre/news/ebola/25-august-2014/en/ (accessed October 16, 2015).

WHO and the Governments of Guinea, Liberia and Sierra Leone (2014). *Ebola Virus Disease Outbreak Response Plan in West Africa, July–December 2014*, July 31. http://who.int/csr/disease/ebola/evd-outbreak-response-plan-west-africa-2014.pdf?ua=1 (accessed September 20, 2016).

Zyck, S.A (2013). *Regional Organizations and Humanitarian Action*. HPG Working Paper, November. http://www.odi.org/sites/odi.org.uk/files/odi-assets/publications-opinion-files/8733.pdf (accessed October 16, 2015).

10 | THE WORLD HEALTH ORGANIZATION AND THE EBOLA EPIDEMIC

Meredeth Turshen and Tefera Gezmu

All agree that the initial response of the international community to the Ebola epidemic in Guinea, Liberia, and Sierra Leone that was first reported in Guinea in March 2014 was lamentably slow. The World Health Organization (WHO) has faced some of the heaviest criticism, leveled by agencies that (with one exception) were no more aggressive than WHO in their reaction: particularly outspoken were UN bodies like the World Bank and the IMF, private voluntary organizations like Médecins Sans Frontières (MSF), and the aid agencies of the US and UK governments (Associated Press 2014; MSF 2014). Some critics are demanding that WHO become a "first-responder" to contagious disease outbreaks, although the UN Office for the Coordination of Humanitarian Affairs was created in 1998 to be precisely that, whereas WHO is primarily meant to provide technical advice, not services. Unlike NGOs, WHO does not run development or medical projects, it does not provide personnel to give direct care; it is an inter-governmental organization that offers advice and technical assistance to ministries of health.

This chapter reviews WHO's response to the Ebola epidemic and to the organization's critics; it explores the meaning of the demand that WHO take the lead coordinating responses to disease outbreaks and other health emergencies. We are interested in the meaning of this demand in light of the history of neoliberal budgetary constraints that donors have placed on WHO; these fiscal restraints have enabled donors to dictate the organization's priorities. Mindful that WHO has played an important role in the improvement of public health around the globe, particularly in low- and middle-income countries, we argue that, rather than divert WHO's mission to a narrow task, high-income countries should increase their contribution to the agency's regular budget so it can carry out its original broad mandates. We base this argument in part on an analysis of conditions on the ground that caused the Ebola outbreak to be so severe.

The World Health Organization

WHO came into existence in 1948 as an inter-governmental specialized agency of the United Nations, taking over the functions of the Office International d'Hygiène Publique (established in 1907), the Health Organization of the League of Nations (established in 1919), and the International Sanitary Bureau (1902). The last is of special significance because after 1948 it became the Pan American Health Organization, WHO's regional office for the Americas, establishing the pattern of autonomous regionalization.[1] The federal design of WHO, granting authority and decision making to regional offices,[2] sets WHO apart from all other UN specialized agencies (Hanreider 2015), and it goes part way towards explaining WHO's slow response to the Ebola epidemic. Some may think of these arrangements as excessive bureaucracy; we think of them as indicative of democracy and accountability.

WHO was organized to achieve its aims through technical collaboration with its members in the areas of health service administration, environmental hygiene, disease eradication, and nutrition. To this end, WHO maintains epidemiological and statistical services, promotes scientific cooperation, proposes international conventions, conducts research, and develops international standards for food, biological, and pharmaceutical products. Its constitution states that one of its 22 functions is "to furnish appropriate technical assistance and, in emergencies, necessary aid upon the request or acceptance of Governments"; but nowhere is WHO designated as the "first responder" in medical emergencies. The International Federation of Red Cross and Red Crescent Societies (ICRC), a humanitarian organization founded in 1919 that carries out relief operations through national societies operating all over the world, has assumed this responsibility.[3] A plethora of private, voluntary, international organizations, some with many decades of experience, now respond to emergencies: the International Rescue Committee (established 1933), OXFAM (1942), Médecins Sans Frontières (1971), and Mercy Corps (1979), to name a very few.

WHO raises its core budget from annual assessments of member states. The budget for 2014–2015 was US$3.9 billion, 77 percent of which had to be financed through voluntary contributions since assessments remained at their 2012–2013 level, representing zero nominal growth and accounting for only 23 percent of the program budget. Other sources of income are donor-controlled trust funds for such donor-selected conditions as AIDS, tropical disease research, and onchocerciasis (river blindness). The regional offices have no opportunity to express their priorities or influence either the selection of conditions or the dispensation of these extra-budgetary funds. This, then, is the background to WHO's response to the epidemic: a decentralized regional organization, a mandate to provide technical assistance to its members, and an inadequate budget that it does not fully control.

WHO responds to the Ebola outbreak

No medicines, vaccines or diagnostics existed to combat Ebola when the outbreak began. The world was caught unprepared in the face of the epidemic, and not for the first time.[4] On August 28, 2014, five months after the first case reports, WHO released the Global Roadmap against Ebola that would cost US$490 million; most of the funds would be dedicated to building treatment centers, hiring staff, and providing safe burials in Guinea, Liberia, and Sierra Leone, the three most affected countries. Days later WHO leaders went to Washington, DC to ask for US$600 million, citing budget constraints that had already limited WHO's presence in West Africa and constituted one reason for its initial failure to detect and contain Ebola (Park 2014). Cuts in WHO's 2014–2015 budget had reduced by half the funds for handling health crises, causing the organization to lose some of the senior staff most qualified to lead a response. Eventually, the US government pledged US$152 million, a fraction of what was required and little beyond what had been cut between 2011 and 2013, when the United States reduced its contribution to WHO's general fund to US$180 million from US$280 million.

As of March 17, 2015, according to the UN Office for the Coordination of Humanitarian Affairs (OCHA 2015), the United States had transferred a little over US$66 million to WHO. In contrast, UNICEF (a semi-autonomous UN agency that has always been headed by a US citizen selected by the US government) received almost US$86 million from the United States (and a further US$78 million from the World Bank). In all, the World Bank distributed almost US$140 million to fight Ebola, as of March 17, 2015, including nearly US$25 million to WHO. The choice of private voluntary partners bears scrutiny: the US government gave more than US$32 million to Partners in Health (PIH), a Boston-based non-profit known for its medical care in Haiti; this sum is equivalent to one-third of PIH's total income in 2013.[5] And, although the International Monetary Fund (IMF) announced that it would give US$430 million to fund the fight against Ebola in Guinea, Liberia, and Sierra Leone (Kentikelenis et al. 2015), nothing was distributed according to the OCHA report cited above.[6]

In other words, WHO's critics, who were in large part those responsible for funding the organization, never gave it the funds needed to respond to the epidemic, preferring other agencies that we would judge were less well positioned than WHO to respond to short-term as well as long-term health care needs in the three countries. Still, some will say this begs the question about what happened in the five months between March and August 2014. By September 22, 2014, 5,864 people were infected and 2,811 had died, according to WHO; according to MSF, 5,900 had died.

The virus first appeared in Guinea in December 2013; by February 2014, when WHO identified it as Ebola, 87 people were sick and 61 of them had died. The initial focal point was the prefecture of Guéckédou, which is a major regional trading center on the borders of both Liberia and Sierra Leone. Guinea notified WHO about its Ebola cases in March, and WHO was soon on the ground, as were MSF and the ICRC.[7] Cases appeared in Liberia at the end of March infecting a dozen people. By May the first cases had arrived in Sierra Leone, and WHO sent some staff to Kenema Government Hospital in June. The outbreak appeared under control several times, only to re-emerge. In early August WHO declared the epidemic an international public health emergency (the third such declaration ever made under the International Health Regulations enacted in 2007). Ironically, that same week in August, the United States announced that it was cutting resources for the project called the Viral Haemorrhagic Fever Consortium, which started in 2010 to study Lassa fever and included scientists from Kenema, Tulane University, and other partners in West Africa and the United States. In late August, WHO and MSF workers began to restock supplies of protective equipment at Kenema Government Hospital as WHO began its pleas for emergency funds. Speaking to the media in December 2014, Dr. Margaret Chan, Director-General of WHO, said: "It is fair to say the whole world, including WHO, failed to see what was unfolding. Of course, with the benefit of hindsight, if you ask me now ... we could have mounted a much more robust response" (quoted in Global Ebola Response Information Centre 2015, 15). It appears that WHO was alert, active, and engaged in combatting the Ebola epidemic, but handicapped by a lack of personnel and funds. Kamradt-Scott (2016) reviewed WHO's management of the 2014 EVD outbreak from March to September 2014 and concluded that the initial response to the crisis was appropriate and reasonable and the criticisms that have emerged are unjustified.

The role of surveillance

Previous outbreaks of Ebola were localized and quickly extinguished, but given West African conditions – including historical and recent interconnectedness among the countries, more frequent travel, and globalized trade – the disease had a much greater chance of spreading more widely. Soon after the initial outbreak of Ebola, it was apparent to those familiar with the region's political and economic conditions that enormous and far-reaching support was urgently needed. It was also clear that local and national health care support systems were either absent or too weak to handle the rate of infection that followed the initial cases. Several publications have discussed the genesis of the outbreak; some have suggested possible approaches on how to address the crisis (Cenciarelli et al. 2015; Vapalahti et al. 2014; Weyer et al. 2015) including revision of the current international response system in order to better address future epidemics in the Global South.

In the matter of the Ebola outbreak in West Africa in 2014, WHO was guided by the International Health Regulations (IHR) committee, which represents an agreement concluded in 2005 among 196 countries to work together for global health security. Led by a department of global capacities alert and response, WHO plays the coordinating role in IHR, developing guidelines, technical materials and training, and fostering networks for sharing expertise and best practices. The IHR Emergency Committee on Ebola first met on August 8, 2014 and declared that the conditions for a Public Health Emergency of International Concern (PHEIC) had been met.[8] The

WHO Director-General endorsed the Committee's (detailed) advice and suggestions and issued them as Temporary Recommendations under IHR (2005) to reduce the international spread of Ebola, effective August 8, 2014 (WHO 2014).

The greatest challenge in resource-limited settings is determining the surveillance necessary to curtail epidemics effectively before they reach the proportions of the 2013–2016 Ebola outbreak. The West African epidemic emphasizes once again the crucial role of a standardized and coordinated approach for investigating disease outbreaks. The lack of an effective surveillance system in the affected countries limited the ability of those involved in controlling the epidemic to evaluate the severity of the event in the context of previous outbreaks or predict potential changes in the characteristics of the Ebola virus (infectivity, pathogenicity, and virulence). Data collection and investigations of the outbreak were not standardized, resulting in data that were incompletely understood. WHO provides a centralized global mechanism to share epidemiological data and is a trusted authority, but the lack of reliable local data confounded attempts to understand regional patterns of transmission.

The lack of reliable information about the risk and severity of the outbreak contributed to the misinformation, panic, confusion, and fear that led to unnecessary public health measures taken by governments around the world. The lack of verifiable facts exaggerated the risk of infection for people living in or coming from Ebola affected countries, which led governments outside the region to ban flights and travel; these restrictions resulted in economic hardships for the affected populations and jeopardized aid plans. The World Bank estimated that the epidemic eroded the gross domestic product of the three nations by $2.2 billion. WHO and the IHR Emergency Committee on Ebola urged members not to create additional barriers to the delivery of much needed assistance. Meanwhile think tanks projected doomsday scenarios that stigmatized Africans about yet another communicable disease, although effective surveillance mechanisms coupled with appropriate responses could have eliminated the fear and hysteria that led to the isolation of millions of people.

The next section of this chapter addresses the contextual factors that contributed to the large number of deaths rather than the epidemiology or clinical aspects of Ebola in Guinea, Liberia, and

Sierra Leone (Agua-Agum et al. 2015a; Team WER 2014). The clinical and epidemiologic descriptions of haemorrhagic diseases are well documented (Bah et al. 2015; Chertow et al. 2014; Ghayourmanesh and Hawley 2014; Kortepeter et al. 2011; Stein 2015). The important context is the regional and international history, which played a critical role in the outbreak in the three West African nations.

The epidemiologic triad and the political economy of the region The epidemiologic triad of disease causation – the interaction of human conditions, the ecosystem of pathogens, and the environment – acted synergistically with other factors to make this outbreak particularly devastating. Commentators frequently mention the collapse of existing health and treatment facilities and the absence of surveillance systems. Surveillance may be the first but it is only one of three essential components of responding to an epidemic: the others are community mobilization and the delivery of appropriate health care. Few commentators recall the extensive population movement and displacement in the region due to the regional wars (1–2 million refugees and internally displaced people in Guinea, Liberia, and Sierra Leone, about 10 percent of these countries' populations). Internal displacement contributed to the overcrowding and unsanitary conditions of urban slums, and in Liberia, the epidemic was worst in Monrovia, the capital city.

Absent from most discussions was the destruction of ecosystems for industrial mining and large-scale commercial agriculture (Wallace and Wallace 2016). Some reports discuss human encroachment on primal forest in the context of population growth, rarely in terms of the changes in climate that have caused increased exposure to and the proliferation of disease-carrying organisms like mosquitos, ticks, and rodents that can pass pathogens from person to person; climate change also contributes to the adaptation and drug resistance of bacteria. Scientists have identified African fruit bats (family-*Pteropodidae*) as the most likely reservoir species of Ebola viruses.[9] Both scientific and eyewitness reports have traced recent Ebola outbreaks to massive migrations of fruit bats into villages just before the disease appeared.[10]

On the other hand, everyone remarks on the poverty and economic destruction consequent to the civil conflicts in West Africa. The damage associated with the armed conflicts of the 1990s – destruction of roads, markets, schools, and hospitals leading to interruption of education, disruption of agriculture and food distribution systems, and the breakdown of public health campaigns – played a substantial role in reducing the immunity of populations. War aggravated the already low levels of immunity to conditions that can be prevented by vaccines, the persistent and chronic malnutrition, and the high levels of endemic disease (tuberculosis, malaria, Lassa fever, and more); this situation, which should have been remedied after the conflicts ended, multiplied the public health impact of Ebola (WHO 2015).

At the height of the epidemic, reports from the disease-affected regions highlighted the plight of countless patients who were refused treatment by ill-equipped medical clinics and hospitals for fear of disease transmission; the sick were forced to return home and possibly spread infection among family members. Initial efforts to control the epidemic were also hampered by shamefully low levels of literacy (female literacy rates are 22.8 percent in Guinea, 32.8 percent in Liberia, and 37.7 percent in Sierra Leone, probably even lower in rural areas). Cultural differences about the causes of illness, how to treat sickness, and how to bury the dead, coupled with persistent doubt about biomedical systems, created barriers to seeking care in hospitals and clinics; people, especially in rural areas, used home remedies or turned to traditional healers.

These historical political, social, and economic circumstances are academic to the people of Guinea, Liberia, and Sierra Leone, as well as to historians of Africa. In contrast, the so-called "Africa experts" in the Global North came out – some in the Western media, others in respected scientific journals – and pointed to the poor health care infrastructure, the deficiently trained health care workforce, and the absent diagnostic facilities and treatment resources as if these internal factors alone were responsible for the rapid spread of the virus (Bebinger 2014; Bloom et al. 2015; Randolph 2015). In fact, it was principally the appalling history of this conflict-laden region and its wretched political economy that accounted for the high morbidity and mortality (Agua-Agum et al. 2015b). A complete picture of why and how the outbreak was able to cause such devastation, especially among women, children, and youth, emerges from the history, politics, and economics of the region (Baker 1984; Black and Sessay 1997; Changula et al. 2014; Fuest 2008; Groseth et al.

2007; Hoffman 2004; Knobloch et al. 1980; Monson et al. 1984; Murphy 2013).

The complaint here is that experts, according to their own statements, were well aware of the circumstantial context of the looming disaster that materialized, yet they said nothing and did little (Chai 2014; Lindblad et al. 2015; Nadeau 2014). With hindsight, the International Crisis Group (ICG 2015, i) admits:

> Despite huge investments in peacekeeping and state building in Liberia and Sierra Leone in the preceding decade and a significant UN and non-governmental organisation (NGO) presence, the region was ill prepared for a health crisis of such magnitude. Broader issues of national reconstruction, particularly in those two countries, combined with the prioritising of specific diseases, such as HIV/AIDS and malaria, contributed to produce stove-piped health sectors with abundant resources for those targeted diseases but resource-strapped health ministries overall that were particularly vulnerable to a health emergency. Aid organisations, with far better resources than the local ministries, also inadvertently undercut attempts at self-sufficiency.

The attitude that African people and governments are inherently incompetent and incapable of dealing with their own socio-economic, political, and health issues pervades the reactions and recommendations coming from the Global North and perpetuates the stigma attached to Africa (Asgary et al. 2015; Fink 2015a). One sees this in the insistence that "governments must agree to regular, independent, external assessment of their core capacities" (Moon et al. 2015, i). Yet these problems, which have ensnared the continent for too long, are the direct consequences of first colonization, then neo-colonialism, and now resource and economic exploitation by the Global North. In the cases of Guinea, Liberia, and Sierra Leone, these problems were evident in conflict diamonds, and the cocoa, coffee, rubber, and timber trades, to name just a few examples of external interference (Bertocchi and Canova 2002; Olsson 2009; Olsson 2007).

Disease control What is needed at this point is the integration of lessons learned and the implementation of a sustainable approach to prevent what has occurred from repeating itself. This brings us back to a primary aspect of infectious disease outbreaks – monitoring and control.[11] According to WHO (2015a), surveillance is the continuous, systematic collection, analysis, and interpretation of health-related data needed for the planning, implementation, and evaluation of public health practice. Surveillance serves as an early warning system for impending public health emergencies and helps track progress towards specified goals, as well as monitor and clarify the epidemiology of health problems. Thus surveillance allows governments to set priorities and inform public health policies and strategies in dealing with future epidemics. WHO's well developed global surveillance activities play a critical role in developing regional and local haemorrhagic virus surveillance networks with primary aims of monitoring disease outbreaks, especially in disease endemic areas, guiding effective planning and responses, and providing data that assists in research and development of vaccines. Why then, has the US Center for Disease Control and Prevention established with the African Union an African CDC, a new public health institute to support African ministries of health and other health agencies in their efforts to prevent, detect, and respond to any disease outbreak (CDC Media Relations 2015)? Instead of strengthening WHO in these roles, the US in effect has created an alternative agency under its control.

Historically WHO regional bodies have done much of the world's disease surveillance. WHO effectively responds to more than 100 disease outbreaks and emergencies each year. The organization has been conducting and publishing surveillance reports, particularly on communicable disease, since its first report in the 1960s (Declich and Carter 1994). Today WHO operates several surveillance programs that it conducts alone or in a joint effort with other international health bodies, including some in Africa (Agua-Agum et al. 2015b; Committee WGR 2013), using existing coordination and implementation mechanisms; in this way WHO and other interested parties compile the best information available and improve the quality of data needed for informed decision making and planning at the national, regional, and global levels. Any call to limit the role of WHO, particularly in low-income settings, amounts to the abandonment of the Third World poor to agencies that are wolves in sheep's clothing. Why then are its critics so keen to redirect the organization's efforts?

The critiques of WHO and the WHO response

A number of recent reports (ICG 2015; Moon et al. 2015) have been published that are critical of WHO and contain extensive recommendations for its reorganization. We see the critiques as embedded in the new global health landscape dominated by private foundations representing the globalization of commercialized medicine. Space does not permit us to reply to each of the recommendations so we have singled out a few that best illustrate the neoliberal approach to the crisis at WHO.

The 22 authors of the report of the Harvard-London School of Hygiene and Tropical Medicine independent panel on the global response to Ebola, under the chairmanship of Peter Piot, Director of the School and Professor of Global Health, London School of Hygiene and Tropical Medicine, represent a range of medical and legal academic and private sector actors.[12] The International Crisis Group, based in Brussels, describes itself as an independent, non-profit NGO committed to preventing and resolving deadly conflict. At the heart of the matter is the recommendation that WHO

> focus on four core functions: supporting national capacity building through technical advice; rapid early response and assessment of outbreaks (including potential emergency declarations); establishing technical norms, standards, and guidance; and convening the global community to set goals, mobilise resources, and negotiate rules. Beyond outbreaks, WHO should maintain its broad definition of health but substantially scale back its expansive range of activities to focus on core functions (to be defined through a process launched by the WHO Executive Board). (Moon et al. 2015, 2)

We understand this to mean that WHO is to be stripped of its constitutional mandate, described above, and reduced to becoming yet another emergency aid organization. It would seem that WHO, far from failing in its original mission, poses a threat to the neoliberal economic program of commercialization of health care.

This recommendation to reduce WHO's activities is followed by explicit directions to the WHO Executive Board:

> mandate good governance reforms, including establishing a freedom of information policy, an Inspector General's office,

> and human resource management reform, all to be implemented by an Interim Deputy for Managerial Reform by July 2017. In exchange for successful reforms, governments should finance most of the budget with untied funds in a new deal for a more focused WHO. Finally, member states should insist on a Director-General with the character and capacity to challenge even the most powerful governments when necessary to protect public health. (Moon et al. 2015, 2)

The ICG echoes this recommendation by insisting on an independent review of the ongoing WHO reform process that will hold officials at the country, regional, and headquarters levels accountable for fully implementing reforms (ICG 2015, iv).

We are especially concerned with another recommendation: to create a Global Health Committee as part of the UN Security Council. Not only does this bypass the World Health Assembly, a far more representative and democratic body than the Security Council, but it also militarizes public health. Ostensibly the purpose is "to expedite high-level leadership and systematically elevate political attention to health issues, recognising health as essential to human security" (Moon et al. 2015, 2). This trend to militarization follows the approach taken to the AIDS epidemic, a course that for too long blocked recognition of the social, economic, and cultural factors relevant to the spread and prevention of HIV.

WHO responds to its critics In December 2014, WHO brought together health and finance ministers, non-state actors, donors, and international technical agencies with the aim of laying the foundation for stronger health systems in the medium- to long-term in the three Ebola-affected countries. But the current state of global health governance makes WHO's work with governments nigh on impossible. Take for example WHO's work in Sierra Leone before the Ebola outbreak. To conceptualize and implement health projects like strengthening health policies, systems, and environment to improve access and quality of services, WHO collaborates with no less than 13 partners working through five mechanisms for coordination.[13] The proliferation of new organizations, institutes, funds, alliances, and centers has created a crowded global health arena. Particularly influential are a self-appointed group of global health leaders known as the H8, which includes the Gates Foundation, the Global Fund for AIDS, Tuberculosis and Malaria, GAVI the Vaccine Alliance, UNAIDS, UNFPA, UNICEF, WHO, and the World Bank. Created in mid-2007, the aim of H8 is (inter alia) to seize opportunities presented by renewed interest in health systems. We understand that to mean opportunities for commercialization.

The Stocking Report (WHO 2015b), an internal evaluation commissioned by WHO, examined three critical areas: the International Health Regulations that govern the declaration of health emergencies, WHO's health emergency response capacity, and WHO's role and cooperation with the wider health and humanitarian systems. Among its recommendations were proposals to give WHO more clout with countries experiencing epidemics, so that they would be persuaded to declare emergencies sooner, and with countries interfering in trade and traffic, so that adverse economic effects might be mitigated. The report anticipated the ICG and LSHTM by asking the UN Secretary-General's high-level panel on the global response to health crises to put global health issues at the center of the global security agenda.

The WHO response to the Stocking Report notes that, to address the gaps in IHR implementation, political support must be forthcoming and resilient health systems must integrate IHR core capacities (WHO 2015c). This in turn necessitates strong leadership and coordination among governments, donors, technical agencies, implementing partners, non-governmental organizations, and communities – over which, we note, WHO has limited control. To fund these initiatives, WHO must turn to the World Bank. In regard to the global security agenda, WHO notes that humanitarian systems have largely operated separately from those dealing with public health emergencies, despite the clearly defined response and coordination architecture of the Interagency Standing Committee.

Conclusions

The need for strong and effective global health leadership is self-evident, and to us WHO is the obvious candidate for this role. But WHO is subject to tidal forces of international politics that push and pull the organization. WHO is under-funded and over-reliant on public private partnerships (arrangements that involve business organizations and civil society) to achieve what governments and the UN cannot manage alone. WHO cannot criticize this unwieldy structure without biting the hands that feed it, since extra-budgetary funds (contributions outside of the annual assessments of its members that constitute regular budgetary funds) now account for some three-quarters of WHO's expenditure. In 2007 the World Bank declared that it, the World Bank, should be the lead global technical agency for health systems policy and suggested that WHO's comparative advantage was not in health systems but in technical aspects of disease control and health facility management (GHW 2 2008, 284). Behind this declaration, we see the World Bank promoting commercialized medicine, and we also hear the accusations made by the US Congress that WHO promotes socialized medicine. Those in agreement with this approach have seized the Ebola epidemic as an opportunity to advance the Bank's agenda.

The failure of countries to invest in global public goods for health is at the center of the international community's neglect of Third World public health, a failure mirrored as weaknesses in WHO. The agency suffers from a lack of political and financial commitment by its members even though they share the global health risks. We agree with the recommendations that governments should finance WHO's entire budget with untied funds, and that aid organizations stop undercutting local ministries' attempts at self-sufficiency.

Notes

1 WHO consists of three constituent bodies: the large, comprehensive World Health Assembly, which meets annually to decide policy and approve the program and budget; the smaller, representative Executive Board, which meets semiannually to prepare the assembly's agenda; and the Secretariat, which is the staff. Unlike other UN specialized agencies, WHO is a decentralized organization. It maintains headquarters in Geneva, Switzerland.

2 The six regional offices are located in Brazzaville, for the African region; in Washington, DC, for the Americas; in Cairo, for the Eastern Mediterranean region; in Copenhagen, for Europe; in New Delhi, for Southeast Asia; and in Manila, for the Western Pacific region.

3 The Red Cross first responded to the Ebola outbreak in Guinea in March 2014 when the initial cases were reported. See "Red Cross Responds to Ebola Outbreak in Guinea, http://www.ifrc.org/en/news-and-media/news-stories/africa/guinea/red-cross-responds-to-ebola-outbreak-in-guinea--65316/ (accessed September 16, 2016).

4 In the 1995 Ebola outbreak in Kikwit, Democratic Republic of the Congo, the diagnosis was established in April and the epidemic was declared in May, at which time the government asked WHO to coordinate the international response (composed

of experts from DRC, WHO, CDC, Institute of Tropical Medicine, Médecins sans Frontières (Belgium), South African Medical Institute, Red Cross, Institut Pasteur (Paris), and Sweden). Epidemiologic surveillance, which involved gathering information through city-wide surveillance, was the cornerstone of the control strategy. Patients were isolated, health workers received protective gear, nurses used barrier techniques, and the dead were buried in plastic bags by trained and equipped volunteers (Muyembe-Tamfum et al. 1999). These were the same measures employed in the West African outbreak; the difference is the scale: in Kikwit (population 400,000), 317 people were affected (245 died).

5 For a critique of MSF in Sierra Leone, see Fink (2015b).

6 The OCHA Financial Tracking Service does not even list this sum as a pledge. For a comprehensive review of OCHA's analysis, see Grépin (2015).

7 See http://observers.france24.com/content/20140324-guinea-struck-new-outbreak-ebola-virus?ns_mchannel=acquisition&ns_source=google&ns_campaign=sem&ns_linkname=editorial&aef_campaign_ref=the_observers_uk_afrique_guinea_-_ebola_guinea_ebola&aef_campaign_date=inconnue&gclid=CPvAtq-ktcQCFWFp7AodfjMAHQ.

8 A timelier IHR response to the Ebola outbreak was hampered by issues around information sharing, the need for clearance at many levels, and affected governments' anxiety about the consequences of notification (subsequently justified by the actions of other countries, airlines, and business leaders). The IHR declaration of a public health emergency served to mobilize resources for the response, but also resulted in many countries implementing additional measures that interfered with international travel and trade, creating severe economic consequences and barriers to receiving necessary personnel and supplies. See WHO: Ebola Interim Assessment Panel: Report by the Secretariat, May 8, 2015, http://apps.who.int/gb/ebwha/pdf_files/WHA68/A68_25-en.pdf?ua=1 (accessed September 16, 2016).

9 http://www.nature.com/nature/journal/v438/n7068/full/438575a.html; http://journals.plos.org/plosone/article?id=10.1371/journal.pone.0002739.

10 http://www.ncbi.nlm.nih.gov/pubmed/19323614.

11 Although its history goes back earlier, surveillance developed in the nineteenth century into the collection and interpretation of health-related data for the purposes of identifying appropriate action in controlling epidemics (Declich and Carter 1994). In the last century, surveillance has gone from its use as a source of data by the national health insurance system in the United Kingdom in 1911 and the first national health survey in the United States in 1935 to the establishment of an epidemiological surveillance unit in the division of communicable diseases at WHO in Geneva in 1965 (Choi and Pak 2001).

12 The universities are Basel, Duke, Edinburgh, Georgetown, Harvard, Hong Kong, Indiana, LSHTM, Simon Fraser, and UC San Francisco; the private sector groups are Action Contre la Faim International – Monrovia, AIDS Healthcare Foundation, Campaign for Good Governance – Sierra Leone, Center for Strategic and International Studies, Chatham House, Clinton Foundation, Community Partners International, Council on Foreign Relations, Médecins Sans Frontières. Note the absence of Guinea.

13 UN Agencies (UNICEF, UNFPA, UNDP, FAO, and WFP), the World

Bank, EU, DfID, Irish Aid, and the ADB; bilateral partners include the EU, ABB, and DfID. The main mechanisms for coordination in the health sector are: Health Sector Coordinating Committee, Inter Agency Coordinating Committee for Reproductive and Child Health, Country Coordination Mechanism, Health Implementing Partners Coordinating Committee, Health Development Partners Forum, and Development Partnership Aid Coordination Committee, ccsbrief_sierra_leone_en.pdf (accessed May 12, 2015).

References

Agua-Agum, J. et al. (2015a). "Ebola Virus Disease among Children in West Africa," *New England Journal of Medicine* 72, 13: 1274–1277.

Agua-Agum, J. et al. (2015b). "West African Ebola Epidemic after One Year: Slowing but Not Yet under Control," *New England Journal of Medicine* 372, 6: 584–587.

Asgary, R., Pavlin, J.A., Ripp, J.A., Reithinger, R., and Polyak, C.S. (2015). "Ebola Policies That Hinder Epidemic Response by Limiting Scientific Discourse," *The American Journal of Tropical Medicine and Hygiene* 92, 2: 240–241.

Associated Press (2014). "After Botching Ebola, WHO to Pick New Africa Boss," *New York Times*, November 3.

Bah, E.I. et al. (2015). "Clinical Presentation of Patients with Ebola Virus Disease in Conakry, Guinea," *New England Journal of Medicine* 372, 1: 40–47.

Baker, K.M. (1984). "Book Review: The Political Economy of West African Agriculture," *African Affairs* 83, 330: 121.

Bebinger, M. (2014). "Boston-Based Partners in Health Leaps into Ebola Crisis." http://www.pih.org/media-coverage/wbur-boston-based-partners-in-health-leaps-into-ebola-crisis (accessed September 16, 2016).

Bertocchi, G. and Canova, F. (2002). "Did Colonization Matter for Growth?: An Empirical Exploration into the Historical Causes of Africa's Underdevelopment," *European Economic Review* 46, 10: 1851–1871.

Black, R. and Sessay, M. (1997). "Forced Migration, Land-use Change and Political Economy in the Forest Region of Guinea," *African Affairs* 96, 385: 587–605.

Bloom, Gerald, MacGregor, Hayley, McKenzie, Andrew, and Sokpo, Emmanuel (2015). *Strengthening Health Systems for Resilience*, Practice Paper in Brief 18. Brighton: Institute of Development Studies.

CDC Media Relations (2015). "African Union and CDC Partner to Launch African CDC." http://www.cdc.gov/media/releases/2015/p0413-african-union.html (accessed September 16, 2016).

Cenciarelli, Orlando et al. (2015). "Ebola Virus Disease 2013–2014 Outbreak in West Africa: An Analysis of the Epidemic Spread and Response," *International Journal of Microbiology* 2015: 1–12.

Chai, Carmen (2014). "First Diagnosed Ebola Case in the North America: What Happened?" *Global News*. http://globalnews.ca/news/1592655/first-diagnosed-ebola-case-in-the-north-america-what-happened/ (accessed September 16, 2016).

Changula, K., Kajihara, M., Mweene, A.S., and Takada, A. (2014). "Ebola and Marburg Virus Diseases in Africa: Increased Risk of Outbreaks in Previously Unaffected Areas?"

Microbiology and Immunology 58, 9: 483–491.

Chertow, D.S., Kleine, C., Edwards, J.K., Scaini, R., Giuliani, R., and Sprecher, A. (2014). "Ebola Virus Disease in West Africa: Clinical Manifestations and Management," *New England Journal of Medicine* 371, 22: 2054–2057.

Choi, B.C. and Pak, A.W. (2001). "Lessons for Surveillance in the 21st Century: A Historical Perspective from the Past Five Millennia," *Sozial- und Praventivmedizin* 46, 6: 361–368.

Committee WGR (2013). *WHO Guidelines Approved by the Guidelines Review Committee. Guidelines for Second Generation HIV Surveillance: An Update: Know Your Epidemic.* Geneva: World Health Organization.

Declich, S. and Carter, A.O. (1994). "Public Health Surveillance: Historical Origins, Methods and Evaluation," *Bulletin of the World Health Organization* 72, 2: 285–304.

Fink, S. (2015a). "Care Differs from American and African with Ebola," *The New York Times*, March 17.

Fink, S. (2015b). "Pattern of Safety Lapses Where Group Worked to Battle Ebola Outbreak," *The New York Times*, April 12.

Fuest, V. (2008). "This Is the Time to Get in Front: Changing Roles and Opportunities for Women in Liberia," *African Affairs* 107, 427: 201–224.

Ghayourmanesh, S.P. and Hawley, H.M. (2014). *Ebola Virus Online: Magill's Medical Guide* (Online Edition), November 23, 2014. https://login.proxy.libraries.rutgers.edu/login?url=http://search.ebscohost.com/login.aspx?direct=true&db=ers&AN=86194072&site=eds-live.

GHW 2 (2008). *Global Health Watch 2*. London: Zed Books.

Global Ebola Response Information Centre (2015). *Making a Difference: The Global Ebola Response: Outlook 2015*. New York: United Nations, January. https://ebolaresponse.un.org/sites/default/files/ebolaoutlook_full.pdf (accessed September 16, 2016).

Grépin, Karen A. (2015). "International Donations to the Ebola Virus Outbreak: Too Little, Too Late?" *B M J – Clinical Research Edition* 350: p.h376; 03 02.

Groseth, A., Feldmann, H., and Strong, J.E. (2007). "The Ecology of Ebola Virus," *Trends in Microbiology* 15, 9: 408–416.

Hanreider, Tine (2015). "The Path-Dependent Design of International Organizations: Federalism in the World Health Organization," *European Journal of International Relations* 21, 1: 215–239.

Hoffman, D. (2004). "The Civilian Target in Sierra Leone and Liberia: Political Power, Military Strategy, and Humanitarian Intervention," *African Affairs* 103, 411: 211–226.

ICG (2015). *The Politics behind the Ebola Crisis*. Africa Report no. 232, October 28. Brussels: International Crisis Group.

Kamradt-Scott, Adam (2016). "WHO's to Blame? The World Health Organization and the 2014 Ebola Outbreak in West Africa," *Third World Quarterly* 37, 3: 401–418.

Kentikelenis, Alexander, King, Lawrence, McKee, Martin, and Stuckler, David (2015). "The International Monetary Fund and the Ebola Outbreak," *The Lancet* 3 (February): e69–e70. http://www.thelancet.com/pdfs/journals/langlo/PIIS2214-109X(14)70377-8.pdf (accessed September 16, 2016).

Knobloch, J., McCormick, J.B., Webb, P.A., Dietrich, M., Schumacher, H.H., and Dennis, E. (1980). "Clinical Observations in 42 Patients with

Lassa Fever," *Tropenmedizin und Parasitologie* 31, 4: 389–398.

Kortepeter, M.G., Bausch, D.G., and Bray, M. (2011). "Basic Clinical and Laboratory Features of Filoviral Hemorrhagic Fever," *Journal of Infectious Diseases* 204 (suppl. 3): S810-6.

Lindblad, R., El Fiky, A., and Zajdowicz, T. (2015). "Ebola in the United States," *Journal of Allergy and Clinical Immunology* 135, 4: 868–871.

Monson, M.H., Frame, J.D., Jahrling, P.B., and Alexander, K. (1984). "Endemic Lassa Fever in Liberia. I. Clinical and Epidemiological Aspects at Curran Lutheran Hospital, Zorzor, Liberia," *Transactions of the Royal Society of Tropical Medicine and Hygiene* 78, 4: 549–553.

Moon, Suerie et al. (2015). "Will Ebola Change the Game? Ten Essential Reforms before the Next Pandemic. The Report of the Harvard-LSHTM Independent Panel on the Global Response to Ebola," *Lancet* 386, 10009 (November 28): 2204–2221.

MSF (2014). *Ebola Response: Where Are We Now?* MSF briefing paper, December. http://www.doctorswithoutborders.org/document/ebola-response-where-are-we-now (accessed September 16, 2016).

Murphy, W.P. (2013). "Book Review: The War Machines: Young Men and Violence in Sierra Leone and Liberia," *African Affairs* 112, 446: 164–165.

Muyembe-Tamfum, J.J., Kipasa, M., Kiyungu, C., and Colebunders, R. (1999). "Ebola Outbreak in Kikwit, Democratic Republic of the Congo: Discovery and Control Measures," *Journal of Infectious Diseases* 179 (suppl. 1): S259–S262.

Nadeau, Barbie Latza (2014). "Europe's Hidden Ebola Cases," *The Daily Beast*, Ocotober 15. http://www.thedailybeast.com/articles/2014/10/15/europe-s-problematic-ebola-patients.html (accessed September 16, 2016).

OCHA, Financial Tracking Service, Ebola Virus Outbreak – Table A: Total funding and outstanding pledges as of March 17, 2015 (Table ref: R10). Compiled by OCHA on the basis of information provided by donors and appealing organizations. http://fts.unocha.org/reports/daily/ocha_R10_E16506_asof___1503172111.pdf.

Olsson, O. (2007). "Conflict Diamonds," *Journal of Development Economics* 82, 2: 267–286.

Olsson, O. (2009). "On the Democratic Legacy of Colonialism," *Journal of Comparative Economics* 37, 4: 534–551.

Park, Alex (2014). Why the World Health Organization Doesn't Have Enough Funds to Fight Ebola," September 8, 2014. http://www.motherjones.com/politics/2014/09/ebola-world-health-organization-budget (accessed March 17, 2015).

Randolph, E. (2015). MSF and WHO Trade Blame Over Slow Global Ebola Response. *Yahoo News*.

Stein, R.A. (2015). "What Is Ebola?" *International Journal of Clinical Practice* 69, 1: 49–58.

Team WER (2014). "Ebola Virus Disease in West Africa: The First 9 Months of the Epidemic and Forward Projections," *New England Journal of Medicine* 371, 16: 1481–1495.

Vapalahti, O., Kallio-Kokko, H., Anttila, V.J., and Lyytikainen, O. (2014). "Ebola : virus, tauti, leviäminen - ja varautuminen Suomessa" [Ebola: Virus, Disease, Transmission: And Preparedness in Finland], *Duodecim* 130, 21: 2163–2177.

Wallace, Rob and Wallace, Rodrick (2016). "Ebola's Ecologies: Agro-Economics and Epidemiology in

West Africa," *New Left Review* 102 (November–December): 1–13.

Weyer, J., Grobbelaar, A., and Blumberg, L. (2015). "Ebola Virus Disease: History, Epidemiology and Outbreaks," *Current Infectious Disease Reports* 17, 5: 480.

WHO (2014). "Statement on the 1st Meeting of the IHR Emergency Committee on the 2014 Ebola Outbreak in West Africa." http://www.who.int/mediacentre/news/statements/2014/ebola-20140808/en/ (accessed September 16, 2016).

WHO (2015). "Global Infectious Disease Surveillance." Fact Sheet no. 200. http://www.who.int/mediacentre/factsheets/fs200/en/ (accessed September 16, 2016).

WHO (2015a). "Public Health Surveillance" [April 30, 2015]. http://www.who.int/topics/public_health_surveillance/en/ (accessed September 16, 2016).

WHO (2015b). "Report of the Ebola Interim Assessment Panel" [the "Stocking Report"], July 7. http://www.who.int/csr/resources/publications/ebola/report-by-panel.pdf?ua=1 (accessed September 16, 2016).

WHO (2015c). *WHO Secretariat Response to the Report of the Ebola Interim Assessment Panel*, August 19. http://www.who.int/csr/resources/publications/ebola/who-response-to-ebola-report.pdf?ua=1 (accessed September 16, 2016).

11 | THE EBOLA EPIDEMIC MOMENT IN US–(WEST) AFRICA RELATIONS

Fodei Batty

Introduction

They say politics makes strange bedfellows. Well, so does disease as evidenced by the multifarious domestic and international coalitions that emerged around the West Africa Ebola epidemic, which reportedly started with an index case of the disease in Guinea in December of 2013 (see Blaize et al. 2014). In the United States, politicians of every stripe put ideological differences aside and coalesced their efforts around addressing the epidemic of Ebola Virus Disease. Democrats and Republicans in the United States Congress often fail to reach a middle ground on a wide range of international and domestic issues. Whether it is the debate over climate change, ratifying the United Nations Arms Trade Treaty, lifting the United States embargo on Cuba, enacting comprehensive gun control, negotiating a nuclear deal with Iran, or fighting the Islamic State in Iraq and Syria, their interests often diverge markedly in the partisan political climate that often engulfs Washington, DC.[1]

Yet, in addressing the Ebola outbreak in West Africa, partisan divides were bridged relatively quickly to approve President Obama's emergency request for funding to lead the efforts against the epidemic. To be clear, although members of both major parties wanted the epidemic addressed swiftly, significant ideological differences were evident in the policy directions they sought. Whereas Republicans preferred quarantines and travel bans from the affected countries, Democrats opted for increased spending on humanitarian and health initiatives. Nevertheless, under a special addition to a funding bill for fiscal year 2015, the US Congress approved various appropriations worth $5.4 billion intended "to prevent, prepare for, and respond to the Ebola virus domestically and internationally."[2] At the same time other public figures, such as Governor Chris Christie of New Jersey, called for extreme measures to quarantine anyone arriving from Ebola-affected West Africa (see, for example, Yan and Botelho 2014). An opinion poll conducted by *ABC News* and *The Washington Post* in October 2014 found that 67 percent of Americans supported restricting entry to the United States by people who have been to countries affected by the Ebola outbreak, in essence seeking the isolation of the region from global interactions.[3] This chapter examines these often conflicting and extraordinary reactions to the first Ebola epidemic in West Africa to reveal several contradictions in the relations between the United States and the region, as well as the inconsistencies inherent in the political economy of our globalized world.

In recent history, no other event has drawn as much attention to discourses of global inequality as what transpired in the wake of the Ebola outbreak in West Africa. In addition to allegations of malfeasance about the origins of the Ebola virus,[4] the epidemic also drew attention to much more tangible concerns about the inconsistencies and contradictions that are prevalent in the operations of the global system.[5] Analyses of the relations between rich industrialized countries of the Global North, such as the United States, and those of the relatively poor countries of the Global South, such as the West African countries of Guinea, Liberia, and Sierra Leone that were most affected by the Ebola epidemic, often cast a picture of disharmonies of interests between the two areas of the world (see for example, Haas and Hird 2013; Brawley 2005; Easterly 2002; Stiglitz 2002; Mshomba 2000). Whether it is addressing climate change, international trade, exploiting natural resources, or bringing alleged violators of human rights to justice, to cite a few examples, the interests of the two areas are said to diverge distinctly so that the rich industrialized countries often gain more from international interactions within the global system, at the expense of the poor countries of the Global South (see for example, Ross and Chan 2002). Many observers claim that the United States and other Western powers establish and dictate their interests in the global system through unfair and disadvantageous policies such as trade laws and other interactions and exchanges which undergird an international capitalist system, in pursuit of hegemonic control over scarce resources (see Wallerstein 1974; Stiglitz 2002).

However, the interactions in question are often fraught with contradictions. The globalized system that is dependent, and functions, on the circulation of resources and people, ostensibly in the interest of the rich industrialized countries of the Global North, frequently struggles to contain such circulation and its consequences. The US Department of State's rather fickle and selective travel advisory system of warnings and alerts that caution Americans about travel to various parts of the world at the slightest provocation are one of the well-known examples of such contradictions in a hyper-securitized post-9/11 global system struggling to cope with the interactions and exchanges it demands.[6]

The reactions in the United States to the Ebola epidemic in West Africa draws attention to one such moment in a system that is designed to facilitate international exchanges and interactions yet, at the same time, appears ill-equipped to address some of the consequences of the circulation upon which it depends. Although the epidemic ultimately became a fleeting moment in the complex relations between the United States and West Africa that stretches back to the beginning of the transatlantic slave trade in the fifteenth century, it was a moment that was quite revealing, nevertheless, and one which, I submit, not only exposed the implications of global inequalities but also complicates the task of isolating and distinguishing between the interests of the Global North from those of the Global South.

Thus, this chapter argues that the inequalities in the interactions within a dynamic global system presents shared consequences for rich and poor countries alike as demonstrated by reactions to the Ebola epidemic. It argues further that this fact was not lost on many policymakers in Washington, DC who, as evidenced by their pronouncements and actions, realized that they could ignore the epidemic at the risk of destabilizing West Africa all over again, which would have imperiled several strategic interests of the United States. This realization convinced many Democrats and Republicans to put ideological differences aside and offer unequivocal support to try to end the epidemic at its source in West Africa.

Beyond a humanitarian concern, many US policymakers were also desperately trying to keep the full consequences of the epidemic at bay. The potential breakdown in law and order under the pressure of dealing with the Ebola outbreak could have fomented new conflicts in a fragile region still recovering from years of devastating civil war.[7] The ensuing chain of reactions could have started refugee flows and the inevitable exodus out of the region that could have spread the full consequence of the epidemic extensively within the global system. Policymakers in Washington, DC, however, were not alone in this realization. Faced with a similar prospect, Britain and France, former colonial hegemons with extensive contacts in the region and host to thousands, if not millions, of Sierra Leoneans and Guineans in the diaspora, which exponentially increased the chances of the virus arriving at their shores beyond the few controlled cases of infected returning health care workers, joined the United States in "a neat balkanization of the response to the epidemic" (see Batty 2015). Each country largely took responsibility for taking care of business in the territory with which it had the strongest colonial ties. Britain sent a small military force to Sierra Leone to construct Ebola Treatment Units (ETUs), France led the response in Guinea, and the United States spearheaded the response in Liberia.

Although the Zika virus is far less deadly and hardly registers as a debilitating disease in adult members of populations, the reactions to its outbreak in Brazil and other countries in South America in 2016 strike a useful contrast with the reactions to the Ebola epidemic. Realizing that Zika was less threatening to their interests, policymakers in the United States or Europe did not offer a similar level of urgency to tackle its outbreak, up to the time of writing this chapter, even though the virus was exerting a significant toll on communities across South America. An alternative view of the reactions to the Zika outbreak in South America could submit that the crisis in the affected countries did not warrant a similar level of urgency as the Ebola epidemic in West Africa because Brazil, Colombia, and other afflicted countries were equipped to handle the outbreak. Such arguments, however, would support the assertion that the United States and other industrialized countries were scrambling to address the shared consequences of global inequities, perpetrated by an unfair capitalist system that has left the health care systems of poorer countries such as Guinea, Liberia, and Sierra Leone woefully ill-equipped to stop the Ebola epidemic from spreading, or handling the crisis that followed.

This chapter draws upon the evidence provided by the reactions to the Ebola epidemic, especially the congressional and presidential responses in the United States to the concern of the American public about the potential spread of the disease within their country, to highlight several contradictions about the interactions and integration that is desired in the global system in the face of persistent inequalities between rich and poor areas within it. The next section discusses how politicians in the United States reacted to the outbreak or manipulated its implications for electoral and other interests. This section is followed by an account of President Obama's efforts in Washington, DC to address the growing crisis by making it one of the lead issues in a summit of African leaders convened by the White House. The third section discusses the implications of the interactions for the Ebola-affected countries of West Africa who are marginalized players in the global system. This is followed by a concluding section that points out the shared consequences of global interactions. Indeed, as the epidemic continued to spread in 2014 and early 2015 it became increasingly complex to differentiate where, in dealing with the disease, the interests of the United States stopped and those of the three most-affected countries in West Africa – Liberia, Sierra Leone, and Guinea – began.

The context of the US response to Ebola

The emergence of the Ebola epidemic in West Africa was one of the major events that shook the global community during this decade. Over several months in the fall of 2014, much of the world was frightened by the prospect of being engulfed in an uncontrollable global disease contagion. Financial markets in the United States and other areas such as Europe reacted to the growing crisis.[8] Images of the hapless victims of the terrible disease splashed across global media captivating television viewers as equally hapless medical staff tried desperately to save what lives they could at great personal risk.

The arrival of Thomas Eric Duncan in the United States, a Liberian visitor infected with Ebola, and his subsequent death in Texas on October 8, 2014 raised the anxiety level in the United States. Duncan, a Liberian citizen, travelled to Texas from Monrovia in Liberia on September 19, 2014 presumably unaware that he was infected with the virus. His arrival in Dallas on September 20, 2014, subsequent admission, and death from the disease a few weeks later on October 8, 2014 complicated the debate within America about how to address the growing crisis. It also led many Americans to question how safe they really were in contradiction with the supposed geographic immunity from the outbreak in the Global South. Thereafter, debates about the inequalities in the global system and the difference in how various people are treated took center stage in the national discourse. By the end of 2014, Ebola's impact on US relations with Africa and, in particular, the West African countries most affected by the epidemic was most visible. The dreaded travel warnings from the State Department issued the strongest warning against travel to the region in spite of the billions of dollars in trade and other interactions between the two areas.

Except for the repatriation of the seriously ill medical missionaries Dr. Kent Brantly and Nancy Writebol from Monrovia to Emory University Hospital in Atlanta Georgia for treatment, Duncan was the first patient to be diagnosed with the Ebola virus disease in the Western hemisphere. The fact that he entered the United States while the Ebola virus was incubating undetected inside him terrified many public figures and ordinary Americans about how quickly someone could traverse between the two areas of the world.

Indeed, technological advancements and capabilities fashioned to expedite travel and increase the circulation of goods and people within the global capitalist system, and considered one of the key indicators of the gap between rich and poor countries, now helped closed the gap between the relative security many felt within the United States, in their imagined insulation from "the world" out there. As far-fetched as it sounded, several public figures went on to draw corollaries between the manner of Duncan's arrival in the United States and the potential for international terrorists to employ a similar strategy. This realization further strengthened numerous calls for the Obama administration to take tougher action against the epidemic and close the country's borders.

In one of the glaring inconsistencies in the operations of an idealized global system and the variations across the various levels of policies upon which such a system is predicated, Duncan was initially refused treatment at a medical facility for lacking basic health insurance even as the US policymakers deliberated sending millions of dollars and troops to West Africa to help combat the virus. How much easier tackling the epidemic would have been had Duncan, or someone in his position, gained access to appropriate care when it mattered and when he needed it? Duncan's unfortunate demise ultimately offered evidence for skeptics of globalism, such as Stiglitz (2002) who claim that poorer citizens of the Global South are treated less well in the international system than citizens of the Global North.

It is now public knowledge that Duncan was treated horribly by the Dallas health facility than standard procedure called for. His family has since sued successfully and settled the suit against the Texas Health Presbyterian Hospital where he lost his life to Ebola (see Moyer 2014). Many observers have suggested that Duncan would have stood a better chance of surviving the disease had he been an American citizen, or had he stayed in the Global South to seek treatment (see Szabo 2014). One cannot fault such speculation when much of the evidence supports such claims. Consider the facts. Two nurses who were treating Duncan and who were accidentally infected by him were successfully treated under specialist care at some of the best facilities around the country for treating dangerous diseases such as Ebola. Both survived. To this day, the only two people known to have died of Ebola on US soil are two individuals from the Global South – Duncan and Dr. Michael Salia, a medical doctor and permanent resident in the United States, who returned to help with the Ebola crisis in his native Sierra Leone during the epidemic, paying dearly with his life for his sacrifices. Dr. Salia was airlifted to Nebraska for medical treatment where he died on November 17, 2014.

Beyond partisanship: the politics of disease in the United States

Following the intense media coverage surrounding Duncan's death from Ebola in Dallas, political machines across the United States went into overdrive seizing upon the climate of fear and uncertainty to fuel various campaigns for elective offices as the country moved towards mid-term elections. One of the first indications that addressing the Ebola epidemic in West Africa will contradict several expectations about the global system were the political campaign ads featuring Ebola that popped up on television screens in the homes of viewers in the United States heading into the mid-term elections of 2014.[9] More than 20 political advertisements for the 2014 mid-term Senatorial and House elections for the US Congress appeared on television, the Internet or other media featuring Ebola. One of the most striking ads came from Republican Senator Pat Roberts of Kansas. In the highlights of the talking points, he called for a "quarantine on West Africa" (Saletan 2014).[10] Across the country, from the liberal state of Vermont in the far northeast to the deeply conservative states of the south such as Alabama, politicians of every shade and stripe appropriated the Ebola epidemic and the sufferings of its victims thousands of miles away in Sierra Leone, Liberia, and Guinea as part of their campaign messages to scare voters into believing that it was in the best interest of the United States to stop Ebola and they, and not their opponents, were the best candidate to get the job done in Washington, DC.

Conservatives and liberals in America who, usually, do not agree on anything regarding foreign or domestic matters reached a consensus on the crisis. Several Republican and Democratic candidates running for US House of Representatives and Senate seats in Congress called for one extreme measure or the other, such as closing the borders of the country or banning travel to and from West Africa. The world suddenly became one, in their view, and events in the previously distant regions of West African now appeared frightfully much closer.

Speaking on the floor of the US Congress, several American lawmakers described the implications and potential consequences of the Ebola epidemic for the United States in stark terms. Republican Congressman Mike Kelly of Pennsylvania, for example, captured "the urgency" of the situation, when he reported on the floor of the US Congress a conversation he held with Dr. Peter Piot, the Belgian doctor who helped discover the Ebola virus in 1976. Among other points in a lengthy address on the crisis, Kelly said:

> [We must contain it to West Africa. We cannot let it get beyond those shores] … It is unthinkable that at this time in human history we are still playing around trying to figure out what we should do. The answer is it better be politically correct or we can't possibly do it. So we are going to risk entire populations. We are going to risk infecting people that have absolutely no contact but come in contact because somebody is able to travel the world freely – somebody wasn't isolated, somebody wasn't quarantined because it doesn't fit our political agenda. This makes no sense. This administration appointed an Ebola czar. That is as far as it went. We have got an Ebola czar. We don't have an Ebola agenda. We don't have an Ebola strategy. We don't have anything to combat this very lethal virus. What is it going to take to wake this country up? And I would just suggest that while it is no longer a headline, it is still very important –

not just to every citizen of this great country, but every citizen of the world. And so the answer is to isolate. The answer is to quarantine.[11]

Following Congressman Kelly, Congressman Louie Gohmert of Texas echoed similar sentiments but went several steps further to describe a doomsday scenario involving the potential weaponization of the Ebola virus, straight out of a Tom Clancy novel.[12] Congressman Gohmert said:

> Mr. Speaker, my dear friend from Pennsylvania (Mr. KELLY) is exactly right. We haven't heard the last of Ebola. It will continue to mutate. It will continue to be a threat. As this President is sending around 3,000 or so of our military members to west Africa – and they have been told they are going to be given gloves and masks and are urged to wash their hands and feet several times a day – basically, what that says is the men and women who have sworn and pledged their lives to protect ours are not going to be adequately protected by this administration. The rules of engagement already put our military at risk, and now, we are going to send them to Ebola-infested countries. The initial report said, initially, our military will not be seeing Ebola patients, but they are certainly going to come into contact with people who have had exposure to Ebola. I recall our President George W. Bush – a good man, a smart man, a witty, clever gentleman, despite what some might say – but he asked after 9/11, in essence, who would have ever dreamed someone would fly a plane into a building like a bomb? My thought immediately was, "Well, actually, Tom Clancy wrote about that several years ago." It was not a radical Islamist as had happened on 9/11/2001. The late Tom Clancy had quite an imagination, but he did his homework in amazing fashion. Some have said his books had too much detail in them, but one of his latter books had research going on in Africa with the strain of monkeys that is the one strain that is believed and has support for having been transferred through the air instead of through liquid body fluids. In the fiction novel, Clancy had somebody working to develop that strain into a mutated strain, since it mutates constantly into one that people could pass through the air, and

> then it was used to infect our military or expose our military and many Americans. Basically, in his fiction novel, that allowed radical Islamists to take over much of the Middle East, while our military had been exposed to Ebola and much of it was quarantined. There are many things Tom Clancy has written about that I hope and pray never happen. That is one of them, but since some things that Tom Clancy's mind dreamed up as a fiction writer novel actually came to fruition, we shouldn't think for a minute that if Clancy could dream it up, our enemies could as well.[13]

These statements, and many others, reflect the primary motivation among policymakers was not a humanitarian concern for saving lives in West Africa, but a desire to keep the virus away from the United States. Paradoxically, conservative Republicans in the US Congress, such as Congressmen Kelly and Gohmert often are among the chief advocates of neoliberal opening of the global system to facilitate free trade. Yet, in addressing Ebola, they appeared reticent in the face of the contradictions and the implications of their arguments calling for restrictions on the free movement of people.

Table 11.1 below presents information on 15 of the 20 Ebola-related bills that were tabled in the US Congress during the 113th Congress from 2013 to 2015. As the information shows, many of the bills were co-sponsored by several Republicans and Democrats. In most cases, the expressed reason for sponsoring the bill was to protect America, its interests, or the interests of its allies from the spread of the epidemic, instead of a humanitarian intervention to save lives in West Africa.

In the US Senate, many speakers took the floor to similarly voice their concerns about the threat the Ebola epidemic posed to people everywhere. On September 11, 2014, Senator Patrick Leahy, a Democrat from Vermont had this to say in the Senate regarding the epidemic:

> Madam President,[14] over the past several months the world's attention has been focused on the Russian invasion of Crimea and fighting in the eastern Ukraine, the explosion of violence in Gaza, the flood of migrant children from Central America, and the horrific death and destruction in Iraq and Syria. In each

TABLE 11.1 Ebola-related Bills in the 113th US Congress, 2013–2015

Number	Title	Sponsors	Co-sponsors	Status
H.Res. 701	Expressing the sense of the House of Representatives that the current outbreak of Ebola in Guinea, Sierra Leone, and Liberia is an international health crisis and is the largest and most widespread outbreak of the disease ever recorded	Rep. Karen Bass (D-CA)	100 (93 Democrats, 7 Republicans)	Referred to Committee on July 31, 2014
S. 2917	Adding Ebola to the FDA Priority Review Voucher Program Act	Sen. Thomas "Tom" Harkin (D-IA)	45 (26 Democrats, 19 Republicans)	Enacted. Signed into law by President Obama on December 16, 2014
H.R. 83	Consolidated and Further Continuing Appropriations Act, 2015	Rep. Donna Christensen (D-VIO)	4 (4 Democrats)	Enacted. Signed into law by President Obama on December 16, 2014. This law provided the funding for the president's special request for Congressional funding to address the Ebola crisis. $5.4 billion was approved as an addition to the original spending bill for fiscal year 2015
H.R. 5710	Ebola Emergency Response Act	Rep. Christopher "Chris" Smith (R-NJ)	5 (4 Democrats, 1 Republican)	Reported by Committee on November 20, 2014
S. 2953	Keeping America Safe from Ebola Act of 2014	Sen. Marco Rubio (R-FL)	5 (5 Republicans)	Referred to Committee on November 20, 2014
H.R. 5746	Keeping America Safe from Ebola Act of 2014	Rep. Mike Kelly (R-PA)	None	Referred to Committee on November 20, 2014

TABLE 11.1 Continued

S. 2942	Infectious Disease Hospital Hubs Act	Sen. Edward "Ed" Markey (D-MA)	1 (1 Republican)	Referred to Committee on November 19, 2014
H.R. 5729	Adding Ebola to the FDA Priority Review Voucher Program Act	Rep. Marsha Blackburn (R-TN)	4 (2 Republicans, 2 Democrats)	This bill was signed by President Obama and enacted as S2917
H.Con.Res. 118	Expressing the sense of Congress that health workers deserve our profound gratitude and respect for their commitments and sacrifices in addressing the Ebola epidemic in West Africa	Rep. David Cicilline (D-RI)	12 (11 Democrats, 1 Republican)	Referred to Committee on November 14, 2014
H.R. 5707	Ebola Response Act of 2014	Rep. Ted Yoho (R-FL)	2 (2 Republicans)	Referred to Committee on November 13, 2014
H.R. 5694	Contain Ebola and Stop the Epidemic Act of 2014	Rep. Dennis Ross (R-FL)	3 (3 Republicans)	Referred to Committee on November 12, 2014
H.R. 5692	Ebola Prevention Act of 2014	Rep. Ted Poe (R-TX)	None	Referred to Committee on November 12, 2014
S.Res. 541	A Resolution recognizing the severe threat that the Ebola outbreak in West Africa poses to populations, governments, and economies across Africa and, if not properly contained, to regions across the globe ...	Sen. Chris Coons (D-DE)	20 (17 Democrats, 3 Republicans)	This resolution was agreed to as a simple resolution on September 18, 2014

Sources: (1) GovTrack.US at https://www.govtrack.us/congress/bills/browse#congress=113&text=Ebola (accessed February 21, 2016); (2) The Library of Congress at https://www.congress.gov/ (accessed February 20, 2016)

> of these places vast numbers of innocent people have suffered terribly, and our own policies and capability to respond have been severely tested. Yet one of the most urgent, difficult, and frightening challenges facing the world today is not the result of armed conflict or ethnic or religious extremism. It is the world's first Ebola epidemic, and it poses a potentially devastating threat to Africa and people everywhere ... The challenges are immense: weak government institutions; dysfunctional public health systems that cannot conduct reliable disease surveillance and response; lack of roads and other basic infrastructure; ethnic and political divisions in societies recovering from war; misconceptions about the disease and low levels of literacy; and inadequate and uncoordinated international aid ... The Congress has a role to play, and I am hopeful that as additional funds are needed we will act responsibly and provide them. I am a cosponsor of S. Res. 541, which recounts the history of this outbreak and the steps that are urgently needed to control it. I commend Senators COONS, DURBIN, MENENDEZ and others who introduced it. This is not a partisan or political issue. It is a public health issue, a moral issue, and one that should unite us all to do what is necessary to defeat this epidemic.[15]

In contrast, the Zika virus scare in South America that followed the Ebola virus in West Africa and has made its way into the United States with more than 20 recorded cases hardly registered more than a few mentions by the Democratic and Republican presidential candidates on the campaign trail seeking their parties' nominations for the 2016 presidential elections.

Ebola steals the show at the United States–Africa Leaders' Summit

Prior to the intensified debates about the epidemic in the halls of Congress and on the campaign trail heading into the US mid-term elections of 2014, President Obama pursued executive action to stop Ebola. On August 4–6, 2014, he hosted a US–Africa Leaders' Summit to which he welcomed leaders from across the African continent to Washington, DC to discuss important issues of mutual concern to America and the African continent such as trade, security, and climate change. Ultimately, the proceedings were overtaken and dominated by the gathering crisis in the Ebola epidemic that was raging in West Africa at the time. Arresting the epidemic soon became *the* main talking point of the summit. The leaders of Sierra Leone and Liberia, Presidents Ellen Johnson Sirleaf and Ernest Koroma, were two of the notable absentees who excused themselves to stay in their respective countries and lead the efforts against the disease. Johnson Sirleaf sent her Vice-President Joseph Boakai in her stead whereas Koroma sent his Foreign Minister, Samura Kamara, to attend on his behalf. Leaders of Eritrea, Central African Republic, Sudan, and Zimbabwe were not invited to the summit because of their poor standing with the United States.

In headlining the summit, President Obama offered the strongest evidence, yet, for the claim of a common interest in addressing inequalities in the global system declaring:

> I do not see the countries and peoples of Africa as a world apart; I see Africa as a fundamental part of our interconnected world – partners with America on behalf of the future we want for all our children. That partnership must be grounded in mutual responsibility and mutual respect.[16]

During the summit, President Obama met with all the African leaders and heads of delegations present for the summit to reiterate the importance of United States–Africa relations and to reassure them of his administration's support for achieving several goals on the African continent. On November 5, 2014, President Obama submitted a formal request to Congress for extraordinary budgetary funding amounting to $6.18 billion dollars to fight the Ebola epidemic (see, for example, Achenbach 2014). The request was received with overwhelming and bipartisan support and much of the funds requested was approved in December 2014 by Congress for a total of $5.4 billion dollars. Additional troops and equipment were subsequently committed to Liberia and the other countries affected by the epidemic, although the mode of deployment was criticized by some observers for mirroring colonial inheritances.

Although this was a special time in the relations between the United States and Africa given President Obama's Kenyan heritage, there is also strong precedence for similar commitment to issues in Africa under the African Growth and Opportunity Act (AGOA) signed by the Clinton administration in 2000, and the President's Emergency Plan For AIDS Relief (PEPFAR) signed into law by George W. Bush in 2008, to list but two examples of initiatives that have tried to walk the line back from the Cold War years when many US policies towards a lot of African countries were hostile and destabilizing. The PEPFAR fund, in particular, is one of the largest international monetary commitments by the United States since the $13 billion dollar Marshall Plan of 1948 pledged to help Europe rebuild following the Second World War. Originally set at $15 billion dollars, and targeted at Africa and the Caribbean, the amount has since exceeded the original figure in re-authorizations by the US Congress.

In addition to the summit organized by the White House, members of Congress held numerous Congressional hearings on the Ebola epidemic in 2014. No less than ten Congressional hearings were held by different Congressional committees and leaders. Each attracted a wide range of ideological actors and testimonies all, remarkably, urging US intervention to help end the epidemic. Seldom do issues succeed in uniting partisan interests for congressional hearings as did the Ebola epidemic. Some members of the ideological right often regard the commitment of US foreign assistance overseas as a waste of taxpayer money. In this instance, however, testimonies delivered to Congressional committees unanimously connected US interests to the interests of the affected countries. Whether out of fear of contagion, a genuine realization that global markets are intricately woven together in the contemporary international system, or for altruistic reasons, previously adversarial neoconservative and global justice coalitions attended the hearings in shows of support for US efforts to address the problem, unlike the scaremongering that had taken place in campaign ads prior to the mid-term elections.

In one particular hearing convened by Senator Thad Cochran, a Republican senator from the conservative southern state of Mississippi on Wednesday, November 12, 2014, over 60 witnesses attended ranging from international non-governmental organizations such as Action Contre La Faim International (ACFI) who advocate global justice issues and the elimination of hunger as a global right, to state and local emergency response agencies such as the St. Louis Area Regional Response System.[17] It was one of the largest congressional hearings in recent times and the testimonies from all independent and government attendees identified common cause with addressing the epidemic in West Africa.

The costs of marginalization

The accounts of how the epidemic of Ebola virus disease in West Africa emerged and how it was transmitted among the infected members of the populations reflected several perspectives on the relations between the United States and West Africa, the contradictions in the global system, and the continuing discourse of inequality in the global system. In spite of much effort by civil society groups, non-governmental organizations, and state officials, rumors emerged in the early stages of the epidemic, and persisted, that Ebola was a human-made virus that was artificially created in a lab in the Western world and unleashed on innocent African populations in order to destroy them. Some accounts pointed to questionable tests of vaccine and laboratory equipment by Tulane University in particular, which was openly announced on the university's website as work being carried out in Sierra Leone since 2007, in collaboration with a bio-pharmaceutical firm known as Tekmira, on behalf of the US military (see Tulane University 2007).

Neither Tulane University nor government officials in the most affected countries ever addressed the rumors, a strategic mistake in my view, which played a key role in exacerbating the epidemic early on. Most victims who believed the rumors that Ebola was an artificially created disease from the West acted on their fears and refused to go to Ebola Treatment Centers until it was often too late to save their lives. Families of deceased victims continued unsafe burial practices believing that the disease did not exist and others refused to seek care when family members showed symptoms of the disease believing that the treatment centers were, in themselves, places of death and medical experimentation by Western interests.

Conversely, Western media interests circulated stories of African's love for bush meat and the perpetuation of outdated cultural practices such as "kissing the dead" as reasons for the intensity with which the disease had decimated their loved ones. Usually respected outlets for the dissemination of scientific findings such as the *New England Journal of Medicine* published incredible accounts of the origins of the Ebola virus in West Africa attributing the cause to a two-year old patient zero in a remote community in Guinea who consumed bats carrying the virus. Later, a revision of the *New England Journal of Medicine*'s account, by a German scientist whose visit to the village was documented by no less a respected global media outlet than the British Broadcasting Corporation, was published to "correct" the narrative as patient zero playing with his friends in the hollow of a tree that contained the droppings of infected bats (see Saez et al. 2014; Roberts 2014), a far more plausible but equally incredulous account of the origins of the epidemic that demonstrates how the production of knowledge and what is considered "the truth" is still heavily skewed by Western influences and interests in the global system (see Chernoh Bah in this volume).

In the account of their work in Sierra Leone found in the archives of their website, Tulane University researchers reported they were testing bioweapons-related equipment for counterterrorism (see Tulane University 2007). This admission raises sufficient cause for anyone to ask why Tulane would conduct a bioweapons test in Sierra Leone of all places. Why did they not take the test to France, Holland, or even the bayous of Louisiana, which have climatic conditions approximating those in Sierra Leone? The answer to the latter question offers evidence for the contradictions that exist in the global system and the continuing discourses on global inequalities. Public policy leaders such as Governor Chris Christie of New Jersey, who called for the quarantining of travelers from West Africa, never questioned why US entities such as Tulane University would conduct a bioterrorism threat test in Sierra Leone but he was prepared to shut that part of the world off from the global system under a controversial policy proposal that was rightly condemned by global rights activists.

In the main, in spite of the pledges from President Obama and other assistance from Western donors that flowed into the countries affected by Ebola after the onset of the epidemic, the studies Tulane University claimed it was conducting in Kenema, eastern Sierra Leone demonstrate that the Global South is still subjugated to actions such as dangerous biological experiments involving human subjects the likes of which are not implemented elsewhere. Counterfactually, it is inconceivable that a university from Sierra Leone will arrive in New Orleans, Louisiana where Tulane University is located and undertake a similar experiment such as the one Tulane University carried out in the years preceding the outbreak, which has led many observers and victims to claim an association between the two events. Even if they had the equipment, the nature of unequal relations between citizens of the two areas precludes such an experiment taking place. It takes the wildest imagination to picture residents of a town in Louisiana consenting to having their blood drawn by a research team from Sierra Leone.

Finally, the explosion of social media has had a significant impact on the relations between the United States and Africa as evidenced by the developments that took place during the Ebola epidemic. Whereas in the past two young people growing up on either side of the Atlantic are likely to never hear of each other in their lifetimes, pen pal programs notwithstanding, nowadays social media such as Facebook, Twitter, Pinterest, YouTube, or Instagram, to list but a few examples, have created all kinds of instantaneous connections across divides that use to exist. At the height of the epidemic in 2014, tweets about victims in Liberia, Sierra Leone, or Guinea were instantly retweeted millions of times across the globe giving voices and faces to victims. In addition, there are also many inspiring stories, as well as negative stereotypes, of connections that have been established between ordinary people from across the United States and Africa that have resulted in meaningful friendships. Some of these connections played key roles in helping address the epidemic as voters called on their elected representatives and urged them to act to end the Ebola epidemic.

Conclusion

In its interactions with West Africa during the Ebola epidemic of 2014 and 2015, US efforts to stop the epidemic went beyond the usual claims of humanitarian intervention of extending assistance to poor countries to addressing the increasingly shared consequences of global inequities. The United States' response to the Ebola epidemic in West Africa, and the responses of other states, challenges the relations between the mostly industrialized countries of the Global North and those of the relatively poor countries of the Global South as one of unequal exchanges in which a disharmony of interests exists between the two areas leading to persistent inequalities in the global system. As evidenced by their pronouncements and directives, policymakers in the Global North addressed the crisis with a sense of urgency, not because they wanted to undertake a humanitarian intervention to save "poor African lives," but to also prevent problems that it could generate for them. They wanted to minimize turmoil in the affected countries and avert a potential refugee crisis, which, among other consequences, could have brought Ebola to their doorsteps through massive outmigration from the region facilitated by diaspora connections in the global system. Urged by their citizens to do something, the governments of the United States, France, the United Kingdom, and many other rich countries committed funds, troops, technical, and medical personnel in a desperate bid to stop Ebola in West Africa.

The extreme measures, such as quarantines that were requested by some policy leaders in the United States draws attention to the contradictions that exist in the global system. Where, ordinarily, many advocate the free movement of goods and services to facilitate the functioning of the global system, the calls to ban travel to and from the West African region in the face of public hysteria over the spread of the virus reflected the hypocrisy at the heart of such expected interactions and the struggle to control what was one of the consequences of the desired circulations in the global system.

There must be a rethinking of the characterization of disharmonies of interest that are said to exist between the rich industrialized countries of the Global North and the poor countries of the Global South. Advancements in technology have helped narrow several social and economic gaps between the two areas of the world, in contradiction with prevailing assumptions that such technological advancements have widened the gaps between the two areas. Duncan's arrival in the United States on a transatlantic flight from Liberia demonstrated clearly how advances in air travel have bridged the distance between the two areas. Social media now creates instantaneous connections between the peoples of the two areas. Thus, cultivating positive-sum relationships between the two areas is also in the best interest of the Global North.

Whether it is within the context of the Ebola epidemic or climate change, for example, previous dichotomies between the interests of the Global North and South are hardly relevant for understanding contemporary realities in the international system. Take the issue of climate change as another example. If theorists of climate change are correct, and mounting evidence from places such as California where a long drought has parched the state to record low water levels over the past three years suggests they are, then the word "tropics" for example, which previously described humid areas of the Global South will be less relevant. It may well be that diseases once thought to survive only in the original tropics of the Global South, for which many universities in the United Kingdom in particular established "departments of Tropical Medicine," will come to also be found in other parts of the Global North in our lifetime, thus urging newer understandings of our global system.

It is also possible that the interactions in the global system around the Ebola epidemic examined in this paper are temporary and that we will see a return to the status quo ante when once the specter of contagion recedes from global discourse. But it is doubtful. The South is an extension of the Global North. Its failures are also the North's failures. As many policymakers in the United States realized, the global system is currently too integrated to easily disentangle the interests of the Global North from those of the Global South.

Notes

1 The Constitution of the United States requires all international treaties and agreements to be ratified by a majority in the US Senate before the country is bound by such agreements. Even after they have been signed by presidents and secretaries of state, many potential agreements, however, are never ratified by the Senate because of partisan interests and divisions. For example, the UN Arms Trade Treaty was signed by Secretary of State John Kerry on behalf of the United States on September 25, 2013. Several years later, it has not been ratified. See the United Nations Office for Disarmament Affairs for information on this treaty: http://www.un.org/disarmament/ATT/.

2 The quotation is from the actual language used in Title VIII of Public Law 113-235 that was signed into law on December 16, 2014.

3 Conducted October 9–12, 2014, the poll by *ABC News* and the *Washington Post* asked "in dealing with the Ebola outbreak, would you support or oppose restricting entry to the United States by people who've been in affected countries?" It found that 29 percent of respondents opposed restricting entry to the United States by individuals who have been to countries affected by the Ebola outbreak. Four percent were unsure, but the majority of people, 67 percent, supported restricting entry.

4 For examples of some of the allegations of malfeasance about the origins of the virus, see Jones and Elbagir (2014).

5 As used here, the global system refers to the extensive political engagements, technological connectivities, personal contacts, and economic integration outlined by A.T. Kearney, Inc. in its annual Global Index published in collaboration with Foreign Policy.

6 The US State Department's travel advisory system offers a system of alerts or warnings cautioning US citizens about travel to various parts of the world. The system can be accessed through the

State Department's website at: https://travel.state.gov/content/passports/en/alertswarnings.html (accessed January 17, 2016).

7 A BBC report, "Ebola-Hit Nations May 'Face Collapse'," published on September 24, 2014, quoted the International Crisis Group to draw attention to the threat of state collapse in Ebola-hit countries and the implications for other areas outside the region.

8 For accounts of how the potential Ebola pandemic affected global market calculations including trading on Wall Street and the electoral prospects of Democrats in Washington, DC heading into the mid-term elections of 2014, see, for example, Lillis and Cirilli (2014). See also Valetkevitch (2014).

9 See, for example, Rucker (2014). See also, CBS News 2014. "Campaigns Citing Ebola, Using Other Fear Tactics," November 3.

10 For a record of such calls, see Saletan (2014).

11 The full transcript of Congressman Kelly's speech "Keeping America Safe from Ebola" is available at: *Congressional Record* 160, 143 (2004): H8149–H8150.

12 For a description of this doomsday scenario involving Ebola, please see: Tom Clancy (1996). *Executive Orders* (New York: Putnam).

13 The full transcript of Congressman Gohmert's speech "Ebola" is available at: *Congressional Record* 160, 143 (2004): H8150.

14 "Madam President," here refers to Senator Mazie K. Hirono (D) Hawaii, who was acting as chair or presiding officer, acting president pro tempore, of the session of Senate in which Senator Leahy delivered his remarks. See note 15 for reference.

15 For a full transcript of Senator Patrick Leahy's speech, see: "The Ebola Crisis," *Congressional Record – Senate* (2004): S5550.

16 The full version of President Obama's speech and transcripts of all the deliberations are available at the White House website, https://www.whitehouse.gov/us-africa-leaders-summit (accessed January 17, 2016).

17 See Senator Thad Cochran (R) Mississippi, on behalf of the United States Senate. 2014. "Senate Committee on U.S. Government Response: Fighting Ebola and Protecting America." Washington D.C. United States Congress.

References

Achenbach, Joel (2014). "Obama Seeks $6 Billion from Congress to Fight Ebola in Africa, United States," *Washington Post*, November 5.

Batty, Fodei (2015). "Surviving Ebola, Surviving Postcolonialism?" *The Postcolonialist*. http://postcolonialist.com/culture/surviving-ebola-surviving-postcolonialism/ (accessed January 17, 2016).

Blaize, Sylvain et al. (2014). "Emergence of Zaire Ebola Virus Disease in Guinea: Preliminary Report," *New England Journal of Medicine*. doi:101056/NEJMoa1404505.

Brawley, Mark R. (2005). *Power, Money, and Trade: Decisions That Shape Global Economic Relations*. North York, Ontario: Broadview Press.

Easterly, William (2002). *The Elusive Quest for Growth: Economists' Adventures and Misadventures in the Tropics*. Cambridge, MA: The MIT Press.

Haas, Peter M. and Hird, John A. (2013). *Controversies in Globalization: Contending Approaches to*

International Relations. Washington, DC: CQ Press.

Jones, Bryony and Elbagir, Nima (2014). "Are Myths Making the Ebola Outbreak Worse?" *CNN*. http://www.cnn.com/2014/08/20/world/africa/ebola-myths/ (accessed January 17, 2016).

Lillis, Mike and Kevin Cirilli. (2014). "Ebola, Wall Street Stock Slide Deepen '14 Gloom for Dems," *The Hill*, October 17.

Moyer, Justin Wm. (2014). "Ebola Victim Thomas Eric Duncan's Family Has Settled Suit with Dallas Hospital," *The Washington Post*, November 12.

Mshomba, Richard E. (2000). *Africa in the Global Economy*. Boulder, CO: Lynne Rienner.

Roberts, Michelle (2014). "First Ebola Boy Likely Infected by Playing in Bat Tree," *BBC*.

Ross, Robert J.S. and Chan, Anita (2002). "From North-South to South-South," *Foreign Affairs* 81, 5: 8–13.

Rucker, Philip (2014). "As Midterm Campaigns Enter Stretch Run, Ebola and Other Twists Set Stage for Drama," *The Washington Post*, October 18.

Saez, Almudena Mari et al. (2014). "Investigating the Zoonotic Origin of the West Africa Ebola Epidemic," *EMBO Molecular Medicine*. doi:10.15252/emmm.201404792.

Saletan, William (2014). "The Ebola Voter: Thirteen Ways Democrats and Republicans Are Exploiting the Virus for Political Gain," *Slate*, October 17.

Stiglitz, Joseph E. (2002). "Globalism's Discontents," *The American Prospect* 13, 1: 1–14.

Szabo, Liz (2014). "Odds Were Stacked against Dallas Ebola Patient," *USA Today*. http://www.usatoday.com/story/news/nation/2014/10/08/science-of-ebola/16922293/ (accessed January 17, 2016).

Tulane University (2007). "New Test Moves Forward to Detect Bioterrorism Threats." http://tulane.edu/news/newwave/101807_bioterrorism.cfm (accessed January 18, 2016).

Valetkevitch, Caroline (2014). "Wall Street Tumbles on Ebola Fears; Small Caps Drop," *Reuters*, October 1.

Wallerstein, I. (1974). *The Modern World System*. New York: Academic Press.

Yan, Holly and Botelho, Greg (2014). "Ebola: Some U.S. States Announce Mandatory Quarantines: Now What?" *CNN*. http://www.cnn.com/2014/10/27/health/ebola-us-quarantine-controversy/index.html (accessed 4, March 2016).

12 | UNMEER AND THE INTERNATIONAL RESPONSE TO THE EBOLA EPIDEMIC

Ismail Rashid

Introduction

For an organization frequently criticized as ineffective and bureaucratic in its decision-making processes, the unity, speed and decisiveness with which the United Nations moved to support a massive upscaling of the international response to the West African Ebola Virus Disease (EVD) outbreak in September 2014 seemed remarkably impressive. Within a few weeks, Secretary-General Ban Ki-moon had constituted a Global Ebola Response Coalition (GERC), appointed a Senior Systems Coordinator for Ebola, activated the United Nations (UN) emergency response mechanism,[1] and proposed the establishment of a United Nations Mission for Ebola Emergency Response (UNMEER).[2] In drumming up support for his actions, Ban Ki-moon declared on September 17, 2014, "Ebola crisis is no longer just a public health crisis, but has become multidimensional, with significant political, social, economic, humanitarian, logistical and security dimensions."[3]

The debates and resolutions that followed in the UN Security Council and General Assembly not only supported Ban Ki-moon's actions, but they were also accompanied by generous pledges of financial, material, and personnel support to UNMEER and to a $1 billion trust fund he had launched to support the requirements and needs of the Ebola-affected countries. The United States placed its full weight behind the Secretary-General's plans and actions. Samantha Power, the United States Permanent Representative to the UN, presided over a congenial Security Council debate of the Ebola crisis, only the second session in the history of the body which had been devoted to a health issue, the first being the HIV AIDS epidemic.[4] In an unprecedented show of global unity, the resolution establishing UNMEER was sponsored by 134 countries, and unanimously supported by all 15 members of the Security Council[5] as well as the General Assembly. The resolution set a record for sponsors; since the establishment of the United Nations no resolution has attracted such a high number of sponsors. At a time when the UN was struggling to find consensus on a myriad of international issues and crises, containing EVD provided an issue that member states could rally around.

But behind this picture-perfect moment of international unity, effusive expressions of solidarity, and generous pledges of support, were very troubling issues. The epidemic had clearly unmasked serious failures in the global governance, in particular, the international institutional management of public health and infectious disease. Though Ban Ki-moon reiterated constantly that he was acting in consultation with Dr. Margaret Chan, the Director-General of the World Health Organization (WHO), the creation of UNMEER had clearly signaled a lack of confidence in her organization. At the very least, it conveyed an astute diplomatic calculation on Ban Ki-moon's part not to uphold WHO as the UN's flagship entity in upscaling the international response to EVD.

That Sierra Leone and Liberia were two of the three countries most affected by the outbreak also raised troubling, though unvoiced, questions about the efficacy of the extensive UN's engagement in these countries. Both countries had been the beneficiaries of extensive United Nations' peacekeeping, state reconstruction, and experimental peacebuilding operations. They had absorbed billions of dollars of international aid and donor support.[6] Sierra Leone, in particular, is frequently touted as a shining example of UN peacekeeping and peacebuilding since it had not relapsed into conflict within the last decade, and had shown progress in its political and economic development.

The creation of the mission clearly highlighted a moment of decisive leadership on the part of Secretary-General Ban Ki-moon that helped galvanized international, regional, and local responses around ending EVD. The performance of mission on the ground was, however, uneven. It did facilitate the influx of valuable human, medical, and material resources as well as contribute to fashioning a stronger sense of purpose, direction, and coordination in an environment of multiple international, national, and local actors. The mission, however, struggled to adjust quickly to a dynamic and fluid environment in which greater flexibility was needed to stop a wily and lethal virus, and in which the needs were so enormous. However, to focus solely on the performance is to elide the greater problem of governance failures, which occasioned the formation of UNMEER, and which the mission left after it wound down in July 2015.

This chapter examines the creation, deployment, and performance of UNMEER within the context of the global, national, and local institutional failures that bracketed its brief existence. It is structured into three broad sections. The first section provides a background – a sort of prehistory – to the upscaling of the international response to the EVD epidemic. It analyzes critically the context of the various levels of failures, which led to the massive UN intervention and the formation of UNMEER. The second section examines the formation, deployment, and performance of UNMEER in the MRU region between September 2014 and July 2015. The final section critically evaluates the performance and significance of the mission.

Contextualizing an epic failure

An unknown virus, local fear, and weak governments The discourse on the emergence of EVD in the MRU area is now well entrenched and uncritically reproduced in nearly all of the writings on the outbreak. It supposedly began with the infection of an infant in Meliandou village in the Guéckédou prefecture of Guinea around December 2013. The disease then appeared in Liberia by April 2014, and had reached the capital cities of Conakry, Monrovia, and Freetown by June 2014. For this chapter, what is important to recall is that until the end of March 2014, when the presence of an EVD outbreak in Guinea was scientifically established, there were no indications that any government, national or international organization was seriously engaged in coming to terms with the new reality let alone putting in measures to combating the disease.

There has been extensive commentary from journalists, scholars, and even public officials on why a small, localized, and containable EVD outbreak became a sub-regional epidemic. The first place that they locate the failure to contain the outbreak is at the local level, where they point out that realization of the deadly nature of the outbreak was slow, and responses to it within the first few months haphazard if not inadequate. They generally attribute this tardiness and inadequacy at the local level to a confection of suspect food choices, cultural beliefs, and social behavior, especially unsafe "funeral practices," which the Ebola virus exploited to move from person to person. It is undeniable that the virus ensnared people and via healing, funerary, and social bonding practices that sought to affirm the humanity and dignity of its victims.[7]

However, some of the indictment of the responses of people and local communities in the MRU countries lacks nuance or empathy, and are laced with racist, sexist, and classist undertones for the local responses to an unknown and terrifying affliction (see Mueller 2014b). Understandably, people and communities in the MRU sub-region initially mistook EVD symptoms for those of other diseases that were prevalent in their sub-region, namely cholera and malaria, which have lower fatality rates (Médecins Sans Frontières 2014, 6). The etiology, virulence, and high morbidity, and the seeming ineffectiveness of the available range of healing options, generated myths and fear of the disease. It did not help that as in other African contexts, EVD began its deadly reign in the region by attacking people on the periphery of state attention, power, and resources.

Even the governments of the three most affected countries conceded that their health systems were riddled with a plethora of problems at the onset of the EVD outbreak. These problems included inadequately resourced health facilities, insufficient medical staff, inexperienced health care workers, insufficient medical equipment, and lax infectious disease protocols (see Abdullah and Kamara, Chapter 5 in this volume; Kieh, Chapter 4 this volume; Bano Barry, Chapter 3 in this volume). There was weak or no capacity for the detection of Ebola, management of infectious disease data, and effective surveillance and tracking of infections. Insufficient medical staff and health care service existed before the outbreak, and there was limited participation of senior health officials in arresting the initial outbreak.[8] It is not surprising that after viewing the havoc wreaked by EVD on infected patients and health care workers, people in Liberia and Sierra Leone viewed government hospitals as "places of death" by the middle of 2014. Overcoming this mistrust of health centers and public health messages became one of the most difficult challenges in the fight to arrest the spread of EVD.

Yet, beneath the tragic local and national failures is also a legacy of ineffectual international interventions in these countries (Kentikelenis et al. 2015). The three MRU countries, especially Sierra Leone and Liberia, had been inundated with expert technical advice, externally inspired policy papers, hurriedly crafted legislations, donor aid, and NGO projects from the 1990s onwards (see Howard, Chapter 1 in this volume). None of these interventions seemed to have improved public health substantially. Similarly, the intoxicating economic growth rates of the pre-Ebola years, inflated by the concentration of foreign investors in the few extractive mining enclaves, donor financial inflows, and remittances of diaspora Sierra Leoneans and Liberians, had neither lifted these countries from the lowest rungs of UNDP HDI nor contributed to the development of robust health systems.

It was not that the MRU governments did not take Ebola seriously once it stalked their territories; they were hobbled by their internal contradictions and incurable dependency on the largesse of the international community. Initially all three governments – constrained by fractured political systems, indecisive leadership, and a broad spectrum of governance problems – prevaricated, denied, or hid cases of the EVD until it was too late. Even when they had the expertise of international agencies and organizations, like Médecins Sans Frontières (MSF), WHO or the US Center for Disease Control and Prevention (CDC), they either did not trust or did not act promptly on the reports they were receiving. The president of Guinea, for example, reportedly accused MSF of exaggerating the outbreak to raise donations in May 2014 (Médecins Sans Frontières 2014, 8). Even though that turned out not to be the case, the accusation is not altogether unfounded since many international organizations have raised millions, if not billions, from tragedies in Africa, real or imagined. Once the true nature of the EVD epidemic became clear to them, the three MRU governments did form national emergency response committees. These committees did put in place measures to control the spread of the infections. However, the initial government denials and prevarications eventually led to the very things they had wished to prevent in the first place: causing public panic, disrupting everyday life, and scaring away foreign investors.[9]

Falling behind the curve The prevarications by the national governments in the MRU area seemed to have been mirrored at the international levels, especially by organizations like WHO and CDC that should have been in the frontline of the response to the outbreak, and by countries with the resources and expertise to support such a response. By the beginning of April 2014, these organizations could not claim ignorance of the existence of EVD in the MRU area. The president of MSF, Dr. Joanne Liu, had conveyed her concerns to WHO leadership in Geneva in early April 2014; her organization had been accused of scaremongering. MSF, later supported by the International Federation of Red Cross and Red Crescent Societies (IFRC), and a few faith-based organizations, Samaritan's Purse in Liberia and World Vision in Sierra Leone, would eventually become thinly-stretched and overwhelmed on the ground in the three countries.[10] Twenty-eight MSF staff contracted the virus; 14 eventually succumbed to EVD (Médecins Sans Frontières 2014).

Time magazine reported that Robert Garry, a Tulane University researcher working in Sierra Leone, also raised the alarm with the US Department of State, but received only lukewarm response (Drehle 2014). CDC, already involved in haemorrhagic viral research in Sierra Leone, only dispatched its first set of epidemic specialists to the sub-region in August 2014, after two Americans, an aid worker and a doctor, had contracted the virus. Indeed, it was only after much domestic hysteria and political posturing, and the glaring absence of three MRU heads of state at the US–Africa Summit at the beginning of August 2014 that US political and financial clout would be fully deployed behind the EVD response effort.

However, as noted by Semiha Abdulmelik (see Chapter 9 of this volume), MSF was not the only Cassandra prophesying an impending health catastrophe to an incredulous global audience, ECOWAS was also part of the warning chorus. Rather incredibly, from late March 2014, when the presence of EVD was confined to a small area, ECOWAS had declared the disease "a serious threat to regional security." The organization subsequently created a solidarity fund which raised US$8 million, and forged an agreement between its own regional health body, the West African Health Organization, WHO, and African Development Bank to support the most affected countries. The AU picked up on ECOWAS efforts, and by August launched African Union Support to Ebola Outbreak in West Africa (ASEOWA) and called forth a brigade of volunteers to respond to the outbreak.

It was not that WHO did not act to find effective responses to the EVD epidemic. From April 2014, WHO dispatched different technical teams to assess the situation, and to work with the health ministries of the various governments on the responses to the outbreak. As noted above, it participated in and organized several meetings, including a major one in Accra in July, done in concert with regional and international partners (GOARN), that spurred the governments of Liberia, Guinea, and Sierra Leone to produce accelerated EVD response plans, with estimates of the required funding. These plans were later included as annexes in the more comprehensive Ebola response roadmap that WHO released at the end of August. The WHO African Regional Director, Dr. Luis Sambo, toured the affected countries to assess the situation and review the ongoing response. Dr. Margaret Chan, the Director-General of WHO, even met the three leaders in Conakry, and together launched a $100 million appeal on August 1, 2014 to help support the rapid response to contain the epidemic.

So why has the response of WHO been criticized as "woefully inadequate," "underwhelming and uninspiring?" (Youde 2015; Drehle 2014). Why did the organization's own independent assessment panel set up in early 2015 to assess its response to the epidemic in West Africa castigate it for having "failed in establishing itself as the authoritative body in the EVD crisis?"[11] The main reasons seemed to have been its failure to take decisive actions at the time it confirmed the outbreak and the consequent delay in declaring a "public health emergency of international concern (PHEIC)," which according to some scholars could have quickly unlocked expertise and resources to contain the outbreak. The organization has been criticized for lacking a sense of urgency until EVD moved out of the MRU zone and appeared in Senegal, Nigeria, and most crucially, reached Spain and the United States, via the infection of two Spanish priests and a nurse, and two Americans citizens working in Liberia. The assessment panel, however, noted that there was plenty of blame to go around, from the counterproductive behavior of people and governments in the region to the shirking of responsibility by WHO member states.[12] By the time WHO released its road map which provided the platform for concerted action (WHO Ebola Response Team 2014), it had fallen woefully "behind the curve." It also underestimated the scale of the health as well as the humanitarian crises that the MRU sub-region was facing by the end of July 2014. Two complex emergencies had intersected – a transnational infectious disease outbreak that needed to be brought under control, and societies across three countries needing extensive social and economic assistance.

The intersection of these emergencies provided the foundation for EVD to be effectively securitized and to get the attention of the world. "Crisis" and "security," two code words etched in the DNA of the organization and indicative of our anxiety-filled contemporary existence, were guaranteed to move the gears of the sluggish UN machinery. The securitization of EVD was a complex discourse-making process; it was not only the spread of disease that became perceived as a global security threat, but the multiplicity of potentially destabilizing threats that the intersection of two complex emergencies could produce within as well as beyond the MRU region (McInnes 2016). The securitization of the outbreak first started with ECOWAS, an organization that had been founded on promise of regional economic integration, but which had become very security-consciousness following peacekeeping forays in Liberia, Sierra Leone, Guinea Bissau, Mali, and *Côte d'Ivoire*. AU echoed ECOWAS' position, hoping to amplify the regional body's concerns to Africa and the world, especially the UN. With its advocacy for military intervention, MSF also contributed to the discourse of securitizing the crisis (Médecins Sans Frontières 2014). The August 2014 letter of the three MRU presidents to Ban Ki-moon, which highlighted the devastating impact of the epidemic and crushing embargoes on their countries, also underlined that Ebola was a security and existential crisis for the sub-region.

By the time Ban Ki-moon spoke to the UN Security Council and Barack Obama, the president of the United States, addressed the UN General Assembly, the discourse of EVD as a security crisis that threatened not only West Africans, but the rest of Africa and the world, had become firmly entrenched in the perceptions of the international community. On September 26, 2014, echoing the emerging consensus at the United Nations, Obama stated "[EVD] ... is more than a health crisis. This is a growing threat to regional and global security ... this disease could cause a humanitarian catastrophe across the region. And in an era where regional crises can quickly become global ones, stopping Ebola is in the interests of all of us" (Drehle 2014). The US president's speech came on the heels of apocalyptic predictions from scientists working at the US CDC that EVD cases in Liberia and Sierra Leone could exceed a million by January 2015, if the global response was not scaled up (Meltzer et al. 2014).[13] It is not surprising then that the language deployed throughout the response to EVD in the MRU region was heavily militarized and securitized.

UNMEER: securitizing Ebola, upscaling the international response

Bending the curve Once WHO had declared a PHEIC on August 8, Ban Ki-moon appointed Dr. David Nabarro, a British physician who had been Executive Director of WHO and UN Systems Coordinator for Avian and Human Influenza, as the UN System Senior Coordinator for Ebola Virus Disease. His job was "to provide overall strategic direction and to assist Governments in the region in addressing the crisis."[14] It also included convening weekly meetings of GERC, an informal group of representatives from governments and organizations tasked with monitoring the response, sharing information, and mobilizing the required resources. The group would confer weekly on these matters until December 2015, when it dissolved. Three weeks later, Ban Ki-moon activated the UN's emergency response mechanism[15] and designated Anthony Banbury, an American and a UN Assistant Secretary-General as the Deputy Ebola Coordinator and Emergency Crisis Manager.[16] Banbury was subsequently designated as the Special Representative of the Secretary-General (SRSG) to head UNMEER.

The expectations of what UNMEER could achieve in a very short timeframe was expansive and ambitious. Ban Ki-moon indicated that the mission "will harness the capabilities and competencies of all the relevant United Nations actors under a unified operational structure to reinforce unity of purpose, effective ground-level leadership and operational direction, in order to ensure a rapid, effective, efficient and coherent response to the crisis."[17] Its five strategic objectives, summarized as STEPP, were to stop the outbreak, treat the infected, ensure essential services, preserve stability, and prevent outbreak in uninfected countries. STEPP was further broken down to 13 mission critical actions that included tracing, treatment, and care of infected people, safe and dignified burials, medical care for responders, provision of food, basic non-Ebola health services, remuneration for workers, provision of the necessary logistics, and social mobilization, and community engagement. The guiding principles behind these actions were expected to be based on close coordination of all UN agencies and the harnessing of their capacities and competencies, assistance to governments of affected countries, catalyzing all resources under a single framework, and ensuring a rapid impact on the ground.

Launched in Accra on October 1, 2014 – ten months after EVD was confirmed in the sub-region – UNMEER made its presence felt through bold pronouncements, high-level tours of duty, and major conferences and official meetings. The head of the mission, SRSG Anthony Banbury, unveiled a 30-60-90 plan, with certain operational targets. Within 30 days, he expected all of the inputs, including staff, finance, and logistics, to be in place. In line with STEPP and Phase I of the WHO's rapid response plan, Banbury envisaged that within 60 days of its operations, UNMEER would be overseeing the isolation and treatment of 70 percent of the infected and burying 70 percent of EVD dead in a safe and dignified manner. This became more popularly known as the 70-70-60 plan. WHO noted that the achievement of this target was important to "bend the curve," namely reduce the rate of new EVD cases. Within 90 days, UNMEER aimed to reach and treat all of those infected with the disease, and to bury every death from the disease in a safe and dignified fashion (WHO 2014, 2). Banbury toured Sierra Leone, Liberia, and Guinea during the first week of October to confer with representatives of UN agencies, national organizations, and other partners with which UNMEER was going to be working.

Meanwhile, Ban Ki-moon confirmed the appointments of Marcel Rudasingwa,[18] a Rwandan and senior United Nations Children's Fund (UNICEF) official as Ebola Crisis Manager for Guinea, Peter Jan Graaff, a Dutch diplomat who had served in WHO and Afghanistan, as Ebola Crisis Manager for Liberia, and Amadu Kamara, a Sierra Leonean serving at the UN Department of Peacekeeping Operations (DPKO) as the Ebola Crisis Manager for Sierra Leone.[19] With the confirmation of these key appointments, UNMEER convened a four-day conference in mid-October, with other UN agencies, to agree on an operational framework that delineated the roles and responsibilities of various organizations in the scaled-up response to the epidemic. UNMEER took on the responsibility for overall crisis management, staffing, and information management as well as logistics. In line with expertise and competences outlined in the OCHA cluster system,[20] the World Food Programme (WFP) took on the role of supporting UNMEER in providing logistics. WHO was expected to focus on case management, case finding, laboratories, contact tracing, and training (with the support of CDC), while the United Nations Development Program (UNDP) was given the responsibility for cash payment coordination. The IFRC would continue to be responsible for safe and dignified burials.[21] Banbury traveled once more to the affected countries to brief the presidents and partners of the framework. Kamara and Rudasingwa also met with the presidents of Sierra Leone and Guinea respectively to discuss the response to the epidemic. Kamara also met with the UN country team, and attended the induction of the 14 district managers in Sierra Leone.[22] By the end of the year, UNMEER had almost 45 field teams under the supervision of these country managers.

UNMEER operations, however, started inauspiciously. The Multi-Partner Trust Fund (MPTF), which should have supported the rapid upscaling of capacities, was severely underfunded, at the commencement of UNMEER operations.[23] The mission also had a shortage of funding, trained medical personnel, and material.[24] Only an urgent appeal from Ban Ki-moon quickened the pace of contributions to push pledges and contributions to US$115 million at the end of October.[25] About 100 UNMEER staff members were on the ground by the end of October, although the mission faced bureaucratic hurdles over recruitment and deployment of certain highly qualified staff. Nonetheless, by the end of 2014, U$140 million had been pledged to the fund. By the time the mission ended in 2015, UNMEER had received US$150 million. The Ebola Trust Fund had over U$1.1 billion by then, even though OCHA estimated the needs and requirements of the affected countries to be around US$1.5bn.[26]

A substantial increase in the deployment of military and civilian personnel, expertise, and materials in the MRU countries followed the commencement of UNMEER operations. Between October and November, the United Kingdom deployed around 900 military personnel, medical staff, and other technical experts in Sierra Leone as well as transportation, medical supplies, and other resources to support their teams and the general response efforts. The British contributed to the construction of treatment facilities, especially at Kerry Town and Moyamba. The United States sent nearly 2,900 military and civilian medical personnel to Liberia between October and December. Like the British, the United States in Liberia focused mainly on the construction of treatment facilities, provision of security, training of health workers, and provision of logistical support (Bricknell et al. 2016). China dispatched 160 doctors, epidemiologists, and nurses to run a treatment center they opened on November 24, 2014. The country also contributed mobile laboratories.[27] Cuba trained and sent 450 doctors and nurses to Guinea, Liberia, and Sierra Leone. South Africa also contributed doctors and laboratories. AU and ECOWAS also scaled up their assistance, with the deployment of 87 Ethiopian medical practitioners and health workers, and pledged to contribute more in 2015.[28]

UNMEER had some immediate and visible impact on the ground. It began issuing daily situational reports, tracking the cumulative EVD infections and death statistics, response efforts, and health situation in the affected countries. The reports also provided highlights of key political and economic developments, human rights resources, resource mobilization efforts, logistical contributions and improvements, public outreach, and education efforts. Production of the UNMEER daily reports continued until UNMEER folded on July 31, and the responsibility was taken over by OCHA. The daily reports provide good indications of the extent to which UNMEER supported the boosting of planning, data collection, and monitoring capacity of the various health ministries and national Ebola response centers and of various organizations. They also give good insights into difficult challenges being confronted by UNMEER and the responders as they sought to turn the tide of the epidemic. The health ministries of the three MRU countries also issued regular reports of Ebola infections, deaths, and survivals, which did not usually agree with those of UNMEER\WHO.

The UNMEER reports present some indication that the operational framework agreed at Accra in mid-October 2014, and the funds being donated were translating into more concrete, coordinated action on the ground. UNICEF established an air coordination cell by mid-October to move medical and other vital equipment from Europe to more than 160 relief organizations in West Africa (Fisher and Brandt 2015, 49). WFP had also set up an air corridor between Accra, Monrovia, Freetown, and Conakry to enable UNMEER to schedule regular flights by the end of October. It also developed forward logistics bases in the different countries to speed up transportation. By November, UNMEER helicopters were transporting blood samples from remote locations.[29] UNICEF, in partnership with several national organizations, scaled up their social mobilization and community engagement activities. UNDP was helping to facilitate regular payments of EVD, and training of community volunteers engaged in prevention campaigns. UNICEF supported routine periodic immunization. OCHA continued to track funds, and coordinate the disbursement to various organizations, agencies, and governments. The synergy between the different organizations could be seen in some response locations. In Port Loko District in Sierra Leone, for example, WHO ran the two community care centers, WHO also managed the Forward Logistics Operating Base. The district had a well-functioning command and control center providing points of contact and coordination between various organizations. UNMEER also strongly supported cross-border cooperation, convening a meeting on December 9, 2014 attended by representatives from Sierra Leone, Guinea, Mali, Nigeria, and UN, ECOWAS, and AU. The mission continued to facilitate such meetings in 2015.

Despite the "surge" in international assistance, the EVD epidemiological landscape remained "complicated," an official euphemism for the fact that the epidemic showed little overall sign of slowing down. In early December 2014, Dr. Margaret Chan noted that the disease was still "running ahead" of efforts to contain it.[30] The chronic problems that had made the outbreak difficult to contain between April and September persisted. There were simply not enough experienced and skilled personnel to meet the needs of the response. The influx of foreign medical personnel and health workers, though crucial, came with problems of training and familiarizing them to a dynamic and difficult environment. Many of the foreign personnel, some of them volunteers, were often on short rotations. UNMEER and other organizations could not recruit sufficient highly trained medical staff because of fear of the disease and other bureaucratic hurdles; it had to concede that it would have to rely more strongly on nationally trained professionals.[31]

The allocation of resources in a dynamic disease environment also posed enormous problems. Some areas, because of easier transportation, were better resourced than others. Equally challenging, initially, was the ability of UNMEER and other responders to quickly shift resources as EVD ebbed in some locales and flared up, sometimes unexpectedly, in others. The demand for treatments and community care centers remained acute in different parts of the affected countries. One of the ironies of the scaled-up response was that some of the new facilities, such as the Chinese and American centers in Monrovia, ended up being too large, and located in areas where the epidemic seemed to be receding. UNMEER conceded that its response strategy would shift to the construction and management of smaller and more dispersed treatment facilities. By the end of the year, and in early 2015 this shift was already occurring.

At the end of 2014, when SRSG Banbury bade farewell to the three MRU presidents, the situation still looked bleak. At the start of December, Banbury indicated that the target of 70-70-60 announced in October had been exceeded in Guinea and Liberia, but that in many places such as western and northern regions of Sierra Leone and parts of Guinea, EVD outbreaks and viral transmission were intensifying.[32] Unexpected and significant flare-ups occurred in different areas, such as the one in Kono District, which forced the Sierra Leone government to enforce a two-week lockdown.[33] In mid-December, the Sierra Leone government effected a Western Area Surge (WAS), an exercise that involved widespread house-to-house searches to locate and treat EVD cases, and educate the public about the disease.[34] Its overall effectiveness was unclear (Benton and Donne 2015), and it did not reveal the expected numbers of new cases.

The year closed with confirmed, probable, and suspected EVD cases at 20,171, and new infections still running high. Public fear, disaffection, and occasional protests against different aspects of the response persisted.[35] Nearly everyone associated with the outbreak – the infected, their families, survivors, orphans, and health workers – were shunned by others.[36] However, on an encouraging note, the pattern of EVD increases had turned out to be much more linear than exponential. The scaled-up intervention had prevented the worst-case scenario that was modeled by the CDC scientists, and figures of overall weekly infections indicate that the curve might have been bent.[37] Furthermore, the fine-tuning and ramping up of training and campaigns slowly increased public understanding of the disease, though intermittent resistance to EVD control efforts continued, especially in Guinea. The handling of corpses, especially those confirmed or suspected to have died of Ebola, started shifting.[38]

Perhaps, most important from the point of view of the international community, the spread of EVD outside the MRU sub-region had effectively been contained.

Hunting down the virus When Ismail Ould Chiekh Ahmed, a Mauritanian started his tenure as SRSG of UNMEER and Abdou Dieng, a Senegalese, took over as Ebola Crisis Manager of Guinea in January 2015, it was clear that the mission had not achieved the goal of reaching and treating 100 percent of EVD cases, and safely burying all EVD dead. Unlike Banbury, Ould Cheikh Ahmed, who had served as Deputy SRSG of the United Nations Support Mission in Libya (UNSMIL) and UNDP Resident Representative in Yemen and Syria, did not specify any targets. He merely underlined that EVD was "a global crisis. We definitely have a difficult time ahead of us, but we can achieve our goal of zero cases." On assuming office, Ould Cheikh Ahmed immediately picked up on the serious problem of coordination posed by the multiplicity of organizations involved in the response. He continued with meetings and consultations with government and organizations within and outside the MRU to ensure better coordination of efforts. The new SRSG was also very much supportive of what WHO characterized as Phase II of the response, which entailed rigorous case management, safe and dignified burials, infection control and prevention, vigilant surveillance, and contact tracing supported by full community engagement (WHO 2015).

To achieve the objectives of this new phase, UNMEER and its partner UN agencies concentrated on consolidating their work in certain areas. UNDP and UNMEER worked with governments to pay wages regularly, and to give hazard pay for health workers dealing with EVD.[39] Additional smaller facilities were constructed to ensure that EVD patients did not have to travel long distances to facilities where they could not receive family or communal pyscho-social support. UNMEER also undertook periodic rapid assessments of treatment facilities, especially in Liberia and Sierra Leone, to help ensure that requisite protocols were being observed and they had sufficient medical and other supplies. The mission continued its support of cross-border meetings and consultations, and assessments and training of agencies and groups participating in cross-border surveillance.[40] Data collection, analysis, and sharing continued to be a priority at international, national, and local levels. In February,

UNMEER released a web-based application Geo-Information Management System in Liberia, to help in this process.[41] The mission and its partners continued to provide logistical support, including satellite forms, mobile phones, ambulances, and pick-up trucks to the various government agencies responding to EVD.

By May 2015, contact tracing in all countries, especially Sierra Leone and Guinea, was around 99 percent. With few exceptions and some ongoing resistance, safe and dignified burials were pursued and strongly enforced by the government. By early 2015, around 254 teams had been trained and deployed, with Sierra Leone at 102 having the highest numbers, Liberia the lowest at 69, and Guinea 83.[42] Over 90 percent of deaths, EVD or not, were collected and buried within 24 hours, usually with the support and oversight of the IFRC.

Towards the end of January 2015, the first signs that EVD might be ebbing was when newly reported cases in all three countries fell below 100. The numbers fluctuated above this level in Guinea and Sierra Leone throughout February and March, but Liberia showed an unmistakable downward trend. In line with the declining numbers, the Ebola treatment facilities, which were furiously constructed at the height of the international "surge," began closing down. On March 20, Liberia did not record any cases, and it began a 42-day countdown to be declared free of EVD. UNMEER's office in Liberia closed down on April 30. Peter Graaff, the ECM for Liberia, acted as head of UNMEER from April 25 until the mission folded on July 31. The abatement of EVD in Liberia led to redeployment of some of its field managers to Guinea. On May 9, 2015, Liberia was declared free of EVD, but the virus reappeared on June 29, and by July, the number of new cases had inched up to six.

Ending EVD in Sierra Leone and Guinea proved much more difficult. The governments of these two countries continued to restrict the movement of people, extending the enforcement of quarantines of communities and regions well into June 2015. Government hospitals and clinics remained closed till then. The cases steadily declined, with some fluctuations in the weekly numbers through the year. Guinea was declared Ebola free only on December 29, 2015, while Sierra Leone was first declared Ebola free on November 7, 2015. The last meeting of GERC took place on December 11, 2015.

The discovery of new Ebola cases meant postponement of the date of declaring Sierra Leone Ebola-free until March 17, 2016,[43] almost two years to date of the confirmation of the presence of the disease in the MRU region. Twelve days later, on March 29, 2016, WHO declared the end of EVD as a PHEIC in West Africa. In all three countries, the national Ebola response centers were phased out and their responsibilities as well as their assets turned over to various ministries. It is estimated that 26,610 people had been infected with EVD, and 11,308 had died. Liberia had the most deaths with 4,806 deaths from 10,666 infections, while Sierra Leone had the highest number of infections at 14, 122 with 3,955 deaths. Guinea, where the outbreak was first identified, reported the lowest number of infections, 3,804, and deaths, 2,536.[44]

Empowered leadership or lumbering distraction: evaluating UNMEER

A mixed effort The initial assessments of the performance of UNMEER have been mixed. Even though critical of its narrow health focus, sidelining of human rights issues, and its inconsistent bottom-up approach, Maryam Deloffre views the achievements of the mission positively. The mission, she points out, showed how "empowered leadership improved coordination, fostered collaboration and improved accountability" in a situation of dire "humanitarian crisis." For her, "On balance, UNMEER was effective in meeting its mission of containing the Ebola virus and achieving zero new cases" (Deloffre 2016, 53). It is undeniable that by the time the mission folded, the EVD epidemic was effectively over, despite the emergence of few cases afterwards.

There is much evidence to show that the presence of UNMEER in West Africa did help to catalyze and coordinate the response against EVD at all levels. With the operational framework laid in Accra, and the regular consultations, more UN agencies did pool and channel their resources more effectively. National and district response centers benefitted from the intervention of the mission. In Sierra Leone, for example, UNMEER facilitated more coordination between the Ministry of Health and Sanitation, and other organizations responding to EVD in the country.[45]

The UN intervention, and the formation of UNMEER, led to significant mobilization of financial resources to support the response, and to meet the needs of the affected countries on a scale which WHO, the AU, and ECOWAS could not have done on their own. Over 50 countries and organizations committed around US$140 million to directly support the mission, and over US$8.2 billion to finance the requirements and needs of the affected countries.[46] The resources mobilized by UNMEER improved the technical and logistical capacities of government health ministries, national response, and district response committees, and organizations to plan, collect, and analyze data, and manage different dimensions of the response.[47] In addition to contributing to the construction, staffing, and equipping of treatment centers and community care centers, the mission also supported a variety of quick impact programs in various communities.[48] Some observers see UNMEER's role in providing logistics support and bringing together various UN, international, and national agencies to combat the outbreak as positive (Fischer and Brandt 2015).

Other scholars and observers are not so sanguine about the positive impact or effectiveness of UNMEER. They point out that since it had limited staffing on the ground and inadequate experience, it was ineffective and its performance did not match expectations. Fink and Belluck (2015) noted that it has been widely criticized as "lumbering, expensive and unfocused." An International Crisis Group (ICG) report maintained that UNMEER represented an additional administrative layer that "did little to clarify the multiple crossing mandates in Ebola affected countries" (International Crisis Group 2015). Unsurprisingly the WHO assessment panel, which recommended the adequate resourcing and strengthening of WHO, did not think it was an appropriate mechanism for future large-scale medical emergencies. They considered it "unwieldy," taking "two critical months" at the height of the crisis to be established. It was not very effective on the ground since it bypassed rather than effectively engaged the UN cluster system.[49] Fisher and Brandt, for example, suggested that existing and more specialized UN organizations such as the Office for the Coordination of Humanitarian Affairs (OCHA) and WHO should have been reinforced and utilized effectively rather than being subsumed to UNMEER (Fischer and Brandt 2015).

Some of this critique has merit. While the presence of UNMEER did help the various UN agencies, and other partner organizations to harmonize their efforts, the mission struggled with coordinating the fairly crowded field of actors engaged in the response. Even SRSG Ould Cheikh Ahmed realized that there were "too many cooks" on the ground. Throughout its duration, UNMEER struggled to keep up with the changing dynamics of the response, right-size its approach, and coordinate activities of not only its UN partners, but also governments and the diverse cast of international, national, and local organizations contributing to response efforts. However, is placing the UNMEER on a balance scale of "success" or "failure" how the mission should be judged or should it be considered more expansively within the context of global governance of recurrent crises, and of vulnerable countries like those in the MRU area?

Postscript or back to the future As preparations for UNMEER gathered pace, the MSF report, *Pushed to the Limit and Beyond: A Year in the Largest Ever Ebola Outbreak*, posed crucial questions that were in the minds of many observers of the unfolding catastrophe: "How did the epidemic spiral so spectacularly out of control? Why was the world so slow to work up to its severity and respond? Was it due to fear, lack of political will, lack of expertise or a perfect storm of all three?" The concluding paragraph wrestled with a possible, but clearly unsatisfactory, explanation:

> "The Ebola outbreak has been often described as a perfect storm: a cross-border epidemic in countries with weak public health systems that had never seen Ebola before," says Christopher Stokes. "Yet this is too convenient an explanation. For the Ebola outbreak to spiral this far out of control required many institutions to fail. And they did, with tragic and avoidable consequences." (Médecins Sans Frontières 2014, 21)

MSF was not the only international organization that blamed the development of the EVD epidemic on institutional failure. In their postmortem of the epidemic, the UN, World Bank, EU, and ADB also posited: "this latest and largest-ever Ebola outbreak has highlighted weaknesses, not just the fragile developing nations but also in the global institutional machinery for identifying and quickly neutralizing health hazards."[50] While institutional failure at all levels cannot be denied, a more honest and fuller analysis would probe into larger structural forces that produced such failures. It is no secret that the structural forces underpinning our current, dominant neoliberal capitalist system generates glaring inequalities and is crises-prone. This dynamic forces institutions, global and local ones, especially those operating in the most vulnerable parts of the world, to function in a similar mode.

As pointed out above, it is perhaps not shocking then, that three of the least developed countries on the UNDP HDI, Sierra Leone, Liberia, and Guinea, should have been in the eye of the storm of this latest round of African regional crisis. The neoliberal development paths and global pseudo-trusteeship that they have been under for the past couple of decades have deepened social inequalities and exacerbated poor governance. As Boozary et al. contend, the virulence of EVD in West Africa (vis-à-vis Western countries) "lies not with the virus, but in the collective failure to ensure the availability of adequate health care staff, resources, and systems required for the delivery of high-quality health care services. The Ebola epidemic has placed the failure into stark relief, exposing the pathology of chronic neglect amid broad global inequalities" (Boozary et al. 2014).

It is difficult not to see the EVD epidemic and its disastrous responses as searing indictments of the peace-building and state-building projects in the MRU sub-region that have been heavily mediated by the UN, IFIs, and a plethora of non-governmental organizations for the past two decades. Even as the crisis was ebbing, those organizations have gone back to the same pattern of creating plans, policies, and programs that are then passed on to the leaders – ostensibly for their rubber-stamping.[51] So, though immensely valuable in the upscaling of efforts to stop the EVD epidemic, it is difficult not to situate UNMEER's presence and achievements within this larger context. It is difficult not to hear the echoes of previous UN interventions, whether through the United Nations Mission in Sierra Leone (UNAMSIL, 1999–2006) or the United Nations Mission in Liberia (UNMIL) (2003–present), in the international response to EVD; the only difference being that these missions stayed for much rebuilding, while UNMEER was temporary and left little to build upon.

Notes

1 The UN Mechanism, first established in 1971 (GA 2816 (XXIV) of December 14, 1971), provides for the organization to respond to requests for humanitarian and emergency assistance to governments. It ensures that within 12 to 48 hours the UN would dispatch a United Nations Disaster Assessment and Coordination team (UNDAC) to assist in damage and needs assessment as well as information and coordination management. The mechanism was reinforced through subsequent resolutions (A 44/236 of December 22, 1989, 45/100 of December 14, 1990, and 48/182 of December 19, 1991). The 1991 resolution, in particular, underscores the leadership of the UN Secretary-General in responding to natural disasters and other emergencies. It also makes provision for the UN Secretary-General to designate a high-level official to work closely with the Secretary-General, other UN agencies, other international organizations, and the affected countries to coordinate the international response.

2 Identical letters dated September 17, 2014 from the Secretary-General addressed to the President of the General Assembly and the President of the Security Council, UN General Assembly\Security Council A/69/389-S/2014/679 September 18, 2014.

3 See ibid.

4 UN Security Council 7268th meeting, Thursday September 18, 2014. S/PV.7268.

5 UN General Assembly A/RES/69/1, September 23, 2014: Resolution adopted by the General Assembly on September 19, 2014 69/1. Measures to contain and combat the recent Ebola outbreak in West Africa.

6 The extension of the mandate of United Nations Mission in Liberia (UNMIL) occurred around the time of these actions. See Security Council 2176 (2014) S/Res/2176/2014.

7 See Annex 2: Planned Response to the Ebola Virus Disease Epidemic in Guinea July–December 2014; Annex 3: Liberia Operational Plan for Accelerated Response to the re-Occurrence of Ebola Epidemic July–December 2014; Annex 4: Sierra Leone Accelerated Ebola Virus Disease Outbreak Response Plan July 2014 in WHO, "WHO Ebola Response Road Map," August 28, 2014.

8 Annex 2: Planned Response to the Ebola Virus Disease Epidemic in Guinea July–December 2014; Annex 3: Liberia Operational Plan for Accelerated Response to the re-Occurrence of Ebola Epidemic July–December 2014; Annex 4: Sierra Leone Accelerated Ebola Virus Disease Outbreak Response Plan July 2014 in WHO, "WHO Ebola Response Road Map," August 28, 2014.

9 WHO, "Report of the Ebola Interim Assessment Panel," July 2015, http://www.who.int/csr/resources/publications/ebola/ebola-panel-report/en/ (accessed October 16, 2016).

10 IFRC played a major role setting up volunteer burial management teams, and public health education. See Mueller (2014a). These teams were initially made of mainly young men, but at the height of the epidemic, they included women, and the teams were renamed safe and dignified burial teams. See "Do It Safely or Don't Do At It All," IFRC, July 20, http://www.ifrc.org/en/news-and-media/news-stories/africa/sierra-leone/do-it-safely-or-dont-do-it-at-all-68833/.

11 The Ebola Interim Assessment Panel ultimately determined that WHO had been hampered by its technocratic culture, lack of reliable data, previous overreaction with the swine flu (H1N1) virus of 2009, reticence in challenging governments, and inexperience with dealing with multi-country disease responses, WHO Ebola Response Assessment Panel. See also Busby and Grépin (2015).

12 Oxfam also agrees that while the WHO leadership should be blamed, UN Member States also "failed to provide active, effective stewardship." See Oxfam (2015).

13 These projections were extensively reported in the American media. See Grady (2014); CBC (2014).

14 Identical letters dated September 17, 2014 from the Secretary-General addressed to the President of the General Assembly and the President of the Security Council, UN General Assembly\Security Council A/69/389-S/2014/679 September 18, 2014.

15 See note 1.

16 David Banbury quit the UN in March 2016. His parting shot was a scathing critique of the bureaucracy, politicking, and minimal accountability in the organization. See "Opinion: I Love the U.N." *New York Times*, March 18, 2016, http://mobile.nytimes.com/2016/03/20/opinion/sunday/i-love-the-un-but-it-is-failing.html?referer=&_r=1 (accessed September 27, 2016).

17 Identical letters dated September 17, 2014 from the Secretary-General addressed to the President of the General Assembly and the President of the Security Council, UN General Assembly\Security Council A/69/389-S/2014/679 September 18, 2014.

18 He passed away on November 17, 2014 in Conakry, Guinea, as a result of causes not related to EVD.

19 UN Ebola Crisis Centre, External Situation Report, October 1, 2014.

20 The UN cluster system evolved with the strengthening of the coordination of emergency humanitarian assistance and creation of the Department of Humanitarian Affairs (DHA) (now United Nations Office for the Coordination of Humanitarian Affairs [OCHA]) by UN General Assembly in December 1991 (A/Res/46/182). Overseen by OCHA, the system ensures good coordination between various UN and non-UN humanitarian agencies during all phases of an emergency response from needs assessment and joint planning to monitoring and evaluation. In 2005, the reform of the system introduced new elements to improve leadership, predictability, capacity, accountability, and partnership. The 11 clusters and their responsibilities, designated by the Inter-Agency Standing Committee are UNICEF (water, sanitation, and hygiene), IFRC and UNHCR (shelter), UNCHR (protection), UNICEF (nutrition), WFP (logistics), WHO (health), WFP and FAO (food security), WFP (emergency telecommunications), UNICEF and Save the Children (education), UND (early recovery), and IOM and UNHCR (camp coordination and camp management).

21 WHO: Ebola Response Roadmap Situation Report, December 24, 2014, 16.

22 UNMEER External Situation Report, October 20, 2014.

23 Global Ebola Coalition Response Call, October 10, 2014, https://ebolaresponse.un.org/sites/default/files/10oct2014.pdf.

24 UNMEER External Situation Report, October 30, 2014.

25 UNMEER External Situation Report, October 17, 2014; see also UNMEER External Situation Report, October 20, 2014.

26 Global Ebola Response Coalition Meeting, October 24, 2014: Issues Discussed and Next Steps, https://ebolaresponse.un.org/sites/default/files/24oct.2014_0.pdf (accessed September 26, 2016).

27 UNMEER External Situation Report, November 17, 2014; UNMEER External Situation Report, November 26, 2014.

28 UNMEER External Situation Report, December 10, 2014.

29 UNMEER External Situation Report, November 24, 2014.

30 UNMEER External Situation Report, December 10, 2014.

31 UNMEER External Situation Report, November 13, 2014.

32 Global Ebola Response Coalition Meeting, December 5, 2014: Issues Discussed and Next Steps, https://ebolaresponse.un.org/sites/default/files/5dec.2014_0.pdf (accessed September 25, 2016).

33 UNMEER External Situation Report, December 11, 2014.

34 Global Ebola Response Coalition Meeting, December 12, 2014: Issues Discussed and Next Steps, https://ebolaresponse.un.org/sites/default/files/12dec.2014_0.pdf (accessed September 25, 2016).

35 UNMEER External Situation Report, December 10, 2014.

36 Global Ebola Response Coalition Meeting, December 5, 2014: Issues Discussed and Next Steps, https://ebolaresponse.un.org/sites/default/files/5dec.2014_0.pdf (accessed September 26, 2016).

37 WHO EBSS/3/2, "Current Context and Challenges; Stopping the Epidemic; and Preparedness in Non-affected Countries and Regions: Report by the Secretariat," January 9, 2015.

38 Banbury attributed this to the employment of expatriate anthropologists specializing in public health and community engagement, which provided technical advice to UN agencies and other organizations. Surveys conducted in December 2014, however, showed only around a third of responders said they would not handle corpses. See "Opinion: I Love the U.N." *New York Times*, March 18, 2016.

39 UNMEER External Situation Report, January 30, 2015.

40 UNMEER External Situation Report, February 11, 2015.

41 UNMEER External Situation Report, February 10, 2015.

42 UN General Assembly A 69/939: Letter dated June 16, from the Secretary-General Addressed to the President of the General Assembly.

43 WHO statement on end of Ebola flare-up in Sierra Leone, March 17, 2016, http://www.who.int/mediacentre/news/statements/2016/end-flare-ebola-sierra-leone/en/ (accessed October 1, 2016).

44 WHO Ebola Data and Statistics: Situation Summary, Data published May 11, 2016, http://apps.who.int/gho/data/view.ebola-sitrep.ebola-summary-20160511?lang=en (accessed October 22, 2016).

45 FGD, Employees of UNMEER Sierra Leone. Special Court, Jomo Kenyatta Road, Freetown, June 22, 2015. Among those who participated were Bintu (Head of Operations), Kinsley L. Ighbor (Public Information Officer), Mohamed Kakay (Associate Coordination Officer), Habiba Wurieh (Associate Coordination Officer).

46 The US provided US$2.1 bn, the UK US$687 m, WB US$1.6 bn, the EC US$955 m, and the ADB US$525 m. Thirteen percent of this fund was expended on Guinea, 20 percent on Sierra Leone, and 31 percent on Liberia, 28 percent was on Ebola-countries, 8 percent on unspecified or other countries.

47 FGD, Sierra Leone. Special Court, June 22, 2015.

48 Ibid.

49 WHO Ebola Interim Assessment Panel, 24.

50 *Recovering from the Ebola Crisis: A Summary Report* (submitted by the United Nations, The World Bank, European Union, and African Development Bank as a contribution to the formulation of National Ebola Recovery Strategies in Guinea, Liberia, and Sierra Leone, 9.

51 The Global Ebola Response Coalition, December 11, 2015: Issues and Next Steps, https://ebolaresponse.un.org/sites/default/files/gerc_57_meeting_note.pdf (accessed October 22, 2016).

References

Benton, Ada and Donne, Kim Yi (2015). "Commentary: International Political Economy and the 2014 West African Ebola Outbreak," *African Studies Review* 58, 1 (April): 223–236.

Boozary, Andrew S., Farmer, Paul E. and Jha, Ashish K. (2014). "The Ebola Outbreak, Fragile Health Systems, and Quality as a Cure," *Viewpoint*, November 12.

Bricknell, Martin, Hodgetts, T., Beaton, K., and McCourt, A. (2016). "Operation GRITROCK: The Defenses Medical Services' Story and Emerging Lessons from Supporting the UK Responses to the Ebola Crisis," *Journal of the Royal Army Medical Corps* 162, 3: 169–175.

Busby, Joshua and Grépin, Karen (2015). "What Accounts for the World Health Organization Failure on Ebola," *Political Science and Politics* 48, 1 (January): 12–13.

CBC (2014). "Ebola Cases Could Reach 500,000 to 1.4 Million in 4 Months: CDC," *CBC News*, September 23. http://www.cbc.ca/news/health/ebola-cases-could-reach-550-000-to-1-4-million-in-4-months-cdc-1.2775185.

Deloffre, Maryam (2016). "Human Security Governance: Is UNMEER the Way Forward," *Global Health Governance* 10, 1: 41–59.

Drehle, David Von (2014). "Global Health: Now Arriving: The Deadly Ebola Virus Lands in America," *Time*, October 13 (Chasing Ebola Issue).

Fink, Sheri and Belluck, Pam (2015). "One Year Later, the Ebola Epidemic Offers Lessons for Next Epidemic," *New York Times*, March 22. http://www.nytimes.com/2015/03/23/world/one-year-later-ebola-outbreak-offers-lessons-for-next-epidemic.html (accessed September 26, 2016).

Fischer, Salome and Brandt, Emilie (2015). *The United Nations and the Global Ebola Response. The UN Emergency Health Mission "UNMEER": Lessons Learned and Recommendations for Similar Future Health Emergencies*. Munich: Grin Verlag.

Grady, Denise (2014). "Ebola Cases Could Reach 1.4 million CDC Estimates," *New York Times*, September 23.

International Crisis Group (2015). *The Politics Behind the Ebola Crisis*. Africa Report no. 232, October 28.

Kentikelenis, Alexander, King, Lawrence, Mckee, Martin, and Stucker, David (2015). "The International Monetary Fund and the Ebola Outbreak," *The Lancet* 3, 2 (February): e69–e70.

McInnes, Colin (2016). "Crisis! What Crisis? Global Health and the 2014–2015 West African Ebola Outbreak," *Third World Quarterly* 37, 3: 388–389.

Médecins Sans Frontières (2014). *Pushed to the Limit and Beyond: A Year into the Largest Ever Ebola Outbreak.*

Meltzer, Martin et al. (2014). "Estimating the Future Number of Cases in the Ebola Epidemic: Liberia and Sierra Leone," *Morbidity and Mortality Weekly Report*, September 26. http://www.cdc.gov/mmwr/preview/mmwrhtml/su6303a1.htm (accessed September 27, 2016).

Mueller, Katherine (2014a). "Burying Ebola's Victims in Sierra Leone," IFRC, July 26. http://www.ifrc.org/en/news-and-media/news-stories/africa/sierra-leone/burying-ebolas-victims-in-sierra-leone-66528/ (accessed September 20, 2016).

Mueller, Katherine (2014b). "Ebola, Snakes and Witchcraft: Stopping the

Deadly Disease in Its Tracks," IFRC, June 24. http://www.ifrc.org/en/news-and-media/news-stories/africa/sierra-leone/ebola-snakes-and-witchcraft-stopping-the-deadly-disease-in-its-tracks-in-west-africa-66215/ (accessed September 20, 2016).

Oxfam (2015). *Improving International Governance for Global Health Emergencies: Lessons from the Ebola Crisis.* Oxfam Discussion Paper, January 2015. https://www.oxfam.org/sites/www.oxfam.org/files/file_attachments/dp-governance-global-health-emergencies-ebola-280115-en.pdf (accessed September 26, 2016).

WHO (2014). "Ebola Briefing: WHO Responses and Challenges to Control the Outbreak," December 1.

WHO (2015). WHO Strategic Response Plan: West African Ebola Outbreak. Geneva: WHO.

WHO Ebola Response Team (2014). "Ebola Virus Disease in West Africa: The First Nine Months of the Epidemic and Forward Projections," *New England Journal of Medicine* 371: 1481–1495. http://www.nejm.org/doi/full/10.1056/NEJMoa1411100?query=featured_home&#t=articleResults (accessed September 27, 2016).

Youde, Jeremy (2015). "The World Health Organization and Responses to Global Health Emergencies," *Political Science and Politics* 48, 1 (January): 11–13.

ABOUT THE EDITORS AND CONTRIBUTORS

Editors

Ibrahim Abdullah was until recently a professor of history at Fourah Bay College, University of Sierra Leone. He has published extensively in the area of African social/labor history and contemporary social change and conflict in West Africa, and is the editor of *Democracy and Terror: The Sierra Leone Civil War* (2004).

Ismail Rashid is professor of history at Vassar College. Among his recent publications are (co-edited with A. Adebajo) *West Africa's Security Challenges* (2004) and (co-edited with Sylvia Ojukutu-Macauley) *The Paradoxes of History and Memory in Postcolonial Sierra Leone* (2013). He currently serves as chair of the Advisory Board of the African Peacebuilding Network of the Social Science Research Council.

Contributors

Semiha Abdulmelik is an alumnus of the African Leadership Centre, and has worked for local and international NGOs, as well as the UN in various capacities. She has undertaken country-level programming work, working with local government, national institutions, and civil society as well as engaging in policy and advocacy in the areas of humanitarian affairs, peace and security, and post-conflict reconstruction, with a wide range of policy and decision makers at the African Union level.

Julia Amos is the Peter J. Braam research lecturer in global wellbeing at Merton College, University of Oxford. She sits on the OxPeace Steering Committee, the British Pugwash Executive Committee, and the Oxford Peace Research Trust, and is a member of the Department of International Development, where she is based as a research associate.

Chernoh Alpha M. Bah is an award-winning journalist and political activist. He is the author of *Neocolonialism in West Africa* (2014) and *The Ebola Outbreak in West Africa: Corporate Gangsters, Multinationals and Rogue Politicians* (2015).

Alpha Amadou Bano Barry is currently rector of the Oprah Winfrey University in Guinea. He is the author of *Les violences collectives en Afrique: le cas Guinéen* (2000) and *La démocratie et le vote en Guinée* (2010).

Fodei Batty is assistant professor of political science at Quinnipac University. He has consulted for a number of international NGOs and previously served as policy analyst in the office of the president of Sierra Leone in the administrations of Presidents Ahmad Tejan Kabbah and Ernest Koroma.

Tefera Gezmu is NIH/NHLBI PRIDE cardiovascular disease scholar, a senior epidemiologist and assistant professor at the Edward J. Bloustein School of Planning and Public Policy and at the RBHS-School of Public Health at Rutgers, the State University of New Jersey. He has worked and taught as well as evaluated numerous public health programs in several South American and African countries. Dr. Gezmu was recently chosen to be a member of a working group in the Northeast Cerebrovascular Disease Consortium (NECC), and is also a member of the Governing Council for the American Public Health Association (APHA), secretary of the Councils of Affiliate at APHA, and the Society for Epidemiologic Research (SER). He has served as the president of the New Jersey Public Health Association (NJPHA) and currently serves the regional representative to APHA. Dr. Gezmu has served as a consultant and board member for several national and global not-for-profit organizations.

Allen M. Howard is professor emeritus of African and global history at Rutgers University. He has published widely on Sierra Leone and Guinea, focusing on cities, ethnicities, and trade and traders. He is a co-editor of *The Spatial Factor in African History: The Relationship of the Social, Material, and Perceptual* (2005).

Aisha Fofana Ibrahim is currently the director of the Institute for Gender Research and Documentation (INGRADOC) at Fourah Bay College, University of Sierra Leone and past president of 50/50 Group, a national women's organization. For the past two decades Dr. Ibrahim's research interests and publications have been in the areas of gender-based violence, gender equality, and women's increased political participation and representation. As a consultant, Dr. Ibrahim provides technical support to the state government and national and international non-governmental organizations in the area of women's empowerment and gender analysis.

Abou Bakarr Kamara currently works as country economist at the International Growth Centre (IGC) – Sierra Leone country office. Prior to working with the IGC, he worked as the director of policy planning and information in the Sierra Leonean Ministry of Health and Sanitation. He has also worked as a policy analyst in the Office of the President with a mandate to drive the implementation of the Government Development Agenda.

George Klay Kieh, Jr. is a professor of political science at the University of West Georgia. Prior to that, he served in various administrative and teaching positions, including dean of the College of Arts and Sciences and professor of political science at the University of West Georgia, dean of international affairs and professor of political science at Grand Valley State University, Michigan, and chair and professor of political science and international studies at Morehouse College, Georgia.

Meredeth Turshen is a professor in the Edward J. Bloustein School of Planning and Public Policy at Rutgers University. She has written five books, including *Women's Health Movements: A Global Force for Change* (2007) and *Gender and the Political Economy of Conflict in Africa: The Persistence of Violence* (2016). Her edited books include *What Women Do in Wartime: Gender and Conflict in Africa* (Zed 1998) and *The Aftermath: Women in Postconflict Transformation* (Zed 2002). She has served on the boards of the Association of Concerned Africa Scholars, the Committee for Health in Southern Africa and the *Review of African Political Economy*, and is on the editorial board of the *Journal of Public Health Policy*.

INDEX

Note: Page numbers followed by *n* indicate an endnote with relevant number; page numbers in bold refer to tables.